STAGE-WISE ADAPTIVE DESIGNS

WILEY SERIES IN PROBABILITY AND STATISTICS

Established by WALTER A. SHEWHART and SAMUEL S. WILKS

A complete list of the titles in this series appears at the end of this volume.

STAGE-WISE ADAPTIVE DESIGNS

SHELEMYAHU ZACKS

WILEY

A JOHN WILEY & SONS, INC., PUBLICATION

Published by John Wiley & Sons, Inc., Hoboken, New Jersey

Published simultaneously in Canada

Library of Congress Cataloging-in-Publication Data:

Zacks, Shelemyahu, 1932–
Stage-wise adaptive designs / Shelemyahu Zacks.
p. ; cm. — (Wiley series in probability and statistics)
Includes bibliographical references and indexes.
ISBN 978-0-470-05095-8 (cloth)
1. Medicine—Research—Statistical methods. 2. Medical statistics. 3. Statistics. I. Title. II. Series.
[DNLM: 1. Models, Statistical. 2. Clinical Trials as Topic. WA 950 Z16s 2009]
R853.S7Z33 2009
610.72—dc22 2008047059

To My Wife, Hanna,
for her love, support,
and encouragement

CONTENTS

Preface

Stage-wise adaptive design for collecting and analyzing data or for forecasting and controlling processes occurs in all areas of statistics. The present book discusses such designs in nine different subject areas. We start with two-stage and sequential sampling for estimation and testing with prescribed precision. We then concentrate on generalized linear models followed by stage-wise sampling procedures in sampling surveys. Adaptive forecasting in the area of time series analysis is presented in some length. The important area of clinical trials is dealt with in two chapters, followed by a chapter on "bandits" problems. Sequential detection of change points is discussed as well as sequential applications in industrial statistics, software reliability, and other related areas.

The material is organized in 10 chapters. The first chapter is a synopsis. The other chapters consist of theoretical results in the literature, mainly taken from papers published by the author and his collaborators. Books can be written on each one of the above-mentioned subject areas. One cannot get too deep in each area in one book. Nevertheless, the chapters provide sufficient background material on each subject. The objective is to introduce the reader to problems of adaptive designs. It is very important to compare the efficiency of different procedures. For this purpose, characteristics of procedures have to be evaluated. Formulas for the exact computations of the operating characteristics of procedures are often developed, rather than just asymptotic approximations. This requires, in many cases, the derivation of the distributions of stopping times, or total sample size of two-stage or sequential procedures. In cases where formulas for the exact computations were not developed, simulation algorithms were applied. Special SPLUS® functions were written for the numerical computations required for tables or graphs. The names of these functions are mentioned in the text or under tables. The actual functions are printed in the Appendix with explanations. These functions can be obtained electronically from Wiley's ftp site for the book (ftp://ftp.wiley.com/public/sci_tech_med/stagewise_designs). All these functions can also run in R. The reader can use these functions to validate computations in the book and for generalization purposes.

The present book is aimed at advanced graduate students and researchers in statistics, biostatistics, and related fields. It is assumed that the reader has basic knowledge in probability theory, the theory of statistical distributions, statistical inference, linear algebra, and mathematical analysis.

Finally, I would like to acknowledge and thank Mrs. Marge Pratt for her excellent typing of the manuscript and my colleagues in the department, especially Professor Anton Schick, for occasional discussions of related material. I would like to thank also the reviewer for important comments on an earlier version of the manuscript.

I do hope that this book will fulfill needs of researchers of new methods and those who apply them.

SHELEMYAHU ZACKS

Binghamton, New York
February 2009

CHAPTER 1

SYNOPSIS

In the present chapter we present an overview of the material in Chapters 2–10.

1.1 MULTISTAGE AND SEQUENTIAL ESTIMATION

Chapter 2 is devoted to the problem of determining the minimal sample size required to attain a prescribed precision, in the estimation of a parameter, or a function of parameters of the parent distribution. Consider, for example, the classical problem of estimating the mean of a normal distribution. Let $X_1, \ldots, X_n$ be independent, identically distributed (i.i.d.) random variables from a normal distribution $\mathcal{N}(\mu, \sigma)$. It is well known that, if the standard deviation σ is known, then a confidence interval for μ, with confidence level $1 - \alpha$, $0 < \alpha < 1$, is given by

$$\bar{X}_n \pm Z_{1-\alpha/2} \frac{\sigma}{\sqrt{n}}, \tag{1.1.1}$$

where $\bar{X}_n = \sum_{i=1}^{n} X_i/n$ is the sample mean and $Z_{1-\alpha/2} = \Phi^{-1}(1 - \alpha/2)$ is the $(1 - \alpha/2)$-quantile of the standard normal distribution $\Phi(\cdot)$. Thus, if one

Stage-Wise Adaptive Designs. By Shelemyahu Zacks

wishes to have a $(1-\alpha)$ level confidence for the mean, μ, with bounded length 2δ, the minimal required sample size is

$$(1.1.2) \qquad n^0(\delta, \sigma) = \left\lfloor \frac{Z^2_{1-\alpha/2}\sigma^2}{\delta^2} \right\rfloor + 1.$$

Here $\lfloor x \rfloor$ denotes the largest integer *smaller* than x. We express the precision of the estimation by the bound 2δ on the length of the confidence interval and its confidence level $1-\alpha$. One can express the precision in terms of an estimation risk, like

$$(1.1.3) \qquad R(\hat{\mu}_n, \mu) = AE_\sigma\{(\hat{\mu}_n - \mu)^2\},$$

where $0 < A < \infty$ is a constant and $\hat{\mu}_n$ is an estimator of μ. For $\hat{\mu}_n = \bar{X}_n$ we have a risk of $A\sigma^2/n$. This risk is bounded by a desired positive constant ω, uniformly in σ, if the sample size is at least

$$(1.1.4) \qquad n^*(\omega, \sigma^2) = \left\lfloor A\frac{\sigma^2}{\omega} \right\rfloor + 1.$$

We see that, in order to control the precision of the estimation, one needs to know the value of the nuisance parameter σ. The question is whether a procedure based on a sample of fixed size n can guarantee a desired precision when σ is *unknown*. Dantzig (1940) has proven that if σ is unknown there exists no such fixed-sample-size procedure. That is, there exists no fixed-width confidence interval for μ, in the normal case, if σ is unknown and the sample size is fixed.

Stein (1945, 1949) was the first one to show that a fixed-width confidence interval for μ in the normal case can be attained by a *two-stage* sampling procedure when σ is unknown. As will be shown, Stein's two-stage procedure is an *adaptive* procedure. It utilizes the results of the first stage to estimate σ and determines the required sample size based on this estimate. We describe this method and prove the result in Section 2.1. This classical result of Stein opened the field for many papers which dealt with various properties of two-stage and multistage procedures. A comprehensive review of the results in the literature is presented in the book *Sequential Estimation* of Ghosh, Mukhopadhyay, and Sen (1997). In Section 2.2 we present generalizations of Stein's procedure and the notions of consistency and asymptotic efficiency of the procedure. The exact distribution of the total (random) sample size is compared to its asymptotic normal distribution. Section 2.3 presents two-stage procedures for estimating the parameters of exponential distributions. We present there the exact distribution of the total sample size, N, and interesting results of Mukhopadhyay and Pepe (2006) and Zacks and Mukhopadhyay (2007) concerning a uniformly bounded risk estimation of the mean, β, of the exponential distribution. In Section 2.4 we present the Chow and Robbins (1965) procedure for a fixed-width confidence interval of a distribution mean, μ, when the variance σ^2 is finite. We also prove there Wald's lemma and present Anscomb theorem on asymptotic normality. Section 2.5 presents a method for the exact determination of the distribution of the sample size in the exponential case and certain other characteristics of the estimators. This is based on a recent paper of Zacks and Mukhopadhyay (2006a). In Section 2.6 we show recent results of Zacks and Mukhopadhyay (2007) for a sequential fixed-width interval estimation of the log-odds in Bernoulli trials. Finally, in Section 2.7 we present the Bayesian formulation of sequential estimation.

The numerical characteristics of two-stage and sequential procedures, like the expected total sample size, the expected value of the estimator, and the risk function, can generally be estimated by simulations. We emphasize and apply, as much as possible, exact numerical evaluation of these characteristics. Recursive numerical algorithms can be developed whenever the stopping variables depend on sums of independent random variables.

1.2 ADAPTIVE DESIGNS FOR GENERALIZED LINEAR MODELS

In Chapter 3 we discuss two types of adaptive design problems. The first is that of *quantal response* experiments in which the observed random variables are binary (Bernoulli trials) and the problem is that of determining the level x of an experimental factor. The second type of problem is that of determining the level x in a linear regression $Y = \alpha + \beta x + \epsilon$ so that Y satisfies certain tolerance requirements. We explain now the two problems in detail. For the quantal response problem, we consider m Bernoulli trials and denote by J_m the number of "successes," where J_m has binomial distribution $\mathcal{B}(m, F(\alpha + \beta x))$. The probability of success, $F(\alpha+\beta x)$, depends on an arbitrary location parameter, α, and a positive parameter, β (the inverse of a scale parameter), where x is a level of experimental factor (stress level, temperature, dosage of toxic material, etc). We will assume that $F(u)$ is a cumulative distribution function (c.d.f.). Thus, $F(\alpha + \beta x)$ is an increasing function of x.

In bioassays F is called a *tolerance distribution* (see Finney, 1964). In modern theory of generalized linear models, F is called a *link function*. The problem is to determine a value of x so that $F(\alpha+\beta x)$ has a certain required property. For example, in bioassays one is often seeking the value of a dose x which causes 50% mortality. This is called the median lethal dose (LD-50). For a given tolerance distribution

$$\text{LD-50} = \frac{F^{-1}(0.5) - \alpha}{\beta}.$$

This required dosage depends on the parameters α and β. Adaptive designs are called for when α and β are *unknown*. The objective is to perform a sequence of trials, estimate the unknown parameters after each stage, and determine the dosage for the next stage to maximize the information on the required LD-50.

In Sections 3.1–3.3 the objective is to determine the sequence of dosages $\{X_n\}$ which will come close to the one which maximizes the Fisher information. More specifically, suppose that $\alpha = 0$ and β is unknown. Given $J_m \sim \mathcal{B}(m, F(\beta x))$, the likelihood function of β is

$$L(\beta; J_m) = F(\beta x)^{J_m}(1 - F(\beta x))^{m-J_m}. \tag{1.2.1}$$

The corresponding score function is

$$\frac{\partial}{\partial \beta} \log L(\beta; J_m) = J_m \frac{x f(\beta x)}{F(\beta x)\bar{F}(\beta x)} - m \frac{x f(\beta x)}{F(\beta x)\bar{F}(\beta x)}, \tag{1.2.2}$$

where $f(u)$ is the density of $F(u)$ and $\bar{F}(u) = 1 - F(u)$. The Fisher information function is the variance of the score function, namely

$$I(\beta; x) = \frac{m x^2 f^2(\beta x)}{F(\beta x)\bar{F}(\beta x)}. \tag{1.2.3}$$

Let u^0 be a maximizer of

$$I(u) = \frac{u^2 f^2(u)}{F(u)\bar{F}(u)}. \tag{1.2.4}$$

If β is known, then the optimal x-value is

$$x^0 = \frac{u^0}{\beta}. \tag{1.2.5}$$

If both α and β are unknown, the Fisher information is the matrix

$$II(\alpha, \beta; x) = \frac{m f^2(\alpha + \beta x)}{F(\alpha + \beta x)\bar{F}(\alpha + \beta x)} \begin{pmatrix} 1 & x \\ x & x^2 \end{pmatrix}. \tag{1.2.6}$$

This matrix is singular. One needs to perform trials at two different x-values in order to estimate both α and β. If one is interested in estimating a given linear combination of α and β, $\omega = \xi\alpha + \eta\beta$, the optimal values of x can be determined by the method of Elfing (see Chernoff, 1972, p. 13). In Section 3.1 we present a special case of this problem. We consider a problem of designing a reliability experiment in which m units (systems) are put on test, and the number of failures in a period of x time units is recorded. The question is how large should x be in order to maximize the Fisher information when the life distribution is exponential. Section 3.2 is devoted to adaptive designs to maximize the Fisher information when at each stage the estimation of unknown parameters is by the method of maximum-likelihood estimation (MLE). Section 3.3 discusses the Bayesian approach for adaptive estimation. The last section is devoted to an inverse regression problem. It is assumed that the observed random variable (r.v.) $Y_x \sim N(\alpha + \beta x, \sigma^2 x^2)$. The γ-quantile of this normal distribution is $Y_\gamma = \alpha + \beta x + \Phi^{-1}(\gamma)\sigma x$, where $\Phi^{-1}(\gamma)$ is the

γ-quantile of the standard normal distribution. If we aim that $Y_\gamma = \eta$, where η is a specified threshold, then the x-value should be

$$x_\gamma = \frac{\eta - \alpha}{\beta + \Phi^{-1}(\gamma)\sigma}. \tag{1.2.7}$$

This x-value depends on the parameters α, β, and σ. Adaptive procedures are discussed for cases where some or all of these parameters are unknown.

Design problems connected with generalized linear models attracted the attention of many researchers. The reader is referred to a recent review paper by Khuri, Mukherjee, Sinha, and Ghosh (2006). Dozens of relevant papers are listed in this review paper.

The Newton–Raphson method for iteratively solving nonlinear equations is introduced in this chapter. Stochastic approximation is discussed in Section 3.5.

1.3 ADAPTIVE METHODS FOR SAMPLING FROM FINITE POPULATIONS

Sampling from finite populations, also called sampling surveys, is an important branch of statistics. Sampling surveys are applied in many branches of science and technology which deal with finite populations. Polling the political or economic attitudes of people, estimating the total corn crop in a given county, estimating the total number of bears in a given region of Alaska, estimating the number of fish in a pond, and testing whether the proportion of non conforming items in a lot is acceptable, for example, are but a small number of applications of the theory and methodology of sampling from finite populations. Chapter 4 is devoted to adaptive methods in sampling from finite populations. Accordingly, we typically draw first an initial sample to estimate certain characteristics of the population, and then on the basis of the results obtained in the initial sample we design a two-stage sampling or a sequential one. In the spirit of the terminology of the first two chapters we use the term two-stage or multistage sampling for what is called in many books "double" or "multiphase" sampling. The term single- or two-stage sampling is used in the literature on sampling surveys in connection with cluster sampling. We hope that this will not cause confusion. There are two main streams in the theory of sampling from finite population. One is that of the design of random procedures for selecting the samples (see Cochran, 1977; Hedayat and Sinha, 1991; Thompson, 1992) and the other is that of modeling (superpopulation) the joint distributions of the variables in the population (see Basu, 1969; Bolfarine and Zacks, 1992; Cassel, Särndal, and Wretman, 1977). The two approaches, design and modeling, are different entirely and the associated adaptive methods are different. For this reason we present in the first section the two theoretical approaches and some basic results. Section 4.2 is devoted to two-stage and sequential estimation of the population mean for attaining a fixed-width confidence interval with coverage probabilities close to the nominal. This section is complimentary to the material of the first two chapters. Section 4.3 deals with the adaptive allocation of the sample in stratified sampling and utilizing these results for a two-stage estimation of the population mean with a prescribed precision. Section 4.4 is devoted to an adaptive procedure for search of special elements of the population. This section presents an interesting procedure developed by Thompson (1992) and discussed also in Thompson and Seber (1996). Their method is called by them "adaptive cluster sampling," but the procedure is only similar to the classical single-stage cluster sampling. Thompson and Seber's methods are suitable for search of a rare species or a rare mineral or elements which tend to congregate in clusters whose location has to be found. Section 4.5 presents a Bayesian sequential procedure for estimating the size of a finite population. How many elements are there? Section 4.6 presents adaptive techniques for testing and rectifying software. There are two approaches in modeling the distribution of the length of time until a fault is found. One approach is called time domain modeling and the other is data domain modeling. Sequential stopping rules are discussed for the length of a test in these two domains. Section 4.7 is devoted to adaptive procedures in sampling acceptance schemes for quality assurance. Finally, Section 4.8 presents dynamic Bayesian prediction of the total value of (a) finite population(s) in a sequence of survey times. This type of dynamic prediction (forecasting) will be discussed in more detail in Chapter 5.

1.4 ADAPTIVE PREDICTION AND FORECASTING IN TIME SERIES ANALYSIS

Let $X_1, X_2, \ldots, X_t$ be the observed values of a time series at time t. We wish to *predict* the future value of X_{t+s}, $s \geq 1$. The future value of X_{t+s} is predicted rather than estimated, since X_{t+s} is a random variable. Denote by $\hat{X}_{t+s}(t)$ the predictor of X_{t+s} at time t, $s \geq 1$. The predictor $\hat{X}_{t+s}(t)$ is a statistic which depends on the observations up to time t. We will denote by $\hat{X}_{t+s}^{(n)}(t)$ a predictor of X_{t+s} based on the last n observations $(X_t, X_{t-1}, \ldots, X_{t-n+1})$, $n \leq t$. The *prediction mean-squared error* (PMSE) of a predictor $\hat{X}_{t+s}^{(n)}(t)$ is

$$\text{PMSE}\{\hat{X}_{t+s}^{(n)}(t)\} = E\{[\hat{X}_{t+s}^{(n)}(t) - X_{t+s}]^2\}. \tag{1.4.1}$$

Notice the difference between the PMSE of a predictor and the MSE of an estimator of a parameter of a distribution.

Generally, we choose a predictor which minimizes the PMSE. Such a predictor will be called *best*, or *minimal, PMSE*. If the structure of the time series is very simple, the best predictor might be a very simple one. In Chapter 5 we derive the best predictors for some time series (T.S.) models. We then present the theory of prediction based on *moving average smoothing*, *exponential smoothing*, and *dynamic linear models*. More specifically, we start with the basic tools of T.S. analysis. We then discuss linear predictors for covariance stationary T.S. We then develop quadratic least squares predictors for nonstationary T.S. These follow by moving average predictors, predictors with exponential discounting and smoothing models for seasonal data. The chapter concludes with dynamic linear models (DLMs) and linear control.

There are many books on T.S. analysis, for example, Box, Jenkins, and Reinsel (1994), Fuller (1996), Anderson (1971), Brillinger (1975), Brockwell and Davis (1991), Chatfield (1975, 1984), Harrison and West (1989), Nelson (1973), Davis and Vinter (1985), and many more. We present here the forecasting algorithms in a unified manner. The emphasis is again on computing algorithms. In the Appendix one can find the SPLUS programs developed for this chapter. Certain formal derivations were done with MAPLE. We illustrate the adaptive algorithms on real-life data collected from various sources. For illustration purposes we use simulated data sets, the Dow Jones daily index for the year 1941, and some data sets which are frequently used in the literature.

1.5 ADAPTIVE SEARCH OF AN MTD IN CANCER PHASE I CLINICAL TRIALS

Clinical trials are designed to test a new drug or a new therapy on human subjects. Clinical trials proceed in phases which have different objectives and are conducted differently. Phase I trials are designed to explore the toxicity and the side effects of a new drug. Typically, the sample consists of 20–80 cancer patients in progressive stages of the disease. The aim is to find the *maximal tolerated dose* (MTD) of the new drug to avoid life-threatening toxicity and other unacceptable side effects. Phase II of clinical trials are generally pilot studies of moderate size concerned with evaluating efficacy and safety of the new drug. The MTD established in Phase I is usually the applied dose in Phase II. Phase III trials are of longer duration. The objective is to compare the new therapeutic treatment to an established standard or to several other treatments, and the presence of long-term side effects is monitored. In this phase, patients are allocated to different treatments by adaptive randomization procedures. Phase IV is that of additional testing of a treatment that has been approved for general use.

In Chapter 6 we discuss various methods of finding the MTD in cancer Phase I clinical trials. The human subjects participating in these trials are generally cancer patients who are in advanced stages of the disease and for whom alternative treatments have failed. For such patients toxicity might be severe. It is therefore desired that no more than one-third of the population of such patients will be induced to life-threatening toxicity. A dose which induces such a toxic reaction is called DLT. Thus, the MTD is often defined as the highest dose utilized in the trial for which 33% of the subjects manifest life-threatening toxicity. In the search for the MTD we will discuss methods which avoid, with high probability, overdosing. This is, however, not a concern in many studies, since the patients participating in cancer Phase I clinical trials are already in life-threatening situations due to the advanced stages of their disease.

There are two approaches to dose escalation in cancer Phase I clinical trials. One is a nonparametric approach, like the up-and-down procedure and isotonic regression estimates. The other one is the modeling approach. The modeling approach connects the dosage to the probability of DLT via a tolerance distribution. Examples will be given later. A dose escalation scheme determines the dose for the nth patient as a function of the previous $(n-1)$ dosages and the observed level of toxicity manifested by the first $(n-1)$ subjects. Generally the trials start at a low dose which is considered "safe." It is desired that the doses assigned to the following patients will be as close as possible to the MTD but below it. This is a challenging problem. Babb, Rogatko, and Zacks (1998) developed a Bayesian procedure, called escalation with overdose control (EWOC), which is designed to fulfill these objectives. For a review of Bayesian methods in cancer Phase I clinical trials, see the article of Babb and Rogatko (2003). We start with a discussion of the up-and-down procedure, since it is the oldest one, and proceed to isotonic regression procedures. We then discuss Bayesian escalation schemes. The Bayesian approach is called for since the number of patients participating in Phase I studies is small, and procedures based on asymptotic results may not be appropriate. The literature on Phase I clinical trials contains dozens if not hundreds of papers. We list a few of these at the end of the chapter.

Six up-and-down procedures were evaluated with respect to the logistic tolerance distribution,

$$F(x;\alpha,\beta) = \frac{\exp(\alpha+\beta x)}{1+\exp(\alpha+\beta x)}.$$

Exact formulas for the expected value of the estimator of the MTD, as well as its MSE and probability of overdosing, were developed. The up-and-down procedures were compared numerically according to these characteristics. The EWOC method was compared by simulations to the continuous-reassessment method (CRM) of O'Quigley, Pepe, and Fisher (1990). We conclude the chapter with discussion of three-stage designs for Phase II clinical trials and discuss also some studies which combine toxicity and efficacy.

1.6 ADAPTIVE AND SEQUENTIAL PROCEDURES IN PHASE III CLINICAL TRIALS

In Chapter 7 we discuss adaptive and sequential procedures which are designed to be implemented in Phase III clinical trials, where the main objective is to test the efficacy of one or more new treatment(s) relative to one or more standard treatments. For this purpose we have to assign patients into two or more groups: the test group(s) and the control group(s). Since clinical trials are performed on human beings by doctors or medical technicians, one of the important problems is that of guarding against creeping bias. To avoid uncontrollable bias, patients are assigned to the various treatments at random, and if at all possible, neither the patients nor the persons who administer the treatments know exactly which treatment they give or receive. This obviously is sometimes impossible. Section 7.1 is devoted to randomizations in clinical trials. In Section 7.2 we discuss several randomization procedures designed to minimize imbalance due to random assignment of patients. Some of these procedures are adaptive. In particular, we discuss the random allocation rule, which is similar to sampling at random without replacement from a finite population. If N patients are assigned sequentially to treatments A or B, according to this rule, it is interesting to notice when one of the two treatments is assigned $N/2$ patients. We develop the distribution of the first time that one of the two treatments gets $N/2$ patients. We show that with high probability this event happens close to the last assignments. After that we discuss the truncated binomial design of Blackwell and Hodges (1957). This is followed by Efron's (1971) biased coin design (1971). Wei's (1977) urn designs are discussed next, and finally we discuss randomization procedures which are response adaptive. Excellent sources of material on randomization procedures in clinical trials are the books by Rosenberger and Lachin (2002) and Hu and Rosenberger (2006).

Section 7.3 is devoted to the sequential estimation of the success probability in Bernoulli trials, having fixed-width confidence intervals. We study analytically the characteristics of the stopping rule and in particular its distribution function. In Section 7.4 we develop a sequential procedure for estimating the success probability of Bernoulli trials with the criterion of *prescribed proportional closeness* of level $1-\alpha$, namely $P\{|\hat{p}_n - p| < \lambda p\} \geq 1-\alpha$, where $0 < \alpha$, $\lambda < 1$. This procedure requires large samples when $p < 1/2$ but gives more meaningful results for small p. In Section 7.5 we present sequential procedures for estimating the difference of the success probabilities of two treatments. Finally, Section 7.6 is devoted to the topic of group sequential testing. These methods are especially important when it is difficult or impractical to apply purely sequential procedures, in which analysis of the results must be done after each patient is treated. An important source of information on group sequential methods is in the book of Jennison and Turnbull (2000). We do not discuss in the present chapter bioequivalence testsbioequivalence tests. These are tests which are designed to establish the equivalence of two different drugs or treatments in terms of patient response. Bioequivalence tests often require different types of designs than the ones discussed in the present chapter. The reader can find a good chapter on this subject in Jennison and Turnbull (2000).

There are hundreds of papers and several dozen books on the design and analysis of clinical trials in particular on multistage or sequential ones. We provide in the bibliography a sample of relevant references.

1.7 SEQUENTIAL ALLOCATION OF RESOURCES: THE ONE-ARMED AND MULTIARMED BANDITS APPLIED TO CLINICAL TRIALS

Consider a "two-armed bandit" slot machine. A gambler has a finite number, N, of coins (dollars) which he or she is ready to spend for fun. At each trial the gambler has to insert a coin either on the left-hand side or on the right. This is the cost, c, of a trial. To simplify, assume that each successful trial yields 10 coins. The left and right arms act independently, with probabilities p_1 or p_2 of success. These probabilities are, however, unknown. How should the gambler play in order to maximize the expected number of successes? This is the classical two-armed bandit problem. We can state the problem in more general terms. Suppose that there are K possible experiments to choose from in each trial. If experiment $\mathcal{E}_j$ ($j = 1, \ldots, K$) is chosen, the reward is a random variable, X_j, having a distribution function F_j. If the same experiment is repeated, the resulting rewards $X_{j_1}, X_{j_2}, \ldots$ are i.i.d. We further assume, for simplicity, that $X_1, X_2, \ldots, X_K$ are mutually independent. A strategy $\boldsymbol{\tau} = (\tau_1, \tau_2, \ldots)$ is a sequence of random variables which assume values in $\{1, 2, \ldots, K\}$. If $\tau_n = j$, $j = 1, \ldots, K$, then the nth trial is on $\mathcal{E}_j$. For a given strategy $\boldsymbol{\tau}$, the *expected total discounted* reward is

$$W(\boldsymbol{\tau}, \boldsymbol{\alpha}) = \sum_{n=1}^{\infty} \alpha_n \sum_{j=1}^{K} E\{I\{\tau_n = j\} \cdot X_{jm_j(n)}\} \tag{1.7.1}$$

where $m_j(n) = \sum_{i=1}^{n} I(\tau_i = j)$ is the number of times $\mathcal{E}_j$ has been chosen during the first n trials. Furthermore, $\boldsymbol{\alpha} = (\alpha_1, \alpha_2, \ldots)$ is called a *discounting sequence*. Generally $\alpha_n \geq 0$ for all $n = 1, 2, \ldots$, and to assure convergence of (1.7.1), when $\max_{1 \leq j \leq K} E\{|X_j|\} < \infty$, we have to require that $\sum_{n=1}^{\infty} \alpha_n < \infty$. In the classical Bernoulli bandits, which will be discussed in Section 8.1, one could use the sequence $\boldsymbol{\alpha}_{n^*} = (1, 1, \ldots, 1, 0, 0, \ldots)$ where the number of 1's at the head of the sequence is the number of possible trials, n^*, and all $\alpha_n = 0$ for $n > n^*$. The geometric sequence $\boldsymbol{\alpha} = (1, \alpha, \alpha^2, \alpha^3, \ldots)$ is especially important, as will be shown later.

For a given $\boldsymbol{\alpha}$ the problem is to find an optimal strategy $\boldsymbol{\tau}^0$ under which $W(\boldsymbol{\tau}, \boldsymbol{\alpha})$ is maximized, that is, $W(\boldsymbol{\tau}^0, \boldsymbol{\alpha}) = \sup_{\boldsymbol{\tau}} W(\boldsymbol{\tau}, \boldsymbol{\alpha})$. The problem is trivial if $F_1, F_2, \ldots, F_K$ are completely known, since in this case the optimal strategy is to choose for each trial the experiment for which $\int x \, dF_j(x)$ is maximal. The general problem, however, is difficult when some or all the distributions $F_1, \ldots, F_K$ are unknown or specified up to some unknown parameters. For example, suppose $F_1, \ldots, F_K$ are exponential distributions, that is, $F_j(x; \lambda_j) = 1 - \exp\{-\lambda_j x\}$, $j = 1, \ldots, K$, and the parameters $\lambda_1, \ldots, \lambda_K$ are unknown. A common approach to attack the problem is a Bayesian one. One has to assume a prior distribution $H(\lambda_1, \ldots, \lambda_K)$ over the parameter space $\Theta = \{\boldsymbol{\lambda} = (\lambda_1, \ldots, \lambda_K) : 0 < \lambda_i < \infty,\ i = 1, \ldots, K\}$. After each trial, the prior distribution is converted to the posterior distribution given the observed data. More specifically, for the present example, the sufficient statistic after n trials is $\mathcal{D}_n = (S^{(1)}_{m_1(n)}, S^{(2)}_{m_2(n)}, \ldots, S^{(K)}_{m_K(n)}; \mathbf{m}(n))$, where $S^{(j)}_{m_j(n)} = \sum_{i=1}^{m_j(n)} X_{ji}$ and $\mathbf{m}(n) = (m_1(n), \ldots, m_K(n))$, where $m_j(n) \geq 0$ is the number of trials on $\mathcal{E}_j$ and $\sum_{j=1}^{K} m_j(n) = n$. Let $\mathcal{F}_n$ denote the σ-field generated by $\mathcal{D}_n$. The class of strategies under consideration is that for which $\tau_n \in \mathcal{F}_{n-1}$ for all $n \geq 1$, and τ_1 is a function of the prior distribution H, while τ_n is a function of the posterior distribution $H_{n-1}(\boldsymbol{\lambda} \mid \mathcal{F}_{n-1})$. Notice that if for some i, $i = 1, \ldots, K$, $m_i(n) = 0$, then $S^{(i)}_0 \equiv 0$. The Bayesian total discounted reward is

$$W(\boldsymbol{\tau}, \boldsymbol{\alpha}, H) = \sum_{n=1}^{\infty} \alpha_n \sum_{j=1}^{K} E_H\{I\{\tau_n(\mathcal{F}_{n-1}, H) = j\} \cdot X_j\}. \tag{1.7.2}$$

The problem is to find an optimal Bayesian strategy $\tau_n(\mathcal{F}_{n-1}, H)$ under which $W(\tau, \boldsymbol{\alpha}, H)$ is maximized, if such a strategy exists.

If the number of trials m^* is finite, an optimal strategy τ^0_H exists and can be found in principle by dynamic programming (see Berry and Friestedt, 1985, p. 24). Generally it is very difficult to obtain, even numerically, the optimal solution. Various approximations are available (see Ross, 1983; Hardwick and Stout, 1995, p. 223). If only F_1 is unknown, while $F_2, \ldots, F_K$ are known, the problem is reduced to the so-called *one-armed bandit* (OAB) problem. Indeed, if $\lambda = \max_{2 \leq j \leq K} E\{X_j\}$ we can consider only two arms: arm 1, A_1, (or experiment $\mathcal{E}_1$) whose distribution F_1 is not completely known; and arm 2, A_2, whose expected reward in each trial is λ. As proven in Berry and Friestedt (1985), if the discount sequence is *regular*, that is,

$$\frac{\alpha_{n+2}}{\alpha_{n+1}} \leq \frac{\alpha_{n+1}}{\alpha_n} \quad \text{for all } n \geq 1, \tag{1.7.3}$$

then the optimal strategy in the OAB is to apply A_1 as long as it is optimal and then switch to A_2 and continue using it as long as the trials continue. Accordingly, the optimal strategy in the OAB problem is reduced to that of an optimal stopping time for the trials on A_1.

In the Bernoulli case of the OAB, the probability θ_1 of success in A_1 is unknown. Let $X_1 = 1, 0$, where $\theta_1 = P(X_1 = 1)$. Then let H be a prior distribution of θ_1. Berry and Friestedt (1985) developed an index $\Lambda(\boldsymbol{\alpha}, H)$ such that, as long as $\Lambda(\boldsymbol{\alpha}, H) > \lambda$, it is optimal to apply A_1. Notice that after n trials on A_1, $n \geq 0$, the posterior distribution of θ_1, given $\mathcal{F}_n$, is substituted for H in $\Lambda(\boldsymbol{\alpha}, H)$.

In Section 8.1 we discuss in some detail the one-armed Bernoulli bandits and give formulas for $\Lambda(\boldsymbol{\alpha}, H)$ and some approximations. In Section 8.2 we discuss the optimal solution of Gittins and Jones (1974), who treated the case of infinite trials and a geometric discount sequence $(1, \alpha, \alpha^2, \ldots)$, $0 < \alpha < 1$. They developed a *dynamic allocation index*, called the *Gittins index*. The values of this index are adapted after each trial for each arm separately. The arm with the maximal index value is the optimal one for the next trial. Section 8.3 is devoted to some approximations proposed for medical trials. In Section 8.4 we present the paper of Lamprecht and Zacks (1998) on Bernoulli OAB with change point in A_1. That is, at some unknown time θ_1 changes to a value $\phi > \lambda$. Finally, in Section 8.5 we present the paper of Zacks (1973) on the optimal design of sequential estimation of the common mean of two normal distributions when one variance is unknown. If we knew which population has a smaller variance, then the optimal design is to sample all observations from this population. When one variance is unknown, the question is how long to sample from the population with unknown variance before switching to take all the remaining observations to the other population. This is a version of the OAB problem.

An important book on the subject is the one mentioned earlier, by Berry and Friestedt (1985), entitled *Bandit Problems*. Another important book is that of Gittins (1989), entitled *Multi-Armed Bandit Allocation Indices*. These books contain dozens of relevant references.

1.8 SEQUENTIAL DETECTION OF CHANGE POINTS

Change-point problems have occupied a central position in statistical research during the last half century and are still a subject for interesting papers. A change point is an epoch at which the distribution of a specified random variable (vector) changes. The interesting problems are those where the epochs of the change points are unknown. Given a sequence of independent random variables $X_1, \ldots, X_n$, it is of interest to test whether they have the same distribution or whether there is a point after which the distributions change their law. More specifically, if $F_1, \ldots, F_n$ are the distributions of $X_1, \ldots, X_n$, is there an index τ such that $F_1 = \cdots = F_\tau$, $F_{\tau+1} = \cdots = F_n$, while $F_\tau \neq F_{\tau+1}$? In this case τ is a change point. Such problems of retrospective testing have been studied in a large number of papers. See Zacks (1983) for a survey of such papers. Chapter 9 is devoted to sequential detection procedures, with the objective of finding such change points as soon as they occur. Such procedures are of special importance for *statistical process control* (SPC). We discuss in this chapter three categories of sequential detection procedure: Bayesian sequential procedures (Sections 9.1 and 9.2), cumulative sums procedures (CUSUM, Section 9.3), and tracking procedures (Section 9.4). The rest of the chapter is devoted to related problems of a sequential nature.

Bayesian sequential stopping rules were studied in the early 1960s by Shiryaev (1963a,b), Bather (1963, 1967), Smith (1975), Zacks and Barzily (1981), Pollak (1985), and others. Recently, there are studies on Bayesian detection of change points in the intensity of a Poisson process by Peskir and Shiryaev (2002), Herbert and Jensen (2004), and Brown and Zacks (2006). CUSUM procedures were introduced in the 1950s by Page (1954, 1955, 1957). There are many papers on this subject. We discuss the asymptotic optimality of CUSUM procedures, as in Lorden (1971) and Pollak (1985). It is more difficult to derive the exact distribution of the stopping times of CUSUM. On this problem we present the results of Zacks (1981, 2004a). See also Woodall (1983, 1984) and Yashchin (1985).

Tracking methods provide current estimates of some parameters of interest of the stochastic process and flag whenever there is evidence of change points. Chernoff and Zacks (1964) have studied the problem of estimating the current mean of a simple normal (Gaussian) process which is subjected to changes in the mean at unknown time points. We provide a development of a Bayesian tracking algorithm, which estimates parameters of the posterior distributions of the means, μ_n $(n = 1, 2, \ldots)$, under the at-most-one-change-point (AMOC) model. Other tracking procedures which are based on adaptive Kalman filtering are cited. In particular see the study of Gordon and Smith (1988). Tracking procedures are discussed in Section 9.3. In Section 9.4 we present some results on recursive methods and change points. Finally, in Section 9.5 we study the problem of detecting faults in software. Each time of such detection is a change point in which the reliability of the software is increasing.

1.9 SEQUENTIAL METHODS IN INDUSTRIAL TESTING, RELIABILITY, AND DESIGN OF EXPERIMENTS

Statistical methods for quality control consist of three categories: sampling acceptance schemes, process control, and robust designs. All three areas of statistical procedures include adaptive methods. In Section 4.7 we present two-stage sampling inspection schemes. In Chapter 10, Section 10.1, we present the important *Wald sequential probability ratio test* (SPRT), for testing whether the quality level of a lot of items or of a process is up to a specified standard. These methods of statistical quality control were developed during World War II and were in common practice since then.

In Section 10.1 we develop the theory and operating characteristics of the Wald SPRT. The exact distribution of the stopping variable is derived for the exponential case. In Section 10.2 we present a few sequential methods to evaluate the operating characteristic function of reliability testing of equipment. In Section 10.3 we discuss additional sequential procedures for design of experiments. Finally, in Section 10.4 we discuss another model of adaptive software reliability testing.

For the various schemes and practices of sampling acceptance by attributes or by variables, including the famous Skip-Lot and other procedures,Skip-Lot procedure see Chapter 9 of Kenett and Zacks (1998).

CHAPTER 2

MULTISTAGE AND SEQUENTIAL ESTIMATION

2.1 STEIN'S TWO-STAGE PROCEDURE

The Stein two-stage procedure, as explained before, was designed to achieve a fixed-width confidence interval for the normal mean, μ, when the standard deviation, σ, is unknown.

The procedure:

Stage I: Draw a random sample of m i.i.d. random variables from $\mathcal{N}(\mu, \sigma)$. Compute the sufficient statistics

$$\bar{X}_m = \frac{1}{m}\sum_{i=1}^{m} X_i, \quad S_m^2 = \frac{1}{m-1}\sum_{i=1}^{m}(X_i - \bar{X}_m)^2.$$

Let $t_{1-\alpha/2}[m-1]$ be the $(1-\alpha/2)$-quantile of the t-distribution with $m-1$ degrees of freedom. Compute the random sample size

$$N_m = \max\left\{\left\lfloor \frac{t^2_{1-\alpha/2}[m-1]S_m^2}{\delta^2}\right\rfloor + 1, m\right\}. \tag{2.1.1}$$

If $N_m = m$, stop sampling and set $\bar{X}_{N_m} = \bar{X}_m$; else go to Stage II.

Stage II: Draw an additional random sample of $N_m - m$ observations: $X_1^*, \ldots, X_{N-m}^*$. Compute $\bar{X}_{N_m} = (X_1 + \cdots + X_m + X_1^* + \cdots + X_{N_m - m}^*)/N_m$. The confidence interval for μ is

$$I_{N_m}(\delta) = (\bar{X}_{N_m} - \delta, \bar{X}_{N_m} + \delta). \tag{2.1.2}$$

We prove now that the coverage probability of $I_{N_m}(\delta)$ is at least $1 - \alpha$.

Theorem 2.1.1 *For all $m \geq 2$,*

$$P_\sigma\{\mu \in I_{N_m}(\delta)\} \geq 1 - \alpha \quad \text{for all} \quad 0 < \sigma < \infty. \tag{2.1.3}$$

Proof: The proof is based on the important result that, in random samples of fixed size, m, from a normal distribution, the sample mean $\bar{X}_m$ and the sample variance S_m^2 are independent (see Seber, 1977, p. 29). Since N_m depends only on S_m^2, the conditional distribution of $X_1^*, \ldots, X_{N_m - m}^*$ given S_m^2 is independent of $\bar{X}_m$. Moreover,

$$P_\sigma\{\bar{X}_{N_m} - \delta \leq \mu \leq \bar{X}_{N_m} + \delta \mid S_m^2\} = 2\Phi\left(\frac{\delta}{\sigma}\sqrt{N_m}\right) - 1 \quad \text{for all} \quad \sigma. \tag{2.1.4}$$

Accordingly,

(2.1.5)

$$\begin{aligned}
P_\sigma\{\bar{X}_{N_m} - \delta \leq \mu \leq \bar{X}_{N_m} + \delta\} &= 2E\left\{\Phi\left(\frac{\delta}{\sigma}\sqrt{N_m}\right)\right\} - 1 \\
&\geq 2E\left\{\Phi\left(\frac{\delta}{\sigma} \cdot t_{1-\alpha/2}[m-1]\frac{S_m}{\delta}\right)\right\} - 1 \\
&= 2P\left\{\frac{N(0,1)}{\sqrt{\chi^2[m-1]/(m-1)}} \right. \\
&\qquad \left. \leq t_{1-\alpha/2}[m-1]\right\} - 1 \\
&= 1 - \alpha,
\end{aligned}$$

where $N(0,1)$ denotes a standard normal random variable and $\chi^2[m-1]$ denotes a chi-squared random variable with $m-1$ degrees of freedom. Also, $N(0,1)/\sqrt{\chi^2[m-1]/(m-1)}$ has a student's t-distribution with $m-1$ degrees of freedom. ■

We develop now the distribution of N_m, which depends according to (2.1.1) on the distribution of S_m^2. Notice that if $m = 2k+1$ then

$$S_m^2 \sim \frac{\sigma^2}{2k}\chi^2[2k] \sim \frac{\sigma^2}{k}G(1,k),$$

where $G(1,k)$ is a random variable having a gamma distribution with scale parameter 1 and shape parameter k. The symbol $\sim$ denotes equivalence of random variables, which means that they have the same distribution. Let $P(j;\mu)$ denote the c.d.f. of the Poisson distribution with mean μ. According to the Poisson–gamma relationship (see Kao, 1977, p. 47)

$$P\{G(1,k) \le x\} = 1 - P(k-1;x) \tag{2.1.6}$$

for all $0 \le x < \infty$. Accordingly, since $t^2_{1-\alpha/2}[2k] = F_{1-\alpha}[1,2k]$,

$$\begin{aligned} P\{N_m = m\} &= P\{G(1,k) \le \lambda_k m\} \\ &= 1 - P(k-1;\lambda_k m), \end{aligned} \tag{2.1.7}$$

where

$$\lambda_k = \frac{\delta^2}{\sigma^2 F_{1-\alpha}[1,2k]} k. \tag{2.1.8}$$

Moreover, for every $n > m$,

$$P\{N_m = n\} = P(k-1;\lambda_k(n-1)) - P(k-1;\lambda_k n). \tag{2.1.9}$$

From this we obtain:

Theorem 2.1.2 *The expected value of N_m is*

$$E\{N_m\} = m + \sum_{n=m}^{\infty} P(k-1;\lambda_k n). \tag{2.1.10}$$

Proof:

$$\begin{aligned} E\{N_m\} &= m - mP(k-1;\lambda_k m) \\ &\quad + \sum_{j=1}^{\infty}(m+j)(P(k-1;\lambda_k(m+j-1)) \\ &\qquad - P(k-1;\lambda_k(m+j))) \\ &= m + \sum_{j=0}^{\infty} P(k-1;\lambda_k(m+j)). \end{aligned}$$

■

The exact coverage probability of the confidence interval is, for $m = 2k+1$,

$$\begin{aligned} \mathrm{CP}(\delta,\sigma) &= 2\sum_{n=m}^{\infty} \Phi\left(\frac{\delta\sqrt{n}}{\sigma}\right) P_\sigma\{N_m = n\} - 1 \\ &= 2\Phi\left(\frac{\delta\sqrt{m}}{\sigma}\right)(1 - P(k-1;\lambda_k m)) \\ &\quad + 2\sum_{n=m+1}^{\infty} \Phi\left(\frac{\delta\sqrt{n}}{\sigma}\right)(P(k-1;\lambda_k(n-1)) \\ &\qquad - P(k-1;\lambda_k n)) - 1. \end{aligned}$$

In Table 2.1 we present some numerical values for $\mathrm{CP}(\delta,\sigma)$ and $E_\sigma\{N_m\}$.

Table 2.1: Coverage Probabilities and Expected Sample Size of Stein's Two-Stage Procedure for $\alpha = 0.05$, $\sigma = 1$.

	$\delta^2 = 0.01$		$\delta^2 = 0.005$	
m	CP	$E\{N_m\}$	CP	$E\{N_m\}$
51	0.95015	403.93	0.95008	800.75
101	0.95015	394.11	0.95008	787.49
151	0.95015	390.92	0.95008	781.34
201	0.95015	389.34	0.95008	778.18
251	0.95015	388.39	0.95008	776.29
301	0.95015	387.78	0.95008	775.02
$n^0(\delta, \sigma)$	—	384.14	—	768.28

We see in Table 2.1 that if the initial sample size is large, but smaller than $n^0(\delta, \sigma)$, then the coverage probability is close to $1 - \alpha$ and $E_\sigma\{N_m\}/n^0(\delta, \sigma)$ is close to 1. The problem is that $n^0(\delta, \sigma)$ is unknown and if $m > n^0(\delta, \sigma)$ then the procedure is wasteful (inefficient).

2.2 MODIFICATIONS TO ATTAIN ASYMPTOTIC EFFICIENCY

A two-stage procedure is called *asymptotically efficient* (of the first order) if

$$(2.2.1) \qquad \lim_{\delta \to 0} \frac{E_\sigma\{N_m\}}{n^0(\delta, \sigma^0)} = 1.$$

The Stein two-stage procedure for any fixed integer m, $2 \leq m < \infty$, is *not* asymptotically efficient. Indeed, from the inequalities

$$(2.2.2) \qquad \frac{F_{1-\alpha}[1, m-1]S_m^2}{\delta^2} < N_m < m + 1 + \frac{F_{1-\alpha}[1, m-1]S_m^2}{\delta^2}$$

we immediately obtain, since $E\{S_m^2\} = \sigma^2$,

$$(2.2.3) \qquad \lim_{\delta \to 0} \frac{E\{N_m\}}{n^0(\delta, \sigma)} = \frac{F_{1-\alpha}[1, m-1]}{\chi^2_{1-\alpha}[1]} > 1.$$

It is clear that if the initial sample size m is sufficiently large then the Stein procedure is almost asymptotically efficient. Indeed, $F_{0.95}[1, 29]/\chi^2_{0.95}[1] = 1.0889$ and $F_{0.95}[1, 149]/\chi^2_{0.95}[1] = 1.01644$. The ratio $F_{1-\alpha}[1, m-1]/\chi^2_{1-\alpha}[1] \searrow 1$ as $m \to \infty$. One needs m to be quite large to attain approximate efficiency.

Ghosh and Mukhopadhyay (1981) suggested to take the size of the first stage as a function of δ, namely

$$m(\delta) = \max\{2, \lfloor A\delta^{-2/(1+\gamma)} \rfloor + 1\}, \tag{2.2.4}$$

where $0 < \gamma < \infty$. In this case, as $\delta \to 0$

$$\lim_{\delta \to 0} \frac{m(\delta)}{n^0(\delta, \sigma^2)} = 0, \tag{2.2.5}$$

and

$$\lim_{\delta \to 0} \frac{F_{1-\alpha}[1, m(\delta) - 1]}{\chi^2_{1-\alpha}[1]} = 1. \tag{2.2.6}$$

We then obtain:

Theorem 2.2.1 *For $m(\delta)$ given by (2.2.4)*

$$P_{\mu,\sigma}\{\mu \in I_{N_{m(\delta)}}(\delta)\} \geq 1 - \alpha \quad \text{for all} \quad \mu, \sigma, \tag{2.2.7}$$

$$\lim_{\delta \to 0} \frac{N_{m(\delta)}}{n^0(\delta, \sigma)} = 1 \quad a.s., \tag{2.2.8}$$

$$\lim_{\delta \to 0} \frac{E\{N_{m(\delta)}\}}{n^0(\delta, \sigma)} = 1, \tag{2.2.9}$$

and

$$\lim_{\delta \to 0} P_{\mu,\sigma}\{\mu \in I_{N_{m(\delta)}}(\delta)\} = 1 - \alpha, \quad \text{all} \quad \mu, \sigma. \tag{2.2.10}$$

Proof: See Ghosh and Mukhopadhyay (1981). ■

A procedure is called *second-order asymptotically efficient* if

$$\overline{\lim_{\delta \to 0}}(E\{N_m\} - n^0(\delta, \sigma)) < \infty. \tag{2.2.11}$$

The Stein procedure, even with $m(\delta)$ as in (2.2.4) is, however, *not* a second-order efficient procedure. Indeed,

(2.2.12)

$$\underline{\lim}_{\delta \to 0}\{E\{N_{m(\delta)}\} - n^0(\delta, \sigma)\} \geq \sigma^2 \underline{\lim}_{\delta \to 0}(F_{1-\alpha}[1, m(\delta) - 1] - \chi^2_{1-\alpha}[1])\delta^{-2} = \infty.$$

To verify this we find that

$$F_{1-\alpha}[1, m(\delta) - 1] - \chi^2_{1-\alpha}[1] = 0\left(\delta \frac{2}{1+\gamma}\right) \quad \text{as} \quad \delta \to 0$$

(see Johnson and Kotz, 1970, p. 102). As we will show later, the second-order asymptotic property holds in a sequential procedure. The question is whether it can hold in a two-stage procedure. Mukhopadhyay and Duggan (1997) showed that if $\sigma > \sigma_L > 0$, where σ_L is a *known* lower bound, and one starts the first stage with $m^*(\delta, \sigma_L)$ observations, where

$$m^*(\delta, \sigma_L) = \max\left\{m_0, \left\lfloor \frac{\chi^2_{1-\alpha}[1]\sigma_L^2}{\delta^2} \right\rfloor + 1\right\}, \tag{2.2.13}$$

then the second-order asymptotic property holds. They actually prove:

Theorem 2.2.2 *For a two-stage procedure, with $\sigma > \sigma_L$ and $m = m^*$ as in (2.2.13)*

$$\eta + o(\delta) \le E_\sigma\{N_{m^*}\} - n^0(\delta, \sigma) \le (\eta + 1) + o(\delta) \tag{2.2.14}$$

as $\delta \to 0$, where

$$\eta = \frac{1}{2}(\chi^2_{1-\alpha}[1] + 1)\left(\frac{\sigma}{\sigma_L}\right)^2. \tag{2.2.15}$$

■

They also proved:

Theorem 2.2.3 *For the two-stage procedure when $\sigma > \sigma_L$, with $m^*(\delta)$ as in (2.2.13),*

$$\frac{N_{m^*} - n^0(\delta, \sigma)}{\sqrt{n^0(\delta, \sigma)}} \xrightarrow{d} N\left(0, 2\left(\frac{\sigma}{\sigma_L}\right)^2\right) \quad \text{as } \delta \to 0. \tag{2.2.16}$$

■

Notice that $m^*(\delta, \sigma_L)$ is smaller than $n^0(\delta, \sigma)$ whenever $\sigma_L < \sigma$. We can compute the distribution of the left-hand side of (2.2.16) exactly, according to formulas (2.1.7)–(2.1.9), in which m and k are given by $m^*(\delta, \sigma_L)$ and $k^*(\delta, \sigma_L) = \lfloor \frac{1}{2}[m^*(\delta, \sigma_L) - 1] \rfloor + 1$. The distribution depends strongly on the ratio σ_L/σ. In Figure 2.1 we illustrate the exact c.d.f. of N_{m^*} and its normal approximation for $\sigma/\sigma_L = 2$, $\alpha = 0.05$, $\delta = 0.1$. The exact distribution was computed with the SPLUS program distN_m.

2.3 TWO-STAGE SAMPLING FROM EXPONENTIAL DISTRIBUTIONS

2.3.1 Fixed-Width Confidence Interval for the Location Parameter of an Exponential Distribution

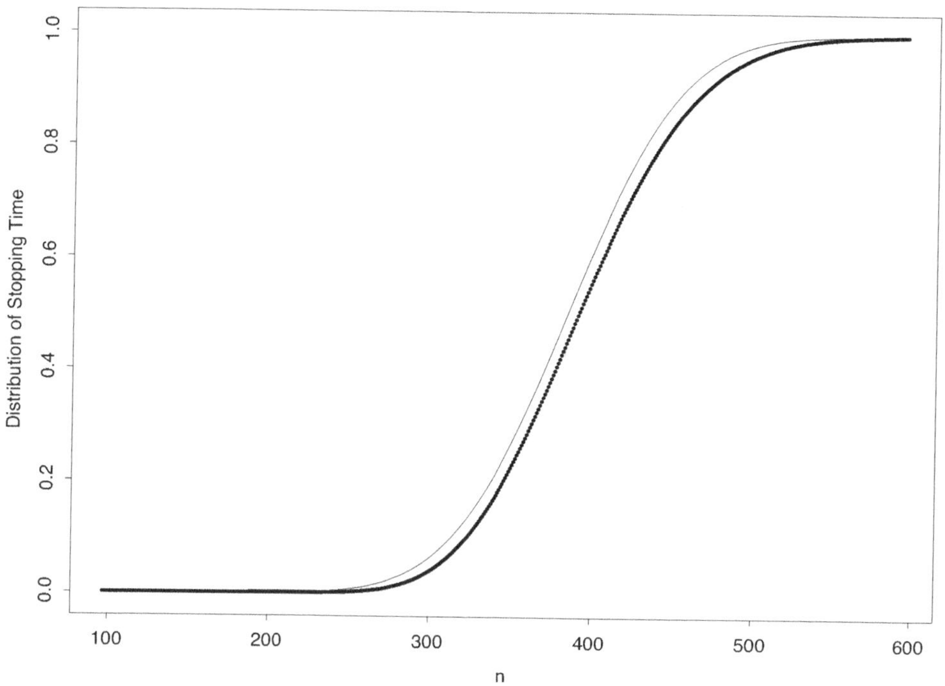

Figure 2.1: Distribution of N_{m^*}, exact (bold) and normal approximation (thin) $\delta = 0.1$, $\alpha = 0.05$, $\sigma_L = 0.5$, $\sigma = 1$.

Let $X_1, X_2, \ldots$ be i.i.d. random variables having an exponential distribution with location parameter μ, $-\infty < \mu < \infty$, and a scale parameter σ, $0 < \sigma < \infty$. We wish to construct a confidence interval for μ of length 2δ having confidence level $1 - \alpha$. We remind the reader (see Zacks, 1971, p. 31) that for a fixed sample of size n the minimal sufficient statistic is $(X_{n:1}, U_n)$, where $X_{n:1} < X_{n:2} < \cdots < X_{n:n}$ is the order statistic and $U_n = \sum_{j=2}^{n}(X_{n:j} - X_{n:1})$. Furthermore, $X_{n:1}$ and U_n are independent,

(2.3.1) $$X_{n:1} \sim \mu + \frac{\sigma}{n} G(1,1)$$

and

(2.3.2) $$U_n \sim \sigma G(1, n-1).$$

Thus, if σ is *known*, the confidence interval $(X_{n:1} - 2\delta, X_{n:1})$ has confidence level $1 - \alpha$ if n is greater or equal to

$$n^0(\delta, \sigma) = (-\log \alpha)\frac{\sigma}{2\delta}. \tag{2.3.3}$$

If σ is *unknown* we can use the Stein two-stage procedure to obtain a confidence interval of level $1 - \alpha$.

Stage I: Take a random sample of size $m \geq 2$. Compute $X_{m:1}$ and the unbiased estimator of σ, $\hat{\sigma}_m = U_m/(m-1)$. Determine the stopping variable

$$N = \max\left\{m, \left\lfloor \frac{F_{1-\alpha}[2, 2(m-1)]\hat{\sigma}_m}{2\delta} \right\rfloor + 1\right\}. \tag{2.3.4}$$

If $N = m$, stop sampling; else go to:

Stage II: Take an additional $N - m$ independent observations. Let $X_{N:1}$ be the minimum value of the combined sample $X_1, \ldots, X_m, X^*_{m+1}, \ldots, X^*_N$. The confidence interval is $(X_{N:1} - 2\delta, X_{N:1})$. Notice that if $N = m$ (stop after the first stage) then $X_{N:1} = X_{m:1}$.

Theorem 2.3.1 *In the above two-stage sampling*

$$P_{\mu,\sigma}\{X_{N:1} - 2\delta < \mu < X_{N:1}\} \geq 1 - \alpha \tag{2.3.5}$$

for all $-\infty < \mu < \infty$ *and* $0 < \sigma < \infty$.

Proof: Since $X_{m:1}$ is independent of $\hat{\sigma}_m$, and given $\hat{\sigma}_m$, $X^*_{m+1}, \ldots, X^*_N$ are conditionally independent of $\hat{\sigma}_m$, it follows that $X_{N:1}$ is conditionally independent of N given $\hat{\sigma}_m$. Thus, since $X_{N:1} > \mu$ almost surely (a.s.),

(2.3.6)

$$\begin{aligned}
P_{\mu,\sigma}\{X_{N:1} - 2\delta < \mu < X_{N:1}\} &= P_{\mu,\sigma}\{X_{N:1} - \mu < 2\delta\} \\
&= P_{\mu,\sigma}\left\{G(1,1) < \frac{N}{\sigma}2\delta\right\} \\
&\geq P_{\mu,\sigma}\left\{G(1,1) < \frac{F_{1-\alpha}[2, 2(m-1)]}{\sigma} \cdot \hat{\sigma}_m\right\} \\
&= P_{\mu,\sigma}\left\{\frac{\chi^2_1[2]/2}{\chi^2_2[2(m-1)]/2(m-1)} < F_{1-\alpha}[2, 2(m-1)]\right\} \\
&= 1 - \alpha \quad \text{for all } \mu, \sigma.
\end{aligned}$$

■

Notice that for an arbitrary fixed m,

$$\lim_{\delta \to 0} \frac{E\{N\}}{n^0(\delta, \sigma)} = \frac{F_{1-\alpha}[2, 2(m-1)]}{\chi^2_{1-\alpha}[2]} > 1. \tag{2.3.7}$$

Thus, as in the normal case, this two-stage procedure is *not* asymptotically first-order efficient. If, however, m is chosen as in (2.2.13), the procedure becomes asymptotically first-order efficient. Moreover, if $\sigma > \sigma_L$, where σ_L is known, then as shown in Mukhopadhyay and Duggan (1997a,b) the procedure can be even asymptotically second-order efficient. The distribution of N can be determined exactly, like in Section 2.1. Define

$$\lambda_m = \frac{2\delta(m-1)}{F_{1-\alpha}[2, 2(m-1)]\sigma}. \tag{2.3.8}$$

Then

$$P\{N = m\} = 1 - P(m-1; \lambda_m m), \tag{2.3.9}$$

and, for $n > m$,

$$P\{N = n\} = P(m-1; \lambda_m(n-1)) - P(m-1; \lambda_m n). \tag{2.3.10}$$

We then obtain, as in (2.1.10),

$$E_\sigma\{N\} = m + \sum_{n=m}^{\infty} P(m-1; \lambda_m n). \tag{2.3.11}$$

The exact coverage probability of the confidence interval is
(2.3.12)

$$\begin{aligned}
\text{CP}(\delta, \sigma) &= P_\sigma\left\{G(1,1) \le \frac{N}{\sigma}2\delta\right\} \\
&= \sum_{n=m}^{\infty} P_\sigma\{N = n\}(1 - e^{-2n\delta/\sigma}) \\
&= (1 - e^{-2\delta m/\sigma}) + (1 - e^{-2\delta/\sigma}) \sum_{n=m}^{\infty} e^{-2\delta n/\sigma} P(m-1; \lambda_m n).
\end{aligned}$$

In Table 2.2 we present the expected sample size and the coverage probability of this two-stage procedure. Notice that both $E\{N\}$ and $\text{CP}(\delta, \sigma)$ depend on δ and σ only through their ratio $\omega = \delta/\sigma$.

Table 2.2: Values of $E_\sigma\{N\}$ and $CP(\delta, \sigma)$ for $\alpha = 0.05$, $\sigma = 1$

	$\delta = 0.01$		$\delta = 0.005$	
m	$E\{N\}$	CP	$E\{N\}$	CP
10	197.98	0.9645	395.44	0.9643
20	171.28	0.9577	342.06	0.9575
50	158.11	0.9534	315.73	0.9532
100	154.11	0.9520	307.72	0.9517
150	156.46	0.9556	305.14	0.9512
$n^0(\delta, \sigma)$	149.79	0.9500	299.58	0.9500

2.3.2 Two-Stage Sampling for a Bounded Risk Point Estimation of the Exponential Parameter

Consider the problem of estimating the scale parameter (the mean) of an exponential distribution. Suppose that $X_1, \ldots, X_n$ is a fixed random sample from an exponential distribution with mean β. The sample mean $\bar{X}_n = \sum_{j=1}^{n} X_j/n$ is a minimal sufficient statistic. It is a uniformly minimum variance unbiased estimator of β. Suppose that the loss function is $L(\hat{\beta}_n, \beta) = A(\hat{\beta}_n - \beta)^2$, where $0 < A < \infty$ and $\hat{\beta}_n$ is an estimator of β. The corresponding quadratic risk of the estimator $\bar{X}_n$ is $R_n(\beta) = A(\beta^2/n)$. This risk function increases to infinity as $\beta \nearrow \infty$. If β is known and we wish to bound the risk by a quantity ω, $0 < \omega < \infty$, we should choose the sample size n to be at least

$$n^*(\omega, \beta) = \frac{A\beta^2}{\omega}. \tag{2.3.13}$$

If β is unknown we cannot determine n sufficiently large, in a single-stage sampling, to guarantee that $R_n(\beta) \le \omega$ for all $0 < \beta < \infty$. Mukhopadhyay and Pepe (2006) proved that if one applies a two-stage sampling with $m \ge 3$ observations in the first stage and uses the stopping variable

$$N_m = \max\left\{m, \left\lfloor \frac{B\bar{X}_m^2}{\omega} \right\rfloor + 1\right\} \tag{2.3.14}$$

and substitutes $B = B^0$, where

$$B^0 = \frac{2m(m+1)A}{(m-1)(m-2)}, \tag{2.3.15}$$

then $R_{N_m}(\beta) \le \omega$ for all $0 < \beta < \infty$.

We will prove later that, for any $0 < B < \infty$, $R_{N_m}(\beta)$ is an analytic function of β, with $\lim_{\beta \to 0} R_{N_m}(\beta) = 0$ and

$$\limsup_{\beta \to \infty} R_{N_m}(\beta) \le \frac{Am^2\omega}{B(m-1)(m-2)}. \tag{2.3.16}$$

This will prove that $R_{N,m}(\beta)$ is uniformly bounded for any $0 < B < \infty$. We will also show that for a given bound ω the maximal risk is close to ω if we take instead of B^0 the value $B^* = 0.565B^0$. These results were obtained by Zacks and Mukhopadhyay (2006b) after observing that B^0 yields $E_\beta\{N_m\} \approx 3n^0(\omega, \beta)$.

As before, define

$$\lambda_n = \frac{m}{\beta}\sqrt{\frac{\omega}{B}}\sqrt{n}. \tag{2.3.17}$$

Then, the distribution of N_m is

$$P_\beta\{N_m = m\} = 1 - P(m-1; \lambda_m) \tag{2.3.18}$$

and for $n \geq m+1$

$$P_\beta\{N_m = n\} = P(m-1;\lambda_{n-1}) - P(m-1;\lambda_n). \tag{2.3.19}$$

Also,

$$E_\beta\{N_m\} = m + \sum_{n=m}^{\infty} P(m-1;\lambda_n). \tag{2.3.20}$$

One can verify that

$$\frac{\partial}{\partial B} E_\beta\{N_m\} = \frac{m}{2\beta}\frac{\omega^{1/2}}{B^{3/2}}\frac{1}{(m-1)!}\sum_{j=0}^{\infty}(m+j)^{1/2}\lambda_{m+j}^{m-1}e^{-\lambda_{m+j}}. \tag{2.3.21}$$

Thus, $E_\beta\{N_m\}$ is a monotone increasing function of B with $\lim_{B\to 0} E_\beta\{N_m\} = m$ and $\lim_{B\to\infty} E_\beta\{N_m\} = \infty$. Stopping at N_m, the estimator of β is $\hat\beta_{N_m} = \bar X_{N_m} = (1/N_m)\sum_{j=1}^{N_m} X_j$. We now develop formulas for $E\{\bar X_{N_m}\}$ and for the risk $R(\bar X_{N_m}, \beta)$. We denote by $p(j;\mu)$ the Poisson probability distribution function (p.d.f.) with mean μ.

Theorem 2.3.2

$$E_\beta\{\bar X_{N_m}\} = \beta\left(1 - \sum_{j=m}^{\infty}\frac{m}{j(j+1)}p(m;\lambda_j)\right). \tag{2.3.22}$$

Proof: Let $\mathcal{F}_m = \sigma(X_1,\ldots,X_m)$ designate the σ-field generated by the random variables in the first stage. Notice that $X_{m+1}, X_{m+2},\ldots$ are independent of $\mathcal{F}_m$. Moreover, $N_m \in \mathcal{F}_m$. Accordingly,

(2.3.23)

$$\begin{aligned} E\{\bar X_{N_m} \mid \mathcal{F}_m\} &= \bar X_m I(N_m = m) + \frac{m}{N_m}\bar X_m I(N_m > m) \\ &\quad + E\left\{\frac{N_m - m}{N_m}\bar X^*_{N-m} I(N_m > m) \mid \mathcal{F}_m\right\} \\ &= \bar X_m I(N_m = m) + \left(\beta + \frac{m}{N_m}(\bar X_m - \beta)\right) I(N_m > m). \end{aligned}$$

We denote by $I(\cdot)$ the indicator variable. Furthermore by the law of the iterated expectation

$$\begin{aligned} E_\beta\{\bar X_{N_m}\} &= E_\beta\{E\{\bar X_{N_m} \mid \mathcal{F}_m\}\} \\ &= E_\beta\{\bar X_m I(N_m = m)\} + \beta P_\beta\{N_m > m\} \\ &\quad + E_\beta\left\{(\bar X_m - \beta)\frac{m}{N_m} I(N_m > m)\right\}. \end{aligned} \tag{2.3.24}$$

The first term on the right-hand side (r.h.s.) of (2.3.24) is

(2.3.25)
$$\begin{aligned} E_\beta\{\bar{X}_m I(N_m = m)\} &= \frac{\beta}{m}\sum_{n=1}^{m}\frac{1}{(m-1)!}\int_{\lambda_{n-1}}^{\lambda_n} x^m e^{-x}\,dx \\ &= \beta\sum_{n=1}^{m}(P(m;\lambda_{n-1}) - P(m;\lambda_n)) \\ &= \beta(1 - P(m;\lambda_m)). \end{aligned}$$

According to (2.3.19), the second term on the r.h.s. of (2.3.24) is

(2.3.26)
$$\beta P_\beta(N_m > m) = \beta P(m-1;\lambda_m).$$

Furthermore,

(2.3.27)
$$\begin{aligned} \beta E_\beta\left\{\frac{m}{N_m} I(N_m > m)\right\} &= \beta\sum_{n=m+1}^{\infty}\frac{m}{n}(P(m-1;\lambda_{n-1}) \\ &\qquad - P(m-1;\lambda_n)) \\ &= \beta\sum_{n=m}^{\infty}\frac{m}{n+1}(P(m-1;\lambda_n) - P(m-1;\lambda_{n+1})) \\ &= \beta\frac{m}{m+1}P(m-1;\lambda_m) \\ &\quad - \beta\sum_{j=m+1}^{\infty}\frac{m}{j(j+1)}P(m-1;\lambda_j). \end{aligned}$$

Similarly,

(2.3.28)
$$\begin{aligned} E_\beta\left\{\frac{m}{N_m}\bar{X}_m I(N_m > m)\right\} &= \beta\sum_{n=m+1}^{\infty}\frac{m}{n}(P(m;\lambda_{n-1}) - P(m;\lambda_n)) \\ &= \beta\frac{m}{m+1}P(m;\lambda_m) \\ &\quad - \beta\sum_{j=m+1}^{\infty}\frac{m}{j(j+1)}P(m;\lambda_j). \end{aligned}$$

Substituting (2.3.25)–(2.3.28) in (2.3.24) we obtain (2.3.22). ∎

The bias of $\bar{X}_{N_m}$ is negative and bounded below. Indeed,

(2.3.29)
$$\text{Bias}(\bar{X}_{N_m};\beta) = -\beta\sum_{j=m}^{\infty}\frac{m}{j(j+1)}p\left(m;\frac{m}{\beta}\sqrt{\frac{\omega}{B}j}\right).$$

By the dominated convergence theorem,

$$\begin{aligned} \lim_{\beta\to\infty}\text{Bias}(\bar{X}_{N_m};\beta) &= -\sum_{j=m}^{\infty}\frac{m}{j(j+1)}\lim_{\beta\to\infty}\beta p\left(m;\frac{m}{\beta}\sqrt{\frac{\omega}{B}j}\right) \\ &= 0. \end{aligned}$$

Similarly

$$\lim_{\beta \to 0} \text{Bias}(\bar{X}_{N_m}; \beta) = 0.$$

Thus, the function (2.3.29) is analytic, and is bounded below. It is decreasing from zero to a minimum and then increasing to zero.

Next, determine the second moment of $\bar{X}_{N_m}$. The conditional expectation of $\bar{X}^2_{N_m}$ is

$$\begin{aligned} E_\beta\{\bar{X}^2_{N_m} \mid \mathcal{F}_m\} &= \bar{X}^2_m I(N_m = m) + \left(\frac{m}{N_m}\right)^2 \bar{X}^2_m I(N_m > m) \\ &\quad + \beta^2 \left(1 + \frac{1}{N_m - m}\right)\left(1 - \frac{m}{N_m}\right)^2 I(N_m > m) \\ &\quad + 2\beta \frac{m}{N_m}\left(1 - \frac{m}{N_m}\right) \bar{X}_m I(N_m > m). \end{aligned} \tag{2.3.30}$$

Taking the expected value of (2.3.30) we find

$$E_\beta\{\bar{X}^2_m I(N_m = m)\} = \beta^2 \left(1 + \frac{1}{m}\right)(1 - P(m+1; \lambda_m)). \tag{2.3.31}$$

Furthermore,

$$\begin{aligned} \beta^2 E_\beta\left\{\frac{N_m - m}{N^2_m} I(N_m > m)\right\} = -\beta^2 \sum_{j=0}^{\infty} \frac{j + (j+m)(j-m)}{(m+j)^2(m+j+1)^2} \cdot \\ \cdot\ P(m-1; \lambda_{m+j}). \end{aligned} \tag{2.3.32}$$

Also,

$$\begin{aligned} E_\beta\left\{\left(\frac{m}{N_m}\right)^2 \bar{X}^2_m I(N_m > m)\right\} &= \beta^2 \frac{m+1}{m} P(m+1; \lambda_m) \\ - \beta^2 \sum_{j=0}^{\infty} &\frac{m(m+1)(2(m+j)+1)}{(m+j)^2(m+j+1)^2} P(m+1; \lambda_{m+j}). \end{aligned} \tag{2.3.33}$$

In addition

$$\begin{aligned} &\beta^2 E_\beta\left\{\left(1 - \frac{m}{N_m}\right)^2 I(N_m > m)\right\} \\ &\quad = \beta^2 \sum_{j=0}^{\infty} \frac{m(2j(m+j) + m + 2j)}{(m+j)^2(m+j+1)^2} \cdot P(m-1; \lambda_{m+j}). \end{aligned} \tag{2.3.34}$$

Finally,

$$\begin{aligned} &2\beta E_\beta\left\{\frac{m}{N_m}\left(1 - \frac{m}{N_m}\right)\bar{X}_m I(N_m > m)\right\} \\ &\quad = 2\beta^2 \sum_{j=0}^{\infty} \frac{m(m^2 - j(j+1))}{(m+j)^2(m+j+1)^2} \cdot\ P(m; \lambda_{m+j}). \end{aligned} \tag{2.3.35}$$

Adding (2.3.31)–(2.3.35), after some algebraic manipulations we obtain the next theorem.

Theorem 2.3.3

$$E_\beta\{\bar{X}^2_{N_m}\} = \beta^2\Bigg[1 + \frac{1}{m} + \sum_{j=0}^{\infty} b_1(j,m)P(m-1;\lambda_{m+j}) + \sum_{j=0}^{\infty} b_2(j,m)p(m;\lambda_{m+j}) + \sum_{j=0}^{\infty} b_3(j,m)p(m+1;\lambda_{m+j})\Bigg], \tag{2.3.36}$$

where

$$b_1(j,m) = -\frac{1}{(m+j)(m+j+1)}, \tag{2.3.37}$$

$$b_2(j,m) = -\frac{2mj(m+j+2)+m(1+3m)}{(m+j)^2(m+j+1)^2}, \tag{2.3.38}$$

and

$$b_3(j,m) = \frac{-m(m+1)(2(m+j)+1)}{(m+j)^2(m+j+1)^2}. \tag{2.3.39}$$

■

We are ready now to obtain the formula for the risk of $\bar{X}_{N_m}$.

Theorem 2.3.4

$$R(\bar{X}_{N_m},\beta) = A\beta^2\Bigg(\frac{1}{m} + \sum_{j=0}^{\infty} b_1(j,m)P(m-1;\lambda_{m+j}) + \sum_{j=0}^{\infty} b_2^*(j,m)p(m;\lambda_{m+j}) + \sum_{j=0}^{\infty} b_3(j,m)p(m+1;\lambda_{m+j})\Bigg), \tag{2.3.40}$$

where

$$b_2^*(j,m) = \frac{m(m-1)(2(m+j)+1)}{(m+j)^2(m+j+1)^2}. \tag{2.3.41}$$

■

Notice that

$$-b_1(j,m) = \frac{1}{m+j} - \frac{1}{m+j+1}, \quad j \geq 0,$$

and

$$b_2^*(j,m) = m(m-1)\left(\frac{1}{(m+j)^2} - \frac{1}{(m+j+1)^2}\right), \quad j \geq 0.$$

Thus, we obtain

$$\sum_{j=0}^{\infty} b_1(j,m) = -\frac{1}{m},$$

$$\sum_{j=0}^{\infty} b_2^*(j,m) = \frac{m-1}{m},$$

$$\sum_{j=0}^{\infty} b_3(j,m) = -\frac{m+1}{m}.$$

Accordingly, the infinite sums in (2.3.40) are absolutely convergent.

In Table 2.3 we present a few risk values as functions of β.

Table 2.3: $\mathbf{R(\bar{X}_{N_m}, \beta)}$ for m = 10, A = 2, ω= 2, B = 3.5

β	1	2	3	4
$R(\bar{X}_N, \beta)$	0.1994	0.5388	1.0808	1.6334

5	6	7	10	∞
1.8814	1.9392	1.9216	1.8034	1.5873

The maximal value of $R(\bar{X}_N, \beta)$ occurs at $\beta = 6.1$ and is $\sup R(\bar{X}_N, \beta) = 1.9396$. The value $B = 3.5$ can be slightly reduced. We have found empirically that if B^0 is the value of B according to (2.1.4) and $B^* = 0.565B^0$, then we get nearly optimal results. A few values are given in Table 2.4. We denote by β^0 the value of β for which $\sup_{0<\beta<\infty} R(\bar{X}_N, \beta)$ is attained under B^* and by R^0 the value of the maximal risk. Here R^∞ denotes the asymptotic risk as $\beta \to \infty$. The formula for R^∞ is given in (2.3.16).

Table 2.4: Maximal and Asymptotic Risk Values, A = 2, ω= 2

m	B^*	β^0	R^0	R^∞
10	3.40	6.2	1.9966	1.6340
15	2.98	6.7	1.9804	1.6594
20	2.78	7.2	1.9688	1.6828
30	2.59	8.1	1.9460	1.7118

We now prove formula (2.3.16).

Theorem 2.3.5 *For all $m \geq 3$,*

(i) $\lim_{\beta \to 0} R(\bar{X}_{N_m}, \beta) = 0$

and

(ii) $\limsup_{\beta \to \infty} R(\bar{X}_{N_m}, \beta) \leq \dfrac{Am^2\omega}{B(m-1)(m-2)}$.

Proof: According to (2.3.40) and (2.3.41),

$$R(\bar{X}_{N_m}, \beta) = A\beta^2[S_1(m, \beta) + S_2(m, \beta) + S_3(m, \beta)], \tag{2.3.42}$$

where

$$S_1(m, \beta) = \sum_{j=0}^{\infty} \frac{1}{(m+j)(m+j+1)}(1 - P(m-1; \lambda_{m+j})), \tag{2.3.43}$$

$$S_2(m, \beta) = \sum_{j=0}^{\infty} b_2^*(j, m)p(m; \lambda_{m+j}), \tag{2.3.44}$$

and

$$S_3(m, \beta) = \sum_{j=0}^{\infty} b_3(j, m)p(m+1, \lambda_{m+j}). \tag{2.3.45}$$

Notice that for each $j \geq 0$,

$$\lim_{\beta \to 0} \lambda_{m+j} = \infty.$$

Hence, by bounded convergence, $\lim_{\beta \to 0} S_1(m, \beta) = 1/m$, $\lim_{\beta \to 0} S_2(m, \beta) = \lim_{\beta \to 0} S_3(m, \beta) = 0$. This proves part (i).

To prove (ii), we show first that

$$\lim_{\beta \to \infty} \beta^2 S_2(m, \beta) = 0. \tag{2.3.46}$$

A similar proof will do for verifying $\lim_{\beta \to \infty} \beta^2 S_3(m, \beta) = 0$. Notice that

$$\begin{aligned} &\beta^2 \sum_{j=0}^{\infty} \frac{m(m-1)(2(m+j)+1)}{(m+j)^2(m+j+1)^2} \frac{\lambda_{m+j}^m}{m!} e^{-\lambda_{m+j}} \\ &= \frac{\omega}{B} m^2 \sum_{j=0}^{\infty} \frac{2(m+j)+1}{(m+j)(m+j+1)^2} p(m-2; \lambda_{m+j}). \end{aligned} \tag{2.3.47}$$

Thus, by bounded convergence, the limit of (2.3.47) as $\beta \to \infty$ is zero. Indeed, $\lim_{\beta\to\infty} p(m-2;\lambda_{m+j}) = \lim_{\mu\to 0} p(m-2;\mu) = 0$ for all $m \geq 3$. This proves (2.3.46). To prove (2.3.43) we write

$$(2.3.48)\qquad S_1(m,\beta) = \sum_{j=0}^{\infty} \frac{1}{(m+j)(m+j+1)} \int_0^{\lambda_{m+j}} \frac{x^{m-1}}{(m-1)!} e^{-x}\, dx.$$

Since $\lambda_{m+j} = (m/\beta)(\omega/B)^{1/2}(m+j)^{1/2}$, $x \leq \lambda_{m+j}$ if and only if $j \geq (x\beta/c)^2 - m$, where $c = m\sqrt{\omega/B}$. Thus
(2.3.49)

$$S_1(m,\beta) = \int_0^{\infty} \left(\sum_{j \geq (x\beta/c)^2 - m} \frac{1}{(m+j)(m+j+1)} \right) \frac{x^{m-1}}{(m-1)!} e^{-x}\, dx.$$

But, since

$$-b_1(j,m) = \frac{1}{m+j} - \frac{1}{m+j+1} = \frac{1}{(m+j)(m+j+1)}$$

yields

$$\sum_{j \geq (x\beta)^2/c^2 - m} \frac{1}{(m+j)(m+j+1)} \leq \frac{c^2}{\beta^2 x^2}.$$

Hence

$$(2.3.50)\qquad \begin{aligned} S_1(m,\beta) &\leq \frac{c^2}{\beta^2} \int_0^{\infty} \frac{x^{m-3}}{(m-1)!} e^{-x}\, dx \\ &= \frac{c^2}{\beta^2 (m-1)(m-2)}. \end{aligned}$$

Thus

$$(2.3.51)\qquad \limsup_{\beta\to\infty} \beta^2 S_1(m,\beta) \leq \frac{m^2\omega}{B(m-1)(m-2)}.$$

This proves part (ii) and establishes (2.3.16). ∎

We show now the effect of using $B^* = 0.565 B^0$ rather than B^0. In Table 2.5 we compare $E_\beta\{N_m\}$.

Table 2.5: Expected Sample Size, A = 2, ω= 2

β	n^*	$m = 10$ $B^0 = 6.11$	$m = 10$ $B^* = 3.45$	$m = 20$ $B^0 = 4.9123$	$m = 20$ $B^* = 2.7754$
5	25	84.5197	47.9874	65.0109	37.4250
10	100	336.6105	190.2503	258.3826	146.2088
15	225	756.7481	427.4375	579.5491	328.3417
20	400	1344.9223	759.4999	1018.0470	583.2278
25	625	2100.9633	1186.4371	1546.6741	909.9776
30	900	3024.1552	1708.2455	2130.3247	1305.3535
35	1225	4112.6597	2324.9073	2738.7111	1762.6207
40	1600	5363.0250	3036.3630	4112.9780	2331.7980
45	2025	7934.5720	4966.9370	5222.5810	2951.0970
50	2500	9238.6210	5954.4650	6447.8550	3643.2120

In Table 2.6 we present the expected sample size and the expected value of the estimator and its risk when $B = B^0$.

Table 2.6: Exact Values of Expected Sample Size, Expected Estimator, and Risk for m = 10, A = 2, β= 5, and B = 6.1111

ω	$n^*(\beta)$	$E\{N_m\}$	$E\{\bar{X}_{N_m}\}$	Risk
2	25.00	84.5348	4.8279	1.10711
1	50.00	168.5558	4.9108	0.52320
0.5	100.00	336.6106	4.9549	0.24642
0.25	200.00	672.7200	4.9774	0.11860
0.10	500.00	1681.0490	4.9909	0.04626
0.05	1000.00	3361.5980	4.9957	0.02293

We see that the choice of B according to (2.1.4) leads to $E\{N_m\}$, which is about 3 times the value of $n^*(\beta) = (A/\omega)\beta^2$. Also the corresponding risk values are about one-half of ω.

Another comparison of the risk values is given in Table 2.7.

Table 2.7: Risk Values, A = 2, ω= 2

	$m = 5$		$m = 10$	
β	$B^0 = 10$	$B^* = 5.65$	$B^0 = 6.1111$	$B^* = 3.45$
1	0.2161	0.2447	0.1800	0.1994
2	0.6972	0.8302	0.4851	0.5416
3	0.9370	1.3873	0.9273	1.0820
4	1.0073	1.6599	1.0945	1.6454
5	1.0158	1.7623	1.1071	1.9039
6	1.0042	1.7978	1.0796	1.9670
7	0.9873	1.7974	1.0485	1.9511
8	0.9701	1.7771	1.0222	1.9116
9	0.9544	1.7547	1.0016	1.8697
10	0.9406	1.7314	0.9857	1.8320
20	0.8735	1.5847	0.9292	1.6728
30	0.8550	1.5343	0.9181	1.6385
50	0.8467	1.5040	0.9125	1.6205
∞	0.8333	1.4749	0.9091	1.6103

Table 2.7 continued

	$m = 20$	
	$B^0 = 4.9123$	$B^* = 2.7754$
1	0.0999	0.1000
2	0.3683	0.3991
3	0.6065	0.7449
4	0.9734	1.0777
5	1.1078	1.5945
6	1.1050	1.8947
7	1.0764	1.9711
8	1.0506	1.9553
9	1.0311	1.9173
10	1.0166	1.8802
20	0.9687	1.7366
30	0.9596	1.7084
50	0.9550	1.6939
∞	0.9524	1.6832

2.4 SEQUENTIAL FIXED-WIDTH INTERVAL ESTIMATION

For estimating the mean of a normal distribution when σ is *unknown*, Ray (1957) was the first one to suggest a *sequential* procedure to obtain a fixed-width interval estimator. Ray suggested the stopping variable

$$(2.4.1) \qquad N^* = \text{smallest odd integer } n \geq 3 \text{ for which } n \geq \frac{\chi^2_{1-\alpha}[1]S_n^2}{\delta^2},$$

where S_n^2 is the sample variance. For each fixed $n = 2m + 1$ $(m \geq 1)$

$$S_n^2 \sim \frac{\sigma^2}{2m}\chi^2[2m] \sim \frac{\sigma^2}{m}G(1, m).$$

Notice that $G(1, m)$ is distributed like the sum of m independent exponentially distributed random variables. Accordingly, the distribution of N^* can be determined as in Section 2.5.2. We remark that Starr (1966) evaluated the characteristics of Ray's procedure numerically by a different method.

We devote the present section to a brief review of later developments of Chow and Robbins (1965), Simons (1968), Woodroofe (1977), and others. For a complete theoretical development, the reader is referred to Ghosh, Mukhopadhyay, and Sen (1997, Chapter 8).

Chow and Robbins (1965) considered the possibility of stopping at any integer, and the sequence of the observed, i.i.d. random variables is any one which satisfies the central limit theorem for random stopping times. For a stopping variable N, the distribution mean, μ, is estimated by $\bar{X}_N = (1/N)\sum_{j=1}^{N} X_j$, and it is required that $\sqrt{N}(\bar{X}_N - \mu)/\sigma$ will converge in distribution to $N(0, 1)$.

See Theorem 2.4.2 (theorem of Anscomb, 1952) below. The Chow and Robbins stopping variable is

$$N = \min\left\{n \geq n_0 : n \geq \frac{\chi^2_{1-\alpha}[1] S_n^2}{\delta^2}\right\}, \tag{2.4.2}$$

The stopping variable has the following properties:

Theorem 2.4.1 *For the stopping variable (2.4.2) and $n^0(\delta, \sigma)$ given in (1.1.2), if $0 < \sigma < \infty$, then*

(i) $P_\sigma\{N < \infty\} = 1$;

(ii) $E_\sigma\{N\} \leq n_0 + 1 + n^0(\delta, \sigma)$;

(iii) $E_\sigma\{N^2\} \leq (n_0 + 1 + n^0(\delta, \sigma))^2 - 2$;

(iv) $N \nearrow \infty$ *a.s. as* $\delta \to 0$;

(v) $N/n^0(\delta, \sigma) \to 1$ *a.s.*;

(vi) $\lim_{\delta \to 0} E_\sigma\{N\}/n^0(\delta, \sigma) = 1$;

(vii) $\lim_{\delta \to 0} P\{\bar{X}_n - \delta < \mu < \bar{X}_N + \delta\} = 1 - \alpha$.

Note: Property (vi) is called *asymptotic efficiency* and property (vii) is called *asymptotic consistency*. Before proving the above theorem, we prove some auxiliary material.

Lemma 2.4.1 (Wald Lemma) *Let $X_1, X_2, \ldots$ be a sequence of i.i.d. random variables with $E\{|X_1|\} < \infty$ and $\mu = E\{X_1\}$. Let N be a stopping variable having a finite expectation. Then*

$$E\left\{\sum_{i=1}^{N} X_i\right\} = \mu E\{N\}. \tag{2.4.3}$$

Proof: Without loss of generality we assume that $X_i > 0$, $i = 1, 2, \ldots$. Accordingly,

$$\begin{aligned} E\left\{\sum_{i=1}^{N} X_i\right\} &= E\left\{\sum_{n=1}^{\infty} I\{N = n\} \sum_{i=1}^{n} X_i\right\} \\ &= \sum_{i=1}^{\infty} E\{X_i I\{N \geq i\}\}. \end{aligned} \tag{2.4.4}$$

By definition of a stopping variable, the random variable $I\{N \geq i\}$ depends only on $\{X_1, \ldots, X_{i-1}\}$. Thus X_i and $I\{N \geq i\}$ are independent for all $i \geq 1$.

We therefore obtain from (2.4.4)

$$
\begin{aligned}
E\left\{\sum_{i=1}^{N} X_i\right\} &= \sum_{i=1}^{\infty} E\{X_i\}E\{I\{N \geq i\}\} \\
&= \mu \sum_{i=1}^{\infty} P\{N \geq i\} \qquad (2.4.5) \\
&= \mu E\{N\}.
\end{aligned}
$$

■

Theorem 2.4.2 (Anscomb's Theorem) *Suppose that $U_1, U_2, \ldots$ is a sequence of i.i.d. random variables such that $E\{U_1\} = 0$ and $E\{U_1^2\} = 1$. Let $S_n = \sum_{i=1}^{n} U_i$. Let $N(t)$ be a stopping variable such that*

$$\frac{N(t)}{t} \xrightarrow[t\to\infty]{p} C, \quad 0 < C < \infty.$$

Then

$$\lim_{t\to\infty} P\left\{\frac{1}{\sqrt{N(t)}} S_{N(t)} \leq x\right\} = \Phi(x), \quad -\infty < x < \infty. \tag{2.4.6}$$

■

The proof of this important theorem can be found in Ghosh, Mukhopadhyay, and Sen (1997, Chapter 2) or Zacks (1971, p. 573).

Proof (Proof of Theorem 2.4.1): By definition of (2.4.2) of N,

$$
\begin{aligned}
P\{N = \infty\} &= \lim_{m\to\infty} P\{N > m\} \\
&\leq \lim_{m\to\infty} P\left\{m < \frac{\chi^2_{1-\alpha}[1]}{\delta^2} S_m^2\right\}.
\end{aligned}
$$

However, by the strong law of large numbers,

$$\lim_{m\to\infty} \frac{\chi^2_{1-\alpha}[1]}{\delta^2} S_m^2 = \frac{\chi^2_{1-\alpha}[1]}{\delta^2}\sigma^2 = n^0(\delta,\sigma) < \infty.$$

Hence $\lim_{m\to\infty} P\{m < [(\chi^2_{1-\alpha}[1])/\delta^2] S_m^2\} = 0$. This proves (i). To prove (ii) and (iii) notice that by (2.4.2)

$$(N-1) \leq \frac{\chi^2_{1-\alpha}[1]}{\delta^2} S_{N-1}^2 + (n_0 - 1)I\{N = n_0\}.$$

Hence

$$
\begin{aligned}
(N-1)(N-2) &\leq (n_0-1)(n_0-2)I\{N = n_0\} \\
&\quad + \frac{\chi^2_{1-\alpha}[1]}{\delta^2} \sum_{i=1}^{N-1} (X_i - \bar{X}_{N-1})^2 \qquad (2.4.7) \\
&\leq (n_0 - 2)N + \sum_{i=1}^{N} (X_i - \mu)^2.
\end{aligned}
$$

Since $E_\sigma\{N\} \leq n_0 + 1 + n^0(\delta, \sigma) < \infty$, we obtain from Wald's lemma that

$$E_\sigma\{N^2 - 3N + 2\} \leq (n_0 - 2 + n^0(\delta, \sigma))E_\sigma\{N\}. \tag{2.4.8}$$

Or

$$\begin{aligned} E_\sigma\{N^2\} &\leq (n_0 + 1 + n^0(\delta, \sigma))E_\sigma\{N\} - 2 \\ &< (n_0 + 1 + n^0(\delta, \sigma))E_\sigma\{N\}. \end{aligned} \tag{2.4.9}$$

Moreover, $E_\sigma\{N^2\} \geq (E_\sigma\{N\})^2$. Hence (ii) is obtained from (2.4.9). Property (iii) is given in (2.4.9). From (ii) we immediately obtain (vi) since $\lim_{\delta \to 0} n^0(\delta, \sigma) = \infty$. Property (iv) is immediate. Also, since

$$\frac{\chi^2_{1-\alpha}}{\delta^2} S_N^2 < N \leq \frac{\chi^2_{1-\alpha}}{\delta^2} S_{N-1}^2 + n_0 \tag{2.4.10}$$

and since $\lim_{\delta \to 0} S^2_{N(\delta)} = \sigma^2$ a.s., we obtain (v) from (2.4.10). Finally, (vii) is obtained from Anscomb's theorem. ■

Simons (1968) proved that if $X_1, X_2, \ldots$ are i.i.d. $N(\mu, \sigma)$, then if $n_0 \geq 3$, there exists an integer $k \geq 0$ such that

$$P_{\mu,\sigma}\{|\bar{X}_{N+k} - \mu| < \delta\} \geq 1 - \alpha \tag{2.4.11}$$

for all μ, σ, α, and δ. For a proof of this result see also Ghosh, Mukhopadhyay, and Sen (1997, p. 255) or Woodroofe (1977).

2.5 DISTRIBUTIONS OF STOPPING VARIABLES OF SEQUENTIAL SAMPLING FROM EXPONENTIAL DISTRIBUTIONS

Zacks and Mukhopadhyay (2006a) showed how to determine the exact distribution of stopping variables based on the sample means from exponential distributions. More precisely, let $X_1, X_2, \ldots$ be a sequence of i.i.d. random variables having an exponential distribution with an unknown mean β, $0 < \beta < \infty$. A typical stopping variable for a point estimation of β is

$$\tilde{N} = \min\{n \geq m : n \geq \tilde{A}\bar{X}_n^\alpha\}, \tag{2.5.1}$$

where $0 < \tilde{A} < \infty$ and $1 \leq \alpha < \infty$. For the sequential estimation procedure of Ray (1957) the stopping variable (2.4.1) can be written as $N^* = 2M + 1$, where

$$M = \min\left\{m \geq m_0 : 2m + 1 \geq \frac{\chi^2_{1-\alpha}[1]}{\delta^2}\bar{X}_m\right\}. \tag{2.5.2}$$

Stopping variable (2.5.2) is a special case of (2.5.1). We derive here the exact distribution of (2.5.1) and later we apply it to determine the exact values of various functionals.

2.5.1 General Theory

Let $\{N(t), t \geq 0\}$ be an ordinary Poisson process with $N(0) = 0$ and intensity of arrivals $\lambda = 1/\beta$. For the properties of an ordinary Poisson process, see Kao (1997, p. 47). Let $\tau_0 \equiv 0$ and $\tau_0 < \tau_1 < \tau_2 < \cdots$ be random times at which $N(t)$ jumps one unit. These are also called arrival times. The interarrival times $T_i = \tau_i - \tau_{i-1}$, $i \geq 1$, are i.i.d. random variables having an exponential distribution with mean β. Let $S_n = \sum_{i=1}^{n} T_i$. The pairs (n, S_n) correspond to $(N(\tau_n), \tau_n)$, $n \geq 1$. If we replace n and $n\bar{X}_n$ in the definition of $\tilde{N}$, (2.5.1), by $N(t)$ and t, we arrive at the related stopping time

$$\tilde{T} = \inf\{t \geq t_m : N(t) \geq \gamma t^{\alpha/(1+\alpha)}\}, \tag{2.5.3}$$

where $\gamma = (A^*)^{1/(1+\alpha)}$. Notice that $\tilde{T}$ is the first time the Poisson process $\{N(t), t \geq 0\}$ jumps above a *concave* boundary $B(t) = \gamma t^{\alpha/(1+\alpha)}$ such that $B(0) = 0$ and $\lim_{t\to\infty} B(t) = \infty$.

For $n \geq m$ we define the time sequence t_n, where $t_n = B^{-1}(n)$. Thus, for $B(t) = \gamma t^{\alpha/(1+\alpha)}$ we have, for $n \geq m$,

$$t_n = \left(\frac{n}{\gamma}\right)^{1+1/\alpha}. \tag{2.5.4}$$

Notice that

$$P\{\tilde{T} = t_m\} = 1 - P(m-1; \lambda t_m). \tag{2.5.5}$$

Indeed, the distribution of $N(t)$ is Poisson with mean λt.

We define recursively the defective p.d.f.

$$g_\lambda(j;t) = P\{N(t) = j, \tilde{T} > t\}. \tag{2.5.6}$$

We start with

$$g_\lambda(j;t_m) = p(j;\lambda t_m), \quad 0 \leq j \leq m-1. \tag{2.5.7}$$

For $t_{n-1} < t \leq t_n$, $n \geq m+1$, we have, for $0 \leq j \leq n-1$,

$$g_\lambda(j;t) = \begin{cases} \sum_{i=0}^{j} g_\lambda(i;t_{n-1}) p(j-i; \lambda(t-t_{n-1})) & \text{if } 0 \leq j \leq n-2, \\ \sum_{i=0}^{n-2} g_\lambda(i;t_{n-1}) p(n-1-i; \lambda(t-t_{n-1})) & \text{if } j = n-1. \end{cases}$$

We can write formula (2.5.7) as

$$g_\lambda(j;t) = \sum_{i=0}^{\min(j,n-2)} g_\lambda(i;t_{n-1}) p(j-i; \lambda(t-t_{n-1})). \tag{2.5.8}$$

Also, when $t_{n-1} < t \leq t_n$, $g_\lambda(j;t) = 0$ for all $j \geq n$. From the definition (2.5.6) we obtain

(2.5.9)
$$P\{\tilde{T} > t\} = \sum_{j \leq \lfloor B(t) \rfloor} g_\lambda(j;t).$$

Notice that $\tilde{N} = N(\tilde{T})$. Accordingly,

(2.5.10)
$$\begin{aligned} P_\beta\{\tilde{N} = m\} &= P_\lambda\{\tilde{T} = t_m\} \\ &= 1 - P(m-1; \lambda t_m), \end{aligned}$$

and for $n \geq m+1$,

(2.5.11)
$$\begin{aligned} P_\beta\{\tilde{N} = n\} &= P_\lambda\{t_{n-1} < \tilde{T} \leq t_n\} \\ &= \sum_{j=0}^{n-2} g_\lambda(j; t_{n-1}) - \sum_{j=0}^{n-1} g_\lambda(j; t_n). \end{aligned}$$

Let $\Delta_n = t_n - t_{n-1}$, $n \geq m+1$. From (2.5.8) and (2.5.10) we obtain:

Theorem 2.5.1 *For $n > m$*

(2.5.12)
$$P_\beta\{\tilde{N} = n\} = \sum_{j=0}^{n-1} g_\lambda(j; t_{n-1})(1 - P(n-1-j; \lambda\Delta_n)) - g_\lambda(n-1; t_{n-1})e^{-\lambda\Delta_n}.$$

■

The density of the stopping time $\tilde{T}$ is

(2.5.13)
$$\Psi_{\tilde{T}}(t;\lambda) = \lambda \sum_{n=m+1}^{\infty} I\{t_{n-1} < t < t_n\} \sum_{j=0}^{n-2} g_\lambda(j; t_{n-1}) \cdot p(n-1-j; \lambda(t - t_{n-1})).$$

This density is obtained by differentiating $P_\lambda\{\tilde{T} > t\}$ with respect to t. With the aid of (2.5.13) we can compute $E\{\bar{X}_{\tilde{T}}\}$ exactly. As proven in Zacks and Mukhopadhyay (2006a):

Theorem 2.5.2 *The rth moment of $\bar{X}_{\tilde{T}}$ is*

(2.5.14)
$$\begin{aligned} E_\lambda\{\bar{X}^r_{\tilde{T}}\} &= \frac{1}{(\lambda m)^r} \cdot \frac{(m+r-1)!}{(m-1)!}(1 - P(m-1+r; \lambda t_m)) \\ &+ r! \sum_{n=m+1}^{\infty} \left(\frac{t_{n-1}}{n}\right)^r \sum_{j=0}^{n-2} g_\lambda(j; t_{n-1}) \sum_{i=0}^{r} \frac{1}{(r-i)!(\lambda t_{n-1})^r} \\ &\cdot \binom{n-j-1+i}{i}(1 - P(n-j+i-1; \lambda\Delta_n)). \end{aligned}$$

■

2.5.2 Characteristics of Ray's Procedure

The stopping variable of Ray's procedure is $N^* = 2M + 1$, where M is given in (2.5.2). The boundary $B(t)$ for the Poisson process $\{M(t), t \geq 0\}$ is

$$B(t) = -\frac{1}{4} + \frac{1}{4}(1 + 8(\chi^2_{1-\alpha}[1]/\delta^2)t)^{1/2}.$$

Notice that this boundary is concave, $B(0) = 0$ and $\lim_{t\to\infty} B(t) = \infty$. Moreover, the root t_m of $B(t) = m$ is $t_m = (\delta^2/\chi^2_{1-\alpha}[1])m(2m+1)$, for $m \geq m_0$. The intensity of $\{M(t), t \geq 0\}$ is $\lambda = 1/\sigma^2$. We obtain

$$P_\lambda\{M = m_0\} = 1 - P(m_0 - 1; \lambda t_{m_0}) \tag{2.5.15}$$

and for $m > m_0$

$$P_\lambda\{M = m\} = \sum_{j=0}^{m-2} g_\lambda(j; t_{m-1}) - \sum_{j=0}^{m-1} g_\lambda(j; t_m). \tag{2.5.16}$$

The expected value of N^* is $E_\lambda\{N^*\} = 2E_\lambda\{M\} + 1$, where

$$E_\lambda\{M\} = m_0 + \sum_{m=m_0}^{\infty} \sum_{j=0}^{m-1} g_\lambda(j; t_m). \tag{2.5.17}$$

Finally, since we are in the normal case, the coverage probability of $(\bar{X}_N \pm \delta)$ is

$$\text{CP}(\sigma, \delta) = 2 \sum_{m=m_0}^{\infty} \Phi\left(\frac{\sqrt{2m+1}\,\delta}{\sigma}\right) P_\sigma\{M = m\} - 1. \tag{2.5.18}$$

In Table 2.8 we present values of $E_\sigma\{N^*\}$ and $\text{CP}(\sigma, \delta)$ for various values of δ and m_0.

Table 2.8: Expected Sample Size and Coverage Probability of Ray's Procedure, $\alpha = .05$, $\sigma = 1$

		$m_0 = 3$		$m_0 = 7$	
δ	$n^0(\delta, \sigma)$	$E\{N^*\}$	CP	$E\{N^*\}$	CP
1.25	2.459	7.018	0.999	15.000	0.999
1.00	3.842	7.211	0.992	15.000	0.999
0.90	4.743	7.478	0.985	15.000	0.999
0.75	6.830	8.439	0.965	15.014	0.996
0.60	10.671	10.957	0.938	15.444	0.981
0.50	15.366	14.706	0.923	17.375	0.958
0.25	61.466	60.161	0.938	60.492	0.941

2.5.3 Risk of Some Sequential Point Estimators

Zacks and Mukhopadhyay (2006a) considered several different loss functions for estimating the mean β of an exponential distribution. We bring here four of these and the corresponding stopping variables. In the following c is a cost of one observation. The first one is

$$L^{(1)}(\hat{\beta}_n, \beta) = A(\hat{\beta}_n - \beta)^2 + cn, \quad 0 < A, c < \infty.$$

The corresponding stopping variable is

$$N^{(1)} = \min\left\{n \geq m : n \geq \left(\frac{A}{c}\right)^{1/2} \bar{X}_n\right\}.$$

The second one is

$$L^{(2)}(\hat{\beta}_n, \beta) = A(\hat{\beta}_n - \beta)^2$$

with a bound w, $0 < w < \infty$. The stopping variable is

$$N^{(2)} = \min\left\{n \geq m : n \geq \frac{A}{w}\bar{X}_n^2\right\}.$$

The third one is

$$L^{(3)}(\hat{\beta}_n, \beta) = A(\hat{\beta}_n - \beta)^2 + c\sum_{i=1}^{n} X_i.$$

The stopping variable is

$$N^{(3)} = \min\left\{n \geq m : n \geq \left(\frac{A}{c}\right)^{1/2} \bar{X}_n^{1/2}\right\}.$$

The corresponding stopping times T_i $(i = 1, 2, 3)$ are obtained when the Poisson process $\{N(t), t \geq 0\}$ crosses above the concave boundaries: $B_1(t) = \gamma_1 t^{1/2}$, $B_2(t) = \gamma_2 t^{2/3}$, and $B_3(t) = \gamma_3 t^{1/3}$. In Table 2.9 we present some characteristics of the estimator $\bar{X}_{N(i)}$ under these stopping rules.

Table 2.9: Expected Sample Size and Expected Values and Risk of Estimators β= 1, A = 10, m = 3

	$N^{(1)}$			$N^{(2)}$		
c	$E\{N\}$	$E\{\hat{\beta}_N\}$	Risk	$E\{N\}$	$E\{\hat{\beta}_N\}$	Risk
0.5	4.712	0.8663	4.1318	3.806	0.8836	3.5822
0.1	9.482	0.8757	2.2889	4.924	0.8357	2.0238
0.05	13.472	0.9015	1.7079	5.860	0.8207	1.7992
0.01	31.882	0.9597	0.7207	11.626	0.8103	1.5101
0.005	44.305	0.9742	0.4834	17.182	0.8274	1.3328

Table 2.9 continued

	$N^{(3)}$		
c	$E\{N\}$	$E\{\hat{\beta}_N\}$	Risk
0.5	4.714	0.9078	4.3304
0.1	10.156	0.9468	2.0467
0.05	14.321	0.9633	1.4368
0.01	31.828	0.9841	0.6354
0.005	44.931	0.9887	0.4486

Derived using program Eval.

We see in Table 2.9 that $N^{(1)}$ and $N^{(3)}$ yield similar results while $N^{(2)}$ is unsatisfactory.

2.6 SEQUENTIAL FIXED-WIDTH INTERVALS FOR THE LOG-ODDS IN BERNOULLI TRIALS

The material in this section is based on the paper of Zacks and Mukhopadhyay (2007).

2.6.1 Problem

Let $J_1, J_2, \ldots$ be a sequence of i.i.d. binary random variables with $P(J_1 = 1) = p$. The MLE of p after n observations is $\hat{p}_n = X_n/n$, where $X_n = \sum_{i=1}^{n} J_i$. The MLE of $\log(\rho)$ is $\log(\hat{\rho}_n) = \log[\hat{p}_n/(1 - \hat{p}_n)]$. Since $\hat{p}_n$ can assume the value 0 or 1 with positive probabilities, we will consider the Haldane (1956) estimator:

$$\log(\hat{\rho}_n) \equiv \log\left(\frac{X_n + 1/2}{n - X_n + 1/2}\right). \tag{2.6.1}$$

The asymptotic distribution of $\log(\hat{\rho}_n)$, as $n \to \infty$, is normal with mean $\log(\rho)$ and variance $1/(np(1-p))$. Accordingly, since $p(1-p) \le 1/4$, we define

$$k \equiv k(\delta) = \left\lfloor \frac{4\chi^2_{1-\alpha}[1]}{\delta^2} \right\rfloor + 1. \tag{2.6.2}$$

In order to construct a fixed-width ($= 2\delta$) confidence interval estimator $(\log(\hat{\rho}_n) - \delta, \log(\hat{\rho}_n) + \delta)$ for $\log(\rho)$ with preassigned approximate coverage at least $1 - \alpha$, Robbins and Siegmund (1974a) considered the following purely sequential stopping variable: One would observe $J_1, J_2, \ldots$ with one additional observation at a time and employ the stopping variable

$$N \equiv N(\delta) = \min\left\{n \ge 1 : n \ge \frac{\chi^2_{1-\alpha}}{\delta^2 \hat{p}_n(1 - \hat{p}_n)}\right\}. \tag{2.6.3}$$

Notice that $N(\delta)$ is well defined and hence p would be estimated by $\widehat{p}_N$, the sample proportion of 1's at termination. Also, $\chi^2_{1-\alpha}[1]/(\delta^2\hat{p}_n(1-\hat{p}_n)) = \infty$ if $\hat{p}_n = 0$ or $\hat{p}_n = 1$. Furthermore, $N(\delta) \geq k$, and since $\lim_{n\to\infty} \hat{p}_n = p$ a.s., we have $P_p\{N(\delta) < \infty\} = 1$ for all $0 < p < 1$. If p were known, the minimal fixed number of trials needed would approximately become

$$n^* \equiv n^*(\delta, p) = \frac{\chi^2_{1-\alpha}[1]}{\delta^2 p(1-p)}. \tag{2.6.4}$$

Robbins and Siegmund (1974a) proved some interesting asymptotic first-order properties, namely,

$$\lim_{\delta\to 0} \frac{N(\delta)}{n^*(\delta,p)} = 1 \text{ in probability} \tag{2.6.5}$$

and

$$\lim_{\delta\to 0} E_p\left\{\frac{N(\delta)}{n^*(\delta,p)}\right\} = 1, \quad \lim_{\delta\to 0} E_p\left\{\frac{n^*(\delta,p)}{N(\delta)}\right\} = 1 \tag{2.6.6}$$

by essentially following the fundamental techniques from Chow and Robbins (1965).

They also proved the asymptotic normality of $\log(\hat{\rho}_{N(\delta)})$ and that of $N(\delta)$ as $\delta \to 0$. The asymptotic normality of $\log(\hat{\rho}_{N(\delta)})$ followed rather easily by combining (2.5) with Anscombe's (1952) random central limit theorem, which holds for an MLE.

2.6.2 Distribution of $N(\delta)$

We know that the sample size should exceed k given by (2.6.2). Hence, one may very well start with k initial observations $J_1, \ldots, J_k$ and then use a slightly revised version of the stopping variable $N(\delta)$ from (2.6.3) as follows: The stopping variable $N(\delta)$ can be expressed, in terms of X_n, as

$$N(\delta) = \min\left\{n \geq k : X_n^2 - nX_n + n\frac{\chi^2_{1-\alpha}[1]}{\delta^2} \leq 0\right\}. \tag{2.6.7}$$

The roots of the quadratic equation inside (2.6.7) are

$$\zeta_{1,2} = \frac{n}{2}\left(1 \pm \sqrt{1 - \frac{k^*}{n}}\right), \tag{2.6.8}$$

where $k - 1 \leq k^* = 4\chi^2_{1-\alpha}[1]/\delta^2 < k$. We thus define the stopping region corresponding to $N(\delta)$ as

$$\left\{(n, X_n) : \frac{n}{2}\left(1 - \sqrt{1 - \frac{k}{n}}\right) \leq X_n \leq \frac{n}{2}\left(1 + \sqrt{1 - \frac{k}{n}}\right)\right\}. \tag{2.6.9}$$

Define the boundaries

$$\overline{B}(n) = \frac{n}{2}\left(1 + \sqrt{1 - \frac{k}{n}}\right), \quad n \geq k, \tag{2.6.10}$$

$$\underline{B}(n) = \frac{n}{2}\left(1 - \sqrt{1 - \frac{k}{n}}\right), \quad n \geq k. \tag{2.6.11}$$

The upper boundary of the stopping region, $\overline{B}(n)$, is strictly increasing in n. The lower boundary $\underline{B}(n)$ is a strictly decreasing function of n. Notice that $\overline{B}(k) = \underline{B}(k) = k/2$, and also

$$\lim_{n\to\infty} \frac{1}{n}\overline{B}(n) = 1 \tag{2.6.12}$$

and

$$\lim_{n\to\infty} \underline{B}(n) = \frac{k}{4}. \tag{2.6.13}$$

Thus,

$$N(\delta) = \min\{n \geq k : \underline{B}(n) \leq X_n \leq \overline{B}(n)\}. \tag{2.6.14}$$

Let $b(j; n, p)$ and $B(j; n, p)$ denote the p.d.f. and c.d.f. of the binomial distribution with parameters (n, p).

Theorem 2.6.1 *For each p, $0 < p < 1$,*

$$P_p\{N(\delta) = k\} = \begin{cases} 0 & \text{if } k = 2m+1, \\ b(m; 2m, p) & \text{if } k = 2m, \end{cases} \tag{2.6.15}$$

and for $n \geq k$

$$P_p\{N(\delta) \leq n\} = 1 - B(\lfloor \underline{B}(n) \rfloor; n, p) - B(\lfloor \underline{B}(n) \rfloor; n, 1-p). \tag{2.6.16}$$

Proof: The event $\{N(\delta) > n\}$ for $n \geq k$ can be written as

$$\{N(\delta) > n\} = \bigcap_{j=k}^{n}\{X_j < \underline{B}(j)\} \cup \bigcap_{j=k}^{n}\{X_j > \overline{B}(j)\}. \tag{2.6.17}$$

Since $X_n \leq X_{n+1}$ for all $n \geq 1$ and $\underline{B}(n)$ is decreasing,

$$P_p\left\{\bigcap_{j=k}^{n}\{X_j < \underline{B}(j)\}\right\} = P\{X_n < \underline{B}(n)\} = B(\lfloor \underline{B}(n) \rfloor; n, p). \tag{2.6.18}$$

Let $Y_n = n - X_n$, $n \geq 1$. Then $Y_n \leq Y_{n+1}$ a.s. for all $n \geq 1$. Furthermore

$$\bigcap_{j=k}^{n} \{X_j > \overline{B}(j)\} = \bigcap_{j=k}^{n} \{j - X_j < j - \overline{B}(j)\}. \tag{2.6.19}$$

Also, $j - \overline{B}(j) = \underline{B}(j)$ for all $j \geq k$. Hence, for all $n > k$,

$$P_p\{N(\delta) > n\} = B(\lfloor \underline{B}(n) \rfloor; n, p) + B(\lfloor \underline{B}(n) \rfloor; n, 1-p). \tag{2.6.20}$$

This proves (2.6.16). We have seen that $\underline{B}(k) = \overline{B}(k) = k/2$. Thus, if $k = 2m+1$, $P_p\{N(\delta) = k\} = 0$. On the other hand, if $k = 2m$, $\lfloor \underline{B}(2m) \rfloor = m - 1$. Hence,

$$\begin{aligned} P_p\{N(\delta) = k\} &= 1 - P_p\{N(\delta) > k\} \\ &= 1 - B(m-1; 2m, p) - B(m-1; 2m, 1-p) \\ &= \sum_{j=m}^{2m} b(j; 2m, p) - \sum_{l=m+1}^{2m} b(l; 2m, p) \\ &= b(m; 2m, p). \end{aligned} \tag{2.6.21}$$

This proves (2.6.15). ■

Using the result from Theorem 2.6.1 we obtain:

Theorem 2.6.2 *The expected value and variance of $N(\delta)$ are*

$$E_p\{N(\delta)\} = k + \sum_{n=k}^{\infty} (B(\lfloor \underline{B}(n) \rfloor; n, p) + B(\lfloor \underline{B}(n) \rfloor; n, 1-p)) \tag{2.6.22}$$

and

$$\begin{aligned} V_p\{N(\delta)\} &= 2 \sum_{n \geq k} (n-k) P_p\{N(\delta) > n\} \\ &\quad + \left(\sum_{n \geq k} P_p\{N(\delta) > n\} \right) \left(1 - \sum_{n \geq k} P_k\{N(\delta) > n\} \right), \end{aligned} \tag{2.6.23}$$

where $P_p\{N(\delta) > n\}$ is given in (2.6.20).

Proof: First,

$$\begin{aligned} E_p\{N(\delta)\} &= k + \sum_{n=k+1}^{\infty} P_p\{N(\delta) \geq n\} \\ &= k + \sum_{n=k}^{\infty} P_p\{N(\delta) > n\}. \end{aligned} \tag{2.6.24}$$

Substituting (2.6.20) in (2.6.24) we obtain (2.6.22).

The second moment of $N(\delta)$ is

$$
\begin{aligned}
E_p\{N^2(\delta)\} &= \sum_{m=k}^{\infty} m^2 P_p\{N(\delta) = m\} \\
&= \sum_{m=k}^{\infty} \left(2\sum_{i=1}^{m} i - m\right) P_p\{N(\delta) = m\} \\
&= 2\sum_{m=k}^{\infty} \left(\sum_{i=1}^{m} i\right) P_p(N(\delta) = m) - E_p\{N(\delta)\} \\
&= k^2 + 2\sum_{m=k}^{\infty} mP_p(N(\delta) > m) + E_p\{N(\delta)\} - k.
\end{aligned} \tag{2.6.25}
$$

Finally, subtracting the square of (2.6.24) from (2.6.25), we obtain (2.6.23). ■

In Table 2.10 we present the values of $E_p\{N(\delta)\}$ and compare them with the means $\bar{X}_{1000}$ of $M = 1000$ simulation runs ± 3 SE$\{\bar{X}_{1000}\}$.

Table 2.10: Exact and Simulated Values of $\mathbf{E_p\{N(\delta)\}}$ with $\boldsymbol{\delta = (0.1)^{1/2}}$, $\boldsymbol{\alpha = 0.05}$, and $\mathbf{k = 154}$

p	Exact	Simulated
0.1	432.974	437.225 ± 5.32
0.3	185.252	184.625 ± 1.11
0.5	155.626	155.645 ± 0.12

Notice that $E_p\{N(\delta)\} = E_{1-p}\{N(\delta)\}$.

In the literature, under sequential estimation, it is customary to define an efficiency index of the sequential procedure as follows:

$$
\text{Eff}(\delta, p) = \frac{E_p\{N(\delta)\}}{n^*(\delta, p)}. \tag{2.6.26}
$$

In Table 2.11 we present this efficiency index.

Table 2.11: Values of $\mathbf{E_p\{N(\delta)\}}$, $\mathbf{n^*(\delta,p)}$, and $\mathbf{Eff(\delta,p)}$ with $\boldsymbol{\delta}=(0.1)^{1/2}$

α	p	$E_p\{N(\delta)\}$	$n^*(\delta,p)$	$\text{Eff}(\delta,p)$
0.05	0.1	432.749	426.832	1.0139
	0.2	243.240	240.093	1.0131
	0.3	185.252	182.928	1.0127
	0.4	161.981	160.062	1.0120
	0.5	155.626	153.660	1.0128
0.01	0.1	743.942	737.211	1.0091
	0.2	418.266	414.681	1.0086
	0.3	318.543	315.948	1.0082
	0.4	278.662	276.454	1.0080
	0.5	267.630	265.396	1.0084

It is clear that the purely sequential procedure over samples on average compared with the fixed sample size $n^*(\delta,p)$ by nearly 1%, uniformly in both p and α.

2.6.3 Functionals of $\hat{\rho}_{N(\delta)}$

At the time of stopping, the value of $X_{N(\delta)}$ is either $\lfloor \overline{B}(N(\delta))\rfloor$ or $\lfloor \underline{B}(N(\delta))\rfloor+1$.

Define

$$\overline{\psi}_p(n)=P_p\{N(\delta)=n, X_{N(\delta)}=\lfloor\overline{B}(N(\delta))\rfloor\} \tag{2.6.27}$$

and

$$\underline{\psi}_p(n)=P_p\{N(\delta)=n, X_{N(\delta)}=\lfloor\underline{B}(N(\delta))\rfloor+1\}. \tag{2.6.28}$$

Notice that $\underline{\psi}_p(k)=\overline{\psi}_p(k)=b(k/2;k,p)$ and that $P_p\{N(\delta)>k\}=P_p\{X_k<k/2\}+P_p\{X_k>k/2\}$. Accordingly,

$$\underline{\psi}_p(n)=B(\lfloor\underline{B}(n-1)\rfloor;n-1,p)-B(\lfloor\underline{B}(n)\rfloor;n,p),\quad n\geq k+1, \tag{2.6.29}$$

and
(2.6.30)

$$\overline{\psi}_p(n)=\begin{cases}1-B(\lfloor\frac{k}{2}\rfloor+1;k,p)-B(\lfloor\underline{B}(k+1)\rfloor;k+1,1-p), & n=k+1,\\ B(\lfloor\underline{B}(n-1)\rfloor;n-1,1-p)-B(\lfloor\underline{B}(n)\rfloor;n,1-p), & n>k+1.\end{cases}$$

The corresponding estimator of ρ is

$$\hat{\rho}_{N(\delta)}=\frac{X_{N(\delta)}}{N(\delta)-X_{N(\delta)}}. \tag{2.6.31}$$

Notice also that $\hat{\rho}_k = 1$. Thus,

$$
\begin{aligned}
E_p\{\hat{\rho}_{N(\delta)}\} = b\left(\frac{k}{2}; k, p\right) + \sum_{n=k+1}^{\infty} \Bigg(& \overline{\psi}_p(n) \frac{\lfloor \overline{B}(n) \rfloor}{n - \lfloor \overline{B}(n) \rfloor} \\
& + \underline{\psi}_p(n) \frac{\lfloor \underline{B}(n) \rfloor + 1}{n - \lfloor \underline{B}(n) \rfloor - 1} \Bigg).
\end{aligned} \tag{2.6.32}
$$

Similarly,

$$
\begin{aligned}
\text{MSE}_p\{\hat{\rho}_{N(\delta)}\} &= E_p\{(\hat{\rho}_{N(\delta)} - \rho)^2\} \\
&= (1-\rho)^2 b\left(\frac{k}{2}; k, p\right) \\
&\quad + \sum_{n=k+1}^{\infty} \Bigg[\overline{\psi}_p(n) \left(\frac{\lfloor \overline{B}(n) \rfloor}{n - \lfloor \overline{B}(n) \rfloor} - \rho \right)^2 \\
&\qquad + \underline{\psi}_p(n) \left(\frac{\lfloor \underline{B}(n) \rfloor + 1}{n - \lfloor \underline{B}(n) \rfloor - 1} - \rho \right)^2 \Bigg].
\end{aligned} \tag{2.6.33}
$$

Finally, the coverage of the confidence interval $(\log(\hat{\rho}_N) - \delta, \log(\hat{\rho}_N) + \delta)$ for $\log(\rho)$ is

$$
\begin{aligned}
\text{CP}_p(\hat{\rho}_{N(\delta)}) &= P_p\{\rho e^{-\delta} \le \hat{\rho}_{N(\delta)} \le \rho e^{\delta}\} \\
&= b\left(\frac{k}{2}; k, p\right) I\{\rho e^{-\delta} \le 1 \le \rho e^{\delta}\} \\
&\quad + \sum_{n=k+1}^{\infty} \Bigg[I\left\{ \rho e^{-\delta} \le \frac{\lfloor \overline{B}(n) \rfloor}{n - \lfloor \overline{B}(n) \rfloor} \le \rho e^{\delta} \right\} \cdot \overline{\psi}_p(n) \\
&\qquad + I\left\{ \rho e^{-\delta} \le \frac{\lfloor \underline{B}(n) \rfloor + 1}{n - 1 - \lfloor \underline{B}(n) \rfloor} \le \rho e^{\delta} \right\} \underline{\psi}_p(n) \Bigg].
\end{aligned} \tag{2.6.34}
$$

In Table 2.12 we present some values of these functionals.

Table 2.12: Expected Value, MSE, and Coverage Probability of $\hat{\rho}_{N(\delta)}$ for $\alpha = 0.05$, $\delta = (0.1)^{1/2}$

p	ρ	$E\{\hat{\rho}_N\}$	MSE	CP
0.1	0.1111	0.1136	0.0004	0.9500
0.3	0.4285	0.4348	0.0049	0.9589
0.5	1.0000	1.0007	0.0369	0.9544
0.7	2.3333	2.3587	0.1414	0.9589
0.9	9.0000	9.0258	2.0814	0.9500

2.7 BAYESIAN SEQUENTIAL ESTIMATION

2.7.1 General Theory

The Bayesian paradigm is adaptive in the sense that, starting from a *prior* distribution of the unknown parameters, after each group of observations, one converts the prior distribution to *posterior* distribution. The posterior distribution after n observations contains the total information we have on the unknown parameters at that stage. More precisely, let $X_1, X_2, \ldots$ be a sequence of i.i.d. random variables having a common p.d.f. $p(x;\theta)$, where θ is an unknown parameter (parametric vector). For the purposes of this discussion we assume here, without loss of generality, that θ is real ($\theta \in \mathbb{R}$). Let $h(\theta)$ be a prior density of θ. This density reflects our belief about the possible values of θ. By Bayes' theorem, the posterior density of θ after observing $X_1, \ldots, X_n$ ($n \geq 1$) is

$$(2.7.1) \qquad h(\theta \mid X_1, \ldots, X_n) = \frac{\prod_{i=1}^{n} f(X_i;\theta)h(\theta)}{\int_{-\infty}^{\infty} \prod_{i=1}^{n} f(X_i;\theta)h(\theta)\, d\theta}.$$

Notice that after n observations the posterior density (2.7.1) can be used as a "prior" for θ for future observations. Indeed,

$$(2.7.2) \qquad h(\theta \mid X_1, \ldots, X_n, X_{n+1}) = \frac{f(X_{n+1};\theta)h(\theta \mid X_1, \ldots, X_n)}{\displaystyle\int_{-\infty}^{\infty} f(X_{n+1};\theta)h(\theta \mid X_1, \ldots, X_n)\, d\theta}.$$

Equation (2.7.2) reflects the adaptive characteristic of the Bayesian paradigm.

Given a loss function $L(\hat{\theta}_n, \theta)$ for estimating θ by an estimator $\hat{\theta}_n$, which depends on $X_1, \ldots, X_n$, the Bayesian estimator is the one minimizing the posterior risk

$$(2.7.3) \qquad \rho_h(\hat{\theta}_n; \mathbf{X}_n) = \int_{-\infty}^{\infty} L(\hat{\theta}_n, \theta)h(\theta \mid \mathbf{X}_n)\, d\theta,$$

where $\mathbf{X}_n = (X_1, \ldots, X_n)$. It is easy to verify that the Bayesian estimator of θ for the squared-error loss function $L(\hat{\theta}_n, \theta) = (\hat{\theta}_n - \theta)^2$ and prior density h is the posterior expectation

$$(2.7.4) \qquad \hat{\theta}_h(\mathbf{X}_n) = \int_{-\infty}^{\infty} \theta h(\theta \mid \mathbf{X}_n)\, d\theta.$$

The corresponding posterior risk $\rho_h(\hat{\theta}_h; \mathbf{X}_n)$ is the posterior variance of θ given $\mathbf{X}_n$.

For the purpose of determining a stopping rule for the sequential estimation we have to include the cost of observations. Also, for any stopping variable N, the Bayesian estimator of θ, when $\{N = n\}$, is the one minimizing the posterior risk (2.7.3).

Define, for $n \geq 1$,

$$U_n(\mathbf{X}_n) = \inf_{\hat{\theta}_n} \int_{-\infty}^{\infty} L(\hat{\theta}_n, \theta) h(\theta \mid \mathbf{X}_n)\, d\theta + nc. \tag{2.7.5}$$

The following is a *dynamic programming* formulation of the optimal stopping rule in the class of stopping variables, which do not allow more than J observations, $0 < J < \infty$:

(i) If $\{N = J\}$, then the corresponding risk is $U_J(\mathbf{X}_J)$.

(ii) If $\{N = J - 1\}$, define

$$V_{J-1}^{(1)}(\mathbf{X}_{J-1}) = \min\{U_{J-1}(\mathbf{X}_{J-1}), E\{U_J(\mathbf{X}_{J-1}, X_J) \mid \mathbf{X}_{J-1}\}\},$$

where $E\{U_J(\mathbf{X}_{J-1}, X_j) \mid \mathbf{X}_{J-1}\}$ is the expected value of $U_J(\mathbf{X}_{J-1}, X_J)$ with respect to the predictive distribution of X_J, given $\mathbf{X}_{J-1}$, namely:

$$p_J^*(x \mid \mathbf{X}_{J-1}) = \int_{-\infty}^{\infty} f(x; \theta) h(\theta \mid \mathbf{X}_{J-1})\, d\theta. \tag{2.7.6}$$

(iii) By backwards induction, define for $j \geq 1$

(2.7.7)
$$V_{J-j}^{(j)}(\mathbf{X}_{J-j}) = \min\{U_{J-j}(\mathbf{X}_{J-j}), E\{V_{J-j+1}^{(j-1)}(X_{J-j}, X_{J-j+1}) \mid \mathbf{X}_{J-j}\}\}.$$

The optimal stopping variable, in this class of truncated stopping rules, is

$$N_J^0 = \min\{n \geq 1 : U_n(\mathbf{X}_n) = V_n^{(J-n)}(\mathbf{X}_n)\}. \tag{2.7.8}$$

It is generally difficult to determine the optimal stopping variable. However, it is straightforward to determine the *one-step look-ahead* variable, which is

$$N^{(1)} = \min\{n \geq 1 : U_n(\mathbf{X}_n) = V_n^{(1)}(\mathbf{X}_n)\}. \tag{2.7.9}$$

This stopping variable is called *myopic*. We remark here that if $U_n(\mathbf{X}_n)$ does not depend on x, for all $n \geq 1$, then the optimal stopping rule is a sample of fixed size

$$n^* = \max\{n \geq 1 : U_n \leq B), \tag{2.7.10}$$

where $0 < B < \infty$ is a given budgetary constraint. There are certain monotonicity conditions under which $N^{(1)}$ is optimal (see Chow, Robbins, and Siegmund, 1971). It is often convenient to apply the theory of Bickel and Yahav (1967, 1968, 1969) on *asymptotically pointwise optimal* (APO) stopping rules. Let $Y_n = \rho_h^0(\mathbf{X}_n)$ be the posterior risk of the Bayesian estimator. A stopping variable $N_A(c)$ is called APO if

$$\lim_{c \to 0} \frac{U_{N_A}(c)}{U_{N(c)}} \leq 1 \quad \text{a.s.} \tag{2.7.11}$$

for any other stopping variable $N(c)$.

Theorem 2.7.1 *If*

(i) $P\{Y_n > 0\} = 1$ *for all* $n \geq 1$ *and*

(ii) $\lim_{n\to\infty} n^{\beta}\rho_h^0(\mathbf{X}_n) = V$ *a.s. (a positive r.v.) for some* $\beta > 0$, *then*

$$N_{\text{APO}}(c) = \inf\left\{n \geq 1 : n \geq \frac{\beta Y_n}{c}\right\} \tag{2.7.12}$$

is APO. ■

An example of a myopic stopping variable which is APO will be given in the next section. For a proof of Theorem 2.7.1 see Ghosh, Mukhopadhyay, and Sen (1997, p. 126).

2.7.2 Estimating the Scale Parameter of the Exponential Distribution

Let $X_1, X_2, \ldots$ be a sequence of i.i.d. random variables having an exponential distribution with mean β. Let $\lambda = 1/\beta$ and suppose that λ has a prior gamma distribution, $\lambda \sim G(\Lambda, \nu)$, that is, $h(\lambda) = (1/\Gamma(\nu)\Lambda^{\nu})\lambda^{\nu-1}e^{-\lambda/\Lambda}$, $0 < \lambda < \infty$. The posterior distribution of λ given $\mathbf{X}_n$ is

$$h(\lambda \mid \mathbf{X}_n) = \frac{(T_n + 1/\Lambda)^{n+\nu}}{\Gamma(n+\nu)}\lambda^{n+\nu-1}e^{-\lambda(T_n+1/\Lambda)}, \quad 0 < \lambda < \infty, \tag{2.7.13}$$

where $T_n = \sum_{i=1}^{n} X_i$. Thus, the Bayesian estimator of $\beta = 1/\lambda$ for the squared-error loss is

$$\begin{aligned} E\{\beta \mid T_n\} &= \int_0^{\infty} \frac{1}{\lambda} h(\lambda \mid \mathbf{X}_n)\, d\lambda \\ &= \frac{\Gamma(n+\nu-1)}{\Gamma(n+\nu)} \cdot \frac{(T_n + 1/\Lambda)^{n+\nu}}{(T_n + 1/\Lambda)^{n+\nu-1}} \\ &= \frac{T_n + 1/\Lambda}{n+\nu-1}. \end{aligned} \tag{2.7.14}$$

Notice that by the strong law of large numbers $E\{\beta \mid T_n\} \to \beta$ a.s. as $n \to \infty$. Moreover, the posterior variance of β is

$$V\{\beta \mid T_n\} = \frac{(T_n + 1/\Lambda)^2}{(n+\nu-1)^2(n+\nu-2)}. \tag{2.7.15}$$

We see that

$$\lim_{n\to\infty} nV\{\beta \mid T_n\} = \beta^2 \quad \text{a.s.} \tag{2.7.16}$$

Given $\mathbf{X}_n$, the *predictive* p.d.f. of X_{n+1} is

(2.7.17)
$$p^*_{n+1}(x \mid \mathbf{X}_n) = \int_0^\infty \lambda e^{-\lambda x} \cdot \frac{(T_n + 1/\Lambda)^{n+\nu}}{\Gamma(n+\nu)} \lambda^{n+\nu-1} \cdot e^{-\lambda(T_n+1/\Lambda)}\, d\lambda$$
$$= \frac{n+\nu}{T_n + 1/\Lambda} \cdot \left(1 + \frac{x}{T_n + 1/\Lambda}\right)^{-(n+\nu+1)}.$$

This is a Pareto density with scale parameter $T_n + 1/\Lambda$ and shape parameter $n+\nu$. After n observations, the predictive expectation of $V\{\beta \mid T_n + X_{n+1}\}$ given $\mathbf{X}_n$ is

(2.7.18)
$$\frac{n+\nu}{T_n + 1/\Lambda} \int_0^\infty \left(1 + \frac{x}{T_n + 1/\Lambda}\right)^{-(n+\nu+1)} \frac{(T_n + 1/\Lambda + x)^2}{(n+\nu)^2(n+\nu-1)} dx$$
$$= \frac{(T_n + 1/\Lambda)^2}{(n+\nu)(n+\nu-1)(n+\nu-2)}.$$

This predictive expectation is smaller than $V\{\beta \mid T_n\}$ for all $n > 2 - \nu$. The difference between the posterior risk, $V\{\beta \mid T_n\}$, after n observations and the predictive expectation of the posterior risk after $n+1$ observations is

(2.7.19)
$$V\{\beta \mid T_n\} - E\{V\{\beta \mid T_n + X_{n+1}\} \mid T_n\} = \frac{(T_n + 1/\Lambda)^2}{(n+\nu)(n+\nu-1)^2(n+\nu-2)}.$$

To construct a reasonable stopping rule one should take into account the cost, c, of each observation. The stopping rule which stops for the first $n > 2 - \nu$ such that (2.7.19) is smaller than c is called a *myopic* stopping rule. We thus consider the stopping variable

(2.7.20)
$$N(c) = \min\left\{n > 2 - \nu : \frac{A(T_n + 1/\Lambda)^2}{(n+\nu)(n+\nu-1)^2(n+\nu-2)} < c\right\},$$

where $0 < A < \infty$. Here, $N(c) \downarrow c$ and $\lim_{c\to 0} N(c) = \infty$ a.s. The stopping variable $N(c)$ is an APO. Notice that for the special case of $\nu = 1$ and $\Lambda = 1$ the stopping variable (2.7.20) becomes

(2.7.21)
$$N(c) = \min\left(n \geq m(\geq 1) : n^2(n^2 - 1) \geq \frac{A(1+T_n)^2}{c}\right\},$$

where m is an initial sample size. An asymptotically equivalent stopping rule, as $c \to 0$, is

(2.7.22)
$$N^*(c) = \min\left(n \geq m(\geq 1) : n \geq \left(\frac{A}{c}\right)^{1/4} (1+T_n)^{1/2}\right\}.$$

The Bayesian estimator of β at stopping is, for $\Lambda = 1$ and $\nu = 1$, according to (2.7.6), $\hat{\beta}_N = (T_N + 1)/N$, which is approximately $\bar{X}_N$. We therefore call the following three functionals the *characteristics of the stopping variable* N: $E\{N\}$, $E\{\bar{X}_N\}$, and Risk $= AE\{(\bar{X}_N - \beta)^2\} + cE\{N\}$. We can compute the exact characteristics of $N(c)$ and $N^*(c)$ by the method of Section 2.5.1 with the concave boundaries

$$B(t) = \frac{1}{2}\left(2 + 2\left(1 + 4\frac{A}{c}(1+t^2)\right)^{1/2}\right)^{1/2} \tag{2.7.23}$$

for (2.7.21) and

$$B^*(t) = \left(\frac{A}{c}\right)^{1/4}(1+t)^{1/2} \tag{2.7.24}$$

for (2.7.22). In Table 2.13 we present the characteristics of $N(c)$ and $N^*(c)$. Notice that $N(c) > N^*(c)$ a.s.

Table 2.13: Characteristics of N(c) and N*(c) for β= 1, A = 10, m = 7, ν= Λ = 1

	$N(c)$			$N^*(c)$		
c	$E\{N\}$	$E\{\bar{X}_N\}$	Risk	$E\{N\}$	$E\{\bar{X}_N\}$	Risk
0.1	11.10	0.9329	1.9950	11.06	0.9324	1.9925
0.05	15.07	0.9408	1.4681	15.03	0.9403	1.4691
0.01	32.41	0.9693	0.6591	32.40	0.9692	0.6593
0.005	45.49	0.9780	0.4617	45.48	0.9780	0.4617

CHAPTER 3

ADAPTIVE DESIGNS FOR GENERALIZED LINEAR MODELS

3.1 EXPONENTIAL EXAMPLE

Consider a reliability experiment where m units (systems) are put on test. It is assumed that the life length (time to failure) of these units are i.i.d. random variables having an exponential life distribution

$$F(x;\beta) = 1 - e^{-x/\beta}, \quad x \geq 0.$$

In the present experiment one cannot record the exact failure time. After x units of time the experimenter comes and counts the number of units, J_m, which failed during the time interval $(0, x]$. Since the failure times are i.i.d.,

$$J_m \sim B(m, 1 - e^{-x/\beta})$$

that is, J_m has a binomial distribution with $P\{J_1 = 1\} = 1 - e^{-x/\beta}$. The maximum-likelihood estimator (MLE) of the expected failure time, β, is

$$\hat{\beta}_m = -\frac{x}{\log(1 - \hat{p}_m)}, \tag{3.1.1}$$

where $\hat{p}_m = J_m/m$. The design problem is to determine x. The asymptotic variance of $\hat{\beta}_m$ (for large m) is the inverse of the Fisher information function (see Sen and Singer, 1993, p. 205).

Let $L(\beta; x, J_m)$ denote the likelihood function of β and $l(\beta; x, J_m) = \log L(\beta; x, J_m)$. The Fisher information function is

$$I_m(\beta; x) = V\left\{\frac{\partial}{\partial\beta} l(\beta; x, J_m)\right\}. \tag{3.1.2}$$

In the present case

$$L(\beta; x, J_m) = (1 - e^{-x/\beta})^{J_m} e^{-(m-J_m)x/\beta} \tag{3.1.3}$$

and

$$l(\beta; x, J_m) = J_m \log(1 - e^{-x/\beta}) - \frac{(m - J_m)x}{\beta}. \tag{3.1.4}$$

Furthermore,

$$\frac{\partial}{\partial\beta} l(\beta; x, J_m) = \frac{x}{\beta^2}\left(m - J_m \frac{1}{1 - e^{-x/\beta}}\right). \tag{3.1.5}$$

Thus, the Fisher information function is

$$I_m(\beta; x) = \frac{m x^2 e^{-x/\beta}}{\beta^4 (1 - e^{-x/\beta})}. \tag{3.1.6}$$

It is straightforward to verify that the value of x which maximizes (3.1.6) is the solution of the equation

$$2(1 - e^{-u}) - u = 0, \tag{3.1.7}$$

where $u = x/\beta$, namely,

$$x^0 \doteq 1.5936\beta. \tag{3.1.8}$$

The problem is that β is unknown. In the present chapter we develop several adaptive procedures which address this problem. We illustrate here the maximum-likelihood method, which will be discussed in more detail in the next section.

We should mention that the present example is discussed also by Chernoff (1972) and Cochran (1973), and it can be traced back to Fisher (1922). Ehrenfeld (1962) considered the problem of finding x to minimize a certain expected loss.

The MLE-adaptive procedure is to take a sequence of independent samples, each one of size m. After each sample to estimate β by the method of the MLE using all available data and, if $\hat{\beta}_n$ is the MLE of β after n samples, determine for the next sample $x_{n+1} = 1.5936\hat{\beta}_n$. The log-likelihood function after n stages (samples) is

$$l_n(\beta) = \sum_{i=1}^{n} \left[J_m^{(i)} \log(1 - e^{-x_i/\beta}) - \frac{x_i}{\beta}(m - J_m^{(i)}) \right]. \tag{3.1.9}$$

The score function is

$$\frac{\partial}{\partial\beta} l_n(\beta) = \frac{m}{\beta^2} \sum_{i=1}^{n} x_i \left(1 - \beta_m^{(i)} \frac{1}{1 - e^{-x_i/\beta}}\right). \tag{3.1.10}$$

Thus, $\hat{\beta}_n$ is the root β of the equation

$$\sum_{i=1}^{n} p_m^{(i)} \frac{x_i}{1 - e^{-x_i/\beta}} = \sum_{i=1}^{n} x_i. \tag{3.1.11}$$

The root β of (3.1.11) can be determined numerically by the Newton–Raphson procedure, which is explained in the next section. We continue sampling in this manner until the values of $\{x_n\}$ stabilize around some value. In Table 3.1 we show simulated values of $\{x_n\}$. In this simulation $\beta = 1$ and the true value of $x^0 = 1.5936$. Each sample is of size $m = 30$. We start with $x_1 = 1.1$. We see that already after the sixth sample all values of x_n are within $x^0 \pm 0.05x^0$.

Table 3.1: Simulated Values of $\mathbf{x_n}$ for $\beta = 1$, m = 30

n	x_n	n	x_n	n	x_n	n	x_n
1	1.100	10	1.613	35	1.627	70	1.603
2	2.183	15	1.535	40	1.628	80	1.614
3	1.814	20	1.674	45	1.622	90	1.602
4	1.808	25	1.676	50	1.631	100	1.617
5	1.803	30	1.661	60	1.580	200	1.590

3.2 ADAPTIVE DESIGNS FOR THE FISHER INFORMATION

We consider binary random variables J_x, where $P\{J_x = 1\} = F(\alpha + \beta x)$. Here F is a (tolerance) distribution function having a density f; α and β are parameters belonging to some parameter space $\Theta \subset \mathbb{R}^{(2)}$; and x is a design variable belonging to a finite closed interval $[x^*, x^{**}]$. We assume here that $0 < \beta < \infty$. Thus F is an increasing function of x. If n trials are performed at the same value of x, then the Fisher information matrix for (α, β) is

$$II(\alpha, \beta; x) = \frac{nf^2(\alpha + \beta x)}{F(\alpha + \beta x)\bar{F}(\alpha + \beta x)} \begin{pmatrix} 1 & x \\ x & x^2 \end{pmatrix}, \tag{3.2.1}$$

where $\bar{F}(\cdot) = 1 - F(\cdot)$. Notice that this matrix is singular, since all the n trials are at the same point x. However, one can estimate, if the point x^0 is chosen, the value of $\alpha + \beta x^0$. Let $u = \alpha + \beta x$. Then the Fisher information function of u is

$$I(u) = \frac{nu^2 f^2(u)}{F(u)\bar{F}(u)}. \tag{3.2.2}$$

If u^0 is a point maximizing $I(u)$, then the optimal value of x is a function of (α, β), namely,

$$x^0 = \frac{u^0 - \alpha}{\beta}. \tag{3.2.3}$$

The example of the previous section is a special case.

In many practical cases in bioassays and other fields, the value of α can be assumed. We therefore consider first the case where $\alpha = 0$ and β is unknown. The adaptive procedure is as follows. We take a sequence of relatively small samples. After the nth stage of sampling the MLE of β, $\hat{\beta}_n$, is determined on the basis of the data from all the n stages. The design point x_{n+1} is determined then as

$$x_{n+1} = \begin{cases} x^* & \text{if } \dfrac{u^0}{\hat{\beta}_n} \leq x^* \\ \dfrac{u^0}{\hat{\beta}_n} & \text{if } x^* < \dfrac{u^0}{\hat{\beta}_n} < x^{**} \\ x^{**} & \text{if } \dfrac{u^0}{\hat{\beta}_n} \geq x^{**}. \end{cases} \tag{3.2.4}$$

As in the previous section, the likelihood function after n stages, where m is the size of each sample, is

$$L_n(\beta; (x_i, J_{x_i}^{(i)}, i = 1, \ldots, n)) = \prod_{i=1}^{n} F(\beta x_i)^{J_{x_i}^{(i)}} \bar{F}(\beta x_i)^{m - J_{x_i}^{(i)}}. \tag{3.2.5}$$

Differentiating the log-likelihood function with respect to β, we obtain that the MLE, $\hat{\beta}_n$, is the root of the equation

$$\sum_{i=1}^{n} (\hat{p}_i - F(\beta x_i)) \frac{x_i f(x; \beta)}{F(x; \beta)\bar{F}(x_i \beta)} = 0, \tag{3.2.6}$$

where $\hat{p}_i = J_{x_i}^{(i)}/m$. Generally we solve Eq. (3.2.6) by the following iterative procedure, called the *Newton–Raphson* procedure. To solve numerically a nonlinear equation $G(\beta) = 0$, consider the following approximation.

Suppose that $\beta^{(1)}$ is a point close to β. Then

$$G(\beta) \cong G(\beta^{(1)}) + (\beta - \beta^{(1)})G'(\beta^{(1)}). \tag{3.2.7}$$

Setting (3.2.7) equal to zero, we get

$$\beta = \beta^{(1)} - \frac{G(\beta^{(1)})}{G'(\beta^{(1)})},$$

where $G'(\beta^{(1)})$ is the derivative of $G(\beta)$ at $\beta^{(1)}$. We then substitute the solution β as the initial solution and solve again. More precisely, if $\beta^{(1)}$ is an initial solution, then

$$\beta^{(i+1)} = \beta^{(i)} - \frac{G(\beta^{(i)})}{G'(\beta^{(i)})}, \quad i \geq 1, \tag{3.2.8}$$

is a sequence of approximations to the root β. We illustrate this procedure by solving Eq. (3.1.7), in which $G(u) = 2(1 - e^{-u}) - u$. Here $G'(u) = 2e^{-u} - 1$. We should be careful not to have $G'(u^{(i)}) = 0$, that is, $u^{(i)} = \log(2) \doteq 0.6931$. Starting with $u^{(1)} = 1$, we get $u^{(2)} = 2$, $u^{(3)} = 1.62888$, $u^4 = 1.59403$, $u^{(5)} = 1.593624$, $u^{(i)} = u^{(5)}$ for all $i \geq 6$. We see that the correct positive solution was obtained in five iterations. The correct positive solution can be obtained if we start with any initial value $u^{(1)} > \log(2)$. If $u^{(1)} < \log(2)$, then the procedure leads to the trivial solution $u_1 = 0$. The Newton–Raphson procedure should be used with discretion!

How can we determine the initial value $\beta^{(1)}$ for the Newton–Raphson solution of Eq. (3.2.6)? Starting with the first sample, the moment equation solution of $F(\beta x_1) = \hat{p}_1$ yields, for $0 < x_1 < \infty$,

$$\hat{\beta}^{(1)} = \frac{F^{-1}(\hat{p}_1)}{x_1}. \tag{3.2.9}$$

At the nth stage of the adaptive procedure, $n \geq 2$, we can start the solution of (3.2.6) with the solution $\hat{\beta}_{n-1}$ of the previous stage. If we cannot assume that $\alpha = 0$, we can estimate and test the significance of α initially in the following manner. Take the first two samples, each one of size m, at $x_1 = x^*$ and $x_2 = x^{**}$. Let $\hat{p}_1$ and $\hat{p}_2$ be the corresponding proportions of 1's. Define $Y_i = F^{-1}(\hat{p}_i)$, $i = 1, 2$. The least squares estimates of α and β are then

$$\hat{\beta}_{\text{LS}} = \frac{Y_2 - Y_1}{x_2 - x_1} \tag{3.2.10}$$

and

$$\begin{aligned} \hat{\alpha}_{\text{LS}} &= \frac{Y_1 + Y_2}{2} - \hat{\beta}_{\text{LS}} \frac{x_1 + x_2}{2} \\ &= \frac{Y_1 + Y_2}{2} - \frac{Y_2 - Y_1}{2} \cdot \frac{x_1 + x_2}{x_2 - x_1}. \end{aligned} \tag{3.2.11}$$

Since $\beta > 0$, $F(\alpha + \beta x_1) < F(\alpha + \beta x_2)$. Thus, $\hat{p}_2$ is stochastically greater than $\hat{p}_1$ and we expect that $Y_2 > Y_1$ and $\hat{\beta}_2 > 0$. If however $\hat{p}_2 \leq \hat{p}_1$, increase the size of the samples until $\hat{p}_2$ stabilizes around $F(\alpha+\beta x_2)$ and $\hat{p}_1$ stabilizes around $F(\alpha+\beta x_1)$. Indeed, by the strong law of large numbers $\hat{p}_i \longrightarrow_{m\to\infty} F(\alpha+\beta x_i)$ a.s. Since Y_1 and Y_2 are independent and the asymptotic variance of Y_i is

(3.2.12)
$$V\{Y_i\} \cong \frac{F(\alpha+\beta x_i)\bar{F}(\alpha+\beta x_i)}{m x_i^2 f^2(\alpha+\beta x_i)},$$

we obtain from (3.2.11) that the standard error (estimated standard deviation) of $\hat{\alpha}_{\text{LS}}$ is

(3.2.13)
$$\text{S.E.}\{\hat{\alpha}_{\text{LS}}\} = \frac{1}{\sqrt{m}}\left[\frac{\hat{p}_1(1-\hat{p}_1)\rho^2}{f^2(\hat{\alpha}_{\text{LS}}+\hat{\beta}_{\text{LS}}x_1)} + \frac{\hat{p}_2(1-\hat{p}_2)}{\rho^2 f^2(\hat{\alpha}_{\text{LS}}+\hat{\beta}_{\text{LS}}x_2)}\right]^{1/2} \cdot (x_2-x_1)^{-1},$$

where $\rho = x_2/x_1$. If $|\hat{\alpha}_{\text{LS}}| < 3$ S.E.$\{\hat{\alpha}_{\text{LS}}\}$ the value of $\hat{\alpha}_{\text{LS}}$ is not significantly different from zero. If $\hat{\alpha}_{\text{LS}}$ is not significant, we proceed with the assumption that $\alpha = 0$ and set $x_3 = u_0/\hat{\beta}_{\text{LS}}$. On the other hand, if $\hat{\alpha}_{\text{LS}}$ is significantly different from zero, we set

$$x_3 = \left.\frac{u^0 - \hat{\alpha}_{\text{LS}}}{\hat{\beta}_{\text{LS}}}\right]_{x^*}^{x^{**}},$$

where $a]_{x^*}^{x^{**}} = x^* I(a \le x^*) + aI(x^* < a < x^{**}) + x^{**}I(a \ge x^{**})$. The following is a simple numerical example.

Suppose that $F(x) = \Phi(x)$, which is the standard normal distribution. Let $\phi(x)$ be the standard density. Here $\alpha = 0$ and $\beta = 1$. The Fisher information function is

(3.2.14)
$$I(u) = \frac{u^2\phi^2(u)}{\beta^2\Phi(u)\Phi(-u)}.$$

This is a symmetric function having two maxima at $u^0 = \pm 1.577$. The statistician does not know that $\alpha = 0$ and $\beta = 1$. The statistician starts the procedure with $x_1 = -1$ and $x_2 = 1$ and $m = 30$. Suppose that $\hat{p}_1 = 0.1667$ and $\hat{p}_2 = 0.8333$. For these values of $\hat{p}_i$ we have $Y_1 = -0.9661$, $Y_2 = 0.9673$. The least squares estimates are $\hat{\alpha}_{\text{LS}} = 0.0004$ and $\hat{\beta}_{\text{LS}} = 0.9667$. The standard error of $\hat{\alpha}_{\text{LS}}$, according to (3.2.13), is S.E.$\{\hat{\alpha}_{\text{LS}}\} = 0.0327$. Hence, $\hat{\alpha}_{\text{LS}}$ is not significant. The statistician continues now under the model with $\alpha = 0$. The third sample is taken with $x_3 = \pm 1.577/0.9667 = \pm 1.631$, that is, either $x_3 = 1.631$ or $x_3 = -1.631$, and so on.

If α is significant but unknown, we estimate at each stage both α and β by the method of MLE. Similar to (3.2.5), the likelihood function after n stages is

(3.2.15)
$$L_n(\alpha,\beta;(x_i, J^{(i)}, i=1,\ldots,n)) = \prod_{i=1}^{n} F(\alpha+\beta x_i)^{J^{(i)}}\bar{F}(\alpha+\beta x_i)^{m-J^{(i)}}.$$

The log-likelihood function is

$$(3.2.16)\quad l_n(\alpha,\beta) = \sum_{i=1}^{n} J^{(i)} \log F(\alpha+\beta x_i) + \sum_{i=1}^{n}(m - J^{(i)}) \cdot \log \bar{F}(\alpha+\beta x_i).$$

Let

$$G_1(\alpha,\beta) = \frac{\partial}{\partial\alpha} l_n(\alpha,\beta), \quad G_2(\alpha,\beta) = \frac{\partial}{\partial\beta} l_n(\alpha,\beta).$$

Let $\boldsymbol{\theta} = (\alpha,\beta)'$ and $\mathbf{G}(\boldsymbol{\theta}) = (G_1(\boldsymbol{\theta}), G_2(\boldsymbol{\theta}))'$. Furthermore, let $D(\boldsymbol{\theta})$ be the matrix

$$D(\boldsymbol{\theta}) = \begin{pmatrix} \frac{\partial}{\partial\alpha}G_1(\boldsymbol{\theta}) & \frac{\partial}{\partial\beta}G_1(\boldsymbol{\theta}) \\ \\ \frac{\partial}{\partial\alpha}G_2(\boldsymbol{\theta}) & \frac{\partial}{\partial\beta}G_2(\boldsymbol{\theta}) \end{pmatrix}.$$

Starting with an initial solution $\boldsymbol{\theta}^{(1)}$ for the system $\mathbf{G}(\boldsymbol{\theta}) \equiv 0$, the Newton–Raphson iterative solution is

$$(3.2.17)\qquad \boldsymbol{\theta}^{(i+1)} = \boldsymbol{\theta}^{(i)} - D^{-1}(\boldsymbol{\theta}^{(i)})\mathbf{G}(\boldsymbol{\theta}^{(i)}), \quad i \geq 1.$$

Obviously, $D(\boldsymbol{\theta}^{(i)})$ should be nonsingular for each $i \geq 1$.

To illustrate the procedure, we present the following example: The distribution F is the logistic. Here the standard distribution is

$$F(u) = \frac{e^u}{1+e^u}, \quad -\infty < u < \infty.$$

The standard density is $f(u) = e^u/(1+e^u)^2$. The Fisher information function is

$$I(\beta; u) = \frac{u^2 e^u}{\beta^2(1+e^u)^2}.$$

This function is symmetric about the origin with maxima at $u^0 = \pm 2.4$. Suppose that both α and β are unknown, but the true values are $\alpha = 1$, $\beta = 3$. For these parameters $x^0 = (2.4 - 1)/3 = 0.47$. In each stage the sample size $m = 50$. Suppose we start with $x_1 = -0.5$ and observe $\hat{p}_1 = 0.416$ and $x_2 = 0.5$ with $\hat{p}_2 = 0.931$. The estimated values of $\hat{\alpha}_n$, $\hat{\beta}_n$, and $\hat{x}_n^0 = (2.4 - \hat{\alpha}_n)/\hat{\beta}_n$ for $n = 2, \ldots, 20$ are given in Table 3.2.

Table 3.2: Estimated Values of $\hat{\alpha}_n$, $\hat{\beta}_n$, and $\hat{x}_n^0$ by MLE Method
$\alpha = 1$, $\beta = 3$, $m = 50$, $x^0 = 0.47$

n	$\hat{x}_n^0$	$\hat{\alpha}_n$	$\hat{\beta}_n$
2	0.500	1.1288	2.9372
3	0.433	1.2901	3.0838
4	0.360	1.1848	3.1041
5	0.391	1.1688	3.0986
6	0.397	1.1566	3.0919
7	0.402	1.0860	3.0354
8	0.432	1.0926	3.0844
9	0.424	1.0754	3.0253
10	0.438	1.0596	2.8392
15	0.453	1.0089	3.0129
20	0.465	0.9356	3.2095

The MLE estimates are quite close to the true values, and the $\hat{x}_n^0$ values are close to x^0 after 20 stages.

In the adaptive procedure, the x-value in the n stage, x_n, is a function of results of the first $(n-1)$st stages. Thus, $\hat{p}_m^{(1)}, \hat{p}_m^{(2)}, \ldots$ are not independent. The question is then whether the MLEs $\hat{\alpha}_n$ and $\hat{\beta}_n$ converge in probability (consistent) as $n \to \infty$ to the true values of α and β. In the following theorem we give the conditions under which $\hat{\beta}_n \to \beta$ in probability, as $n \to \infty$, in a one-parameter model ($\alpha = 0$). Assume that $0 < \beta_L \leq \beta \leq \beta_U < \infty$ and $x \in [x^*, x^*]$. Then $u = \beta x \in [u^*, u^{**}]$ where $u^* = x^* \beta_L$ and $u^{**} = x^{**}\beta_U$.

Theorem 3.2.1 *Assume that*

(i) $0 < \delta \leq F(u^*) < F(u^{**}) < 1$;

(ii) $\inf_{u^* \leq u \leq u^{**}} f(u) \geq \eta > 0$;

(iii) $\sup_{u^* \leq u \leq u^{**}} f(u) \leq f^* < \infty$;

(iv) $f(u)$ *is continuously differentiable and* $-\infty < \inf_u f'(u) \leq \sup_u f'(u) < \infty$; *then*

$$\hat{\beta}_n \xrightarrow[n\to\infty]{p} \beta$$

and

$$\sqrt{n}(\hat{\beta}_n - \beta) \xrightarrow[n\to\infty]{d} N\left(0, I^{-1}\left(\beta; \frac{u^0}{\beta}\right)\right). \tag{3.2.18}$$

■

For a proof, see S. Zacks (1996, p. 158). M.K. Khan (1984) studied adaptive designs on discrete sets $\{x_0, \ldots, x_k\}$, where $x_0 = x^*$, $x_k = x^{**}$, and $x_i = x^* + (i/k)(x^{**} - x^*)$, $i = 1, \ldots, k$. He proved consistency and asymptotic normality.

3.3 ADAPTIVE BAYESIAN DESIGNS

Adaptive Bayesian designs in N stages are designs in which after each stage the posterior distribution of the unknown parameter is determined on the basis of the observed results and the remaining experimental levels are determined so as to maximize the expected payoff (utility) or minimize the total expected loss of the remaining stages. As in the previous section, we assume here that m Bernoulli trials are performed at each stage, with probability of success $F(x/\sigma)$, where $x \in [x^*, x^{**}]$ and σ is an unknown parameter, $0 < \sigma < \infty$. Let $H(\sigma)$ denote a prior c.d.f. of σ having a density function $h(\sigma)$ on $(0, \infty)$. Notice that $\sigma = 1/\beta$.

The likelihood function of σ after n stages $L_n(\sigma)$ is given by Eq. (3.2.5). The posterior p.d.f. of σ after n stages is

$$h_n(\sigma) = \frac{h(\sigma)L_n(\sigma)}{\displaystyle\int_0^\infty h(\sigma)L_n(\sigma)\,d\sigma}. \tag{3.3.1}$$

The experimental level for the nth stage X_n is a function of the observations in the previous stages, that is, $X_n \in \mathcal{F}_{n-1}$, $n \geq 1$, where X_1 depends only on the prior distribution of σ and $\mathcal{F}_{n-1}$ denotes the σ-field generated by the first $(n-1)$ observed random variables. Accordingly, the objective is to maximize $E_H\left\{\sum_{n=1}^N I(\sigma; X_n)\right\}$, where $I(\sigma; x)$ is the Fisher information. As in the previous section, let $X_n = u^0\hat{\sigma}_n$ $n \geq 1$, where $\hat{\sigma}_n \in \mathcal{F}_{n-1}$ is a posterior estimator of σ. For a finite number of stages, N, define

$$M_N(x) = x^2 E_H\left\{\frac{f^2(x/\sigma)}{F(x/\sigma)\bar{F}(x/\sigma)} \mid \mathcal{F}_{N-1}\right\}. \tag{3.3.2}$$

The optimal design level, X_N^0, is the argument, in $[x^*, x^{**}]$, maximizing $M_N(x)$. Recursively we define, for each $j = 1, 2, \cdots, N-1$,
(3.3.3)

$$M_{N-j}(x) = x^2 E_H\left\{\frac{f^2(x/\sigma)}{F(x/\sigma)\bar{F}(x/\sigma)} + M_{N-j+1}(X_{N-j+1}^0) \mid \mathcal{F}_{N-j-1}\right\}$$

and X_{N-j}^0 is the argument in $[x^*, x^{**}]$ maximizing $M_{N-j}(x)$.

Generally it is impossible to obtain explicit expressions for X_n^0.

In some situations, like clinical trials, two-stage designs may be preferable to multistage designs due to feasibility constraints. There are many papers in the literature in which the Bayesian adaptive sequence is not optimal but is given by $\left[X_n = u^0\hat{\sigma}_n\right]_{x^*}^{x^{**}}$ (see, e.g., Chevret 1993), where $\hat{\sigma}_n$ is the Bayesian estimator of σ for the squared-error loss, that is, the posterior mean

$$\hat{\sigma}_n = \frac{\displaystyle\int_0^\infty \sigma h(\sigma)L_n(\sigma)\,d\sigma}{\displaystyle\int_0^\infty h(\sigma)L_n(\sigma)\,d\sigma}. \tag{3.3.4}$$

We should comment in this connection that due to the complexity of the likelihood function $L_n(\sigma)$, when the x levels vary, the evaluation of $\hat{\sigma}_n$ by Eq. (3.3.4) generally requires delicate numerical integration.

There are two ways to evaluate the integrals in (3.3.4). One is by simulation, and the other one is by numerical integration. Since $h(\sigma)$ is a density function, the numerator of (3.3.4) is the expected value $E_H\{XL_n(X)\}$, where X is a random variable having a distribution H with density h. For sufficiently large M, $E_H\{XL_n(X)\}$ is approximated by $(1/M)\sum_{i=1}^{M} X_i L_n(X_i)$, where $X_1, X_2, \ldots, X_M$ are drawn at random by Monte Carlo simulation from the distribution H. Similarly $E_H\{L_n(X)\} \simeq (1/M)\sum_{j=1}^{M} L_n(X_j)$.

The second method is by numerical integration. First, by changing the variable σ to $u = 1/(1+\sigma)$, $\sigma = 1/u - 1$ and $d\sigma = (1/u^2)\, du$. Hence

$$
\begin{aligned}
\int_0^{\infty} \sigma h(\sigma) L_n(\sigma)\, d\sigma &= \int_0^1 \frac{1-u}{u^3} h\left(\frac{1-u}{u}\right) L_n\left(\frac{1-u}{u}\right) du \\
&\cong \sum_{i=1}^{8} w_i \frac{1-u_i}{u_i^3} L_n\left(\frac{1-u_i}{u_i}\right) h\left(\frac{1-u_i}{u_i}\right).
\end{aligned} \tag{3.3.5}
$$

Similarly,

$$
\begin{aligned}
\int_0^{\infty} h(\sigma) L_n(\sigma)\, d\sigma &= \int_0^1 \frac{1}{u^2} h\left(\frac{1-u}{u}\right) L_n\left(\frac{1-u}{u}\right) du \\
&\cong \sum_{i=1}^{8} w_i \frac{1}{u_i^2} h\left(\frac{1-u_i}{u_i}\right) L_n\left(\frac{1-u_i}{u_i}\right).
\end{aligned} \tag{3.3.6}
$$

The weights w_i and abscissas u_i are given by those of Gaussian integration of moments (see Abramowitz and Stegan, 1968, p. 921):

i	w_i	u_i
1	0.0506	0.0199
2	0.1112	0.1017
3	0.1569	0.2372
4	0.1813	0.4083
5	0.1813	0.5917
6	0.1569	0.7628
7	0.1112	0.8983
8	0.0506	0.9801

We illustrate these two methods numerically.

Suppose again that $F(x/\sigma) = e^{x/\sigma}(1 + e^{x/\sigma})^{-1}$ is the logistic distribution with a scale parameter σ. For simplicity we consider only one stage with sample size $m = 30$. We suppose also that the true value of σ is 1. Thirty Bernoulli trials at $x = 2.4$ gave $J_{30} = 28$. Let $\beta = 1/\sigma$. The likelihood function of β is then

$$L(\beta) = \frac{\exp(67.2\beta)}{(1+\exp(2.4\beta))^{30}}. \tag{3.3.7}$$

We assign β a prior $G(1/2, 2)$ distribution having a density $h(\beta) = 4\beta e^{-2\beta}$.
The Bayesian estimator of β is then

$$\hat{\beta}_B = \frac{\displaystyle\int_0^\infty \beta^2 \exp\{65.2\beta - 30\log(1+e^{2.4\beta})\}\, d\beta}{\displaystyle\int_0^\infty \beta \exp\{65.2\beta - 30\log(1+e^{2.4\beta})\}\, d\beta}. \tag{3.3.8}$$

Define

$$G_1(\beta) = \beta \exp\{67.2\beta - 30\log(1+e^{2.4\beta})\}$$

and

$$G_2(\beta) = \exp\{67.2\beta - 30\log(1+e^{2.4\beta})\}.$$

We draw at random M values of β from $G(1/2, 2)$ independently and estimate $\hat{\beta}_B$ by

$$\hat{\beta}_{B,M} = \frac{\sum_{i=1}^M G_1(\beta_i)}{\sum_{i=1}^M G_2(\beta_i)}.$$

Some simulation results are given in Table 3.3.

Table 3.3: Monte Carlo Estimates of $\hat{\beta}_B$

M	100	500	1,000	5,000	10,000
$\hat{\beta}_{B,M}$	1.0738	1.0627	1.0404	1.0311	1.0315

Derived using program Bayesim2.

For the Gaussian numerical integration we define

$$A_1(u) = \frac{(1-u)^2}{u^4} \exp\left\{65.2 \cdot \frac{1-u}{u} - 30\log\left(1+\exp\left\{2.4\frac{1-u}{u}\right\}\right)\right\}$$

and $A_2(u) = [u/(1-u)]A_1(u)$. We then have

$$\hat{\beta}_B \simeq \frac{\sum_{i=1}^8 w_i A_1(u_i)}{\sum_{i=1}^8 w_i A_2(u_i)} = 1.18740.$$

(The computations of the numerical integration were performed by the program bayesnum.) It seems that in the present example the simulations gave more accurate results.

Suppose that n stages ($n \geq 1$) of sampling at points $(X_1, \ldots, X_n)$ gave the data $(J^{(1)}, \ldots, J^{(n)})$. The likelihood of β for the logistic distribution is

$$L_n(\beta; (x_i, J^{(i)}, i = 1, \ldots, n)) = \frac{\exp\left\{\beta \sum_{i=1}^n x_i J^{(i)}\right\}}{\exp\left\{m \sum_{i=1}^n \log(1 + e^{\beta x_i})\right\}}.$$

The Bayesian estimator of β after n stages is

$$\hat{\beta}_n = \frac{\int_0^\infty \beta h(\beta) \exp\left\{\beta \sum_{i=1}^n x_i J^{(i)} - m \sum_{i=1}^n \log(1 + e^{\beta x_i})\right\} d\beta}{\int_0^\infty h(\beta) \exp\left\{\beta \sum_{i=1}^n x_i J^{(i)} - m \sum_{i=1}^n \log(1 + e^{\beta x_i})\right\} d\beta}.$$

After estimating β by $\hat{\beta}_n$, we determine X_{n+1} as $X_{n+1} = 2.4/\hat{\beta}_m$. In Table 3.4 we present the results of such Bayesian adaptive procedure with 20 stages and samples of size $m = 30$.

Table 3.4: Values of $\mathbf{x_n}$, $\mathbf{J^{(n)}}$ and $\hat{\boldsymbol{\beta}}_{\mathbf{n}}$, $\mathbf{n = 1, \ldots, 20}$, with $\mathbf{m = 30}$, $\boldsymbol{\beta} = \mathbf{1}$.

n	x_n	$J^{(n)}$	$\hat{\beta}_n$	n	x_n	$J^{(n)}$	$\hat{\beta}_n$
1	2.00	25	0.7909	11	2.62	28	0.9629
2	3.03	27	0.7176	12	2.49	28	0.9589
3	3.18	30	0.8703	13	2.50	28	0.9297
4	2.75	29	0.9593	14	2.58	27	0.9751
5	2.50	24	1.0194	15	2.46	28	0.9682
6	2.35	29	0.8910	16	2.47	25	0.9940
7	2.69	28	0.9463	17	2.41	30	0.9186
8	2.53	26	0.9734	18	2.61	27	0.9942
9	2.46	26	0.9434	19	2.41	28	0.9658
10	2.54	29	0.9150	20	2.48	28	0.9664

Derived using programs adaptiveBS, adaptiveBayes, bayesim2.

3.4 ADAPTIVE DESIGNS FOR INVERSE REGRESSION

3.4.1 Non-Bayesian Adaptive Designs

Consider the following tolerance problem. Let Y_x be a normal random variable having mean $\beta_0 + \beta_1 x$, $\beta_1 > 0$ and variance $\sigma_x^2 = \sigma^2 x^2$. It is desired that $Y_x \leq \eta$ with probability γ, where η is a specified threshold. The largest value of x satisfying this requirement is

$$x_\gamma(\boldsymbol{\theta}) = \frac{\eta - \beta_0}{\beta_1 + \sigma Z_\gamma}, \tag{3.4.1}$$

where $\boldsymbol{\theta} = (\beta_0, \beta_1, \sigma)$ and $Z_\gamma = \Phi^{-1}(\gamma)$ is the γth quantile of the standard normal distribution. If the parameters $(\beta_0, \beta_1, \sigma)$ are known, the optimal x

level is x_γ. When the parameters are unknown, we consider adaptive designs, in which x levels are applied sequentially on groups or on individual trials. We consider here sequential designs in which one trial is performed at each stage. Let $\{X_n; n \geq 1\}$ designate the design levels of a given procedure. It is known a priori that $-\infty < x^* < x_\gamma(\boldsymbol{\theta}) < x^{**} < \infty$. Thus, all design levels X_n are restricted to the closed interval $[x^*, x^{**}]$. We further require that the random variables X_n will satisfy

$$P_{\boldsymbol{\theta}}\{X_n \leq x_\gamma(\boldsymbol{\theta})\} \geq 1 - \alpha \tag{3.4.2}$$

for all $\boldsymbol{\theta} = (\beta_0, \beta_1, \sigma)$ and all $n \geq 1$. This requirement is called the *feasibility requirement.* We wish also that the sequence $\{X_n\}$ will be consistent, that is,

$$\lim_{n\to\infty} P_{\boldsymbol{\theta}}\{|X_n - x_\gamma(\boldsymbol{\theta})| > \epsilon\} = 0 \tag{3.4.3}$$

for any $\epsilon > 0$ and $\boldsymbol{\theta}$. In some cases we can also prove that a feasible sequence $\{X_n^0\}$ is optimal in the sense that

$$\sum_{n=1}^{N} E_{\boldsymbol{\theta}}\{(x_\gamma(\boldsymbol{\theta}) - X_n^0)^+\} \leq \sum_{n=\gamma\theta}^{N} E_{\boldsymbol{\theta}}\{(x_\gamma(\boldsymbol{\theta}) - X_n)^+\} \tag{3.4.4}$$

for $N \geq 1$, where $\{X_n\}$ is any other feasible sequence and where $a^+ = \max(a, 0)$.

In the present section we present some of the results of Eichhorn (1973, 1974) and Eichhorn and Zacks (1973, 1981). See also the review article of Zacks and Eichhorn (1975).

To start, let us consider the special case where β_0 and σ are known. In this case the conditional distribution of $(Y_n - \beta_0)/X_n$, given X_n, is that of a $N(\beta_1, \sigma^2)$ a.s. Hence, the random variables $U_n = (Y_n - \beta_0)/X_n$ are i.i.d. $N(\beta_1, \sigma^2)$ and

$$\hat{\beta}_1^{(n)} = \frac{1}{n}\sum_{i=1}^{n} \frac{Y_i - \beta_0}{X_i}, \quad n \geq 1, \tag{3.4.5}$$

is the best unbiased estimator of β_1. A $1-\alpha$ upper confidence limit for β_1 is $\hat{\beta}_1^{(n)} + Z_{1-\alpha}(\sigma/\sqrt{n})$.

Theorem 3.4.1 *The sequence defined by*

$$X_{n+1} = \xi_n\Big]_{x^*}^{x^{**}}, \tag{3.4.6}$$

where

$$\xi_n = \frac{\eta - \beta_0}{\hat{\beta}_1^{(n)} + (Z_{1-\alpha}/\sqrt{n} + Z_\gamma)\sigma}, \quad n \geq 1, \tag{3.4.7}$$

is feasible, strongly consistent, and optimal.

Proof: The feasibility is due to the fact that

$$P_{\boldsymbol{\theta}}\left\{\beta_1 \leq \hat{\beta}_1^{(n)} + \frac{\sigma Z_{1-\alpha}}{\sqrt{n}}\right\} = 1 - \alpha$$

for all $\boldsymbol{\theta}$. Strong consistency is due to the fact that $\hat{\beta}_1^{(n)} \longrightarrow^{\text{a.s.}} \beta_1$. The optimality is proven using the uniformly most accurate (UMA) property of $\hat{\beta}_1^{(n)} + Z_{1-\alpha}\sigma/\sqrt{n}$, which means (see Lehmann, 1959, p. 177) that for any other $1-\alpha$ upper confidence limit for β_1, say $\tilde{\beta}_{1,\alpha}^{(n)}$, and $\epsilon > 0$,

$$P_{\boldsymbol{\theta}}\left\{\hat{\beta}_1^{(n)} + \frac{\sigma Z_{1-\alpha}}{\sqrt{n}} \geq \beta_1 + \epsilon\right\} \leq P_{\boldsymbol{\theta}}\{\tilde{\beta}_{1,\alpha}^{(n)} \geq \beta_1 + \epsilon\} \tag{3.4.8}$$

for all $\boldsymbol{\theta}$. Let

$$\xi' = \frac{\eta - \beta_0}{\beta_1 + \epsilon + \sigma Z_\gamma} \quad \text{and} \quad y = x_\gamma(\boldsymbol{\theta}) - \xi'.$$

Let

$$\tilde{X}_n = \frac{n - \beta_0}{\tilde{\beta}_{1,\alpha}^{(n)} + \sigma Z_\gamma}.$$

Then, from (3.4.8) one obtains that, for all $y > 0$,

$$P_{\boldsymbol{\theta}}\{x_\gamma(\boldsymbol{\theta}) - X_n \geq y\} \leq P_{\boldsymbol{\theta}}\{x_\gamma(\boldsymbol{\theta}) - \tilde{X}_n \geq y\}.$$

Finally,

$$\begin{aligned} E_{\boldsymbol{\theta}}\{(x_\gamma(\boldsymbol{\theta}) - X_n)^+\} &= \int_0^\infty P_{\boldsymbol{\theta}}\{x_\gamma(\boldsymbol{\theta}) - X_n \geq y\}\, dy \\ &\leq \int_0^\infty P_{\boldsymbol{\theta}}\{x_\gamma(\boldsymbol{\theta}) - \tilde{X}_n \geq y\}\, dy \\ &= E_\theta\{(x_\gamma(\theta) - \tilde{X}_n)^+\} \end{aligned}$$

for all $n \geq 1$. This proves the optimality of $\{X_n\}$ given by Eqs. (3.4.6) and (3.4.7). ■

When the slope β_1 and σ are known, we can obtain a feasible, strongly consistent, and optimal design by similar methods (see Zacks and Eichhorn, 1975). On the other hand, when both β_0 and β_1 are unknown, we can obtain a feasible, consistent design but not optimal in the previous sense. Roughly speaking, one cannot estimate β_0 and β_1 if all observations are at one fixed value of x. In the adaptive procedure, to assure consistency, one needs to assume that

$$\sum_{i=1}^n \left(\frac{1}{X_i} - \frac{1}{n}\sum_{i=1}^n \frac{1}{X_i}\right)^2 \to \infty \quad \text{as} \quad n \to \infty.$$

Let $R_i = Y_i/X_i$ and $V_i = 1/X_i$, $i = 1, 2, \ldots$. After n trials, let $\mathbf{X}^{(n)} = (X_1, X_2, \cdots, X_n)$,

$$\bar{R}_n = \frac{1}{n}\sum_{i=1}^{n} R_i, \qquad \bar{V}_n = \frac{1}{n}\sum_{i=1}^{n} V_i,$$

$$\text{SSD}_V = \sum_{i=1}^{n} V_i^2 - n\bar{V}_n^2, \quad Q_n = \sum_{i=1}^{n} V_i^2$$

and

$$\text{SPD}_{\text{VR}} = \sum_{i=1}^{n} V_i R_i - n\bar{V}_n\bar{R}_n.$$

Notice that $R_i \mid X_i \sim N(\beta_1 + \beta_0 V_i, \sigma^2)$, $i = 1, 2, \ldots$. Indeed $E(Y_i/X_i \mid X_i) = (\beta_0 + \beta_1 X_i)/X_i = \beta_1 + \beta_0 V_i$. Let $\hat{\beta}_{0,n}$ and $\hat{\beta}_{1,n}$ be the least squares estimators of β_0 and β_1 for the linear regression

$$R_i = \beta_1 + \beta_0 V_i + e_i, \quad i = 1, \ldots, n \tag{3.4.9}$$

where $e_1, \ldots, e_n$ are i.i.d. $N(0, \sigma^2)$ random variables independent of $\mathbf{X}^{(n)}$. Accordingly,

$$\begin{aligned}\hat{\beta}_{0,n} &= \frac{\text{SPD}_{VR}}{\text{SSD}_V}, \\ \hat{\beta}_{1,n} &= \bar{R}_n - \hat{\beta}_{0,n}\bar{V}_n.\end{aligned} \tag{3.4.10}$$

Given $\mathbf{X}^{(n)}$, the conditional distribution of $(\hat{\beta}_{0,n}, \hat{\beta}_{1,n})$ is bivariate normal with mean (β_0, β_1) and covariance matrix

$$\Sigma(\mathbf{X}^{(n)}) = \sigma^2 \begin{bmatrix} \dfrac{1}{\text{SSD}_V} & -\dfrac{\bar{V}_n}{\text{SSD}_V} \\[2ex] -\dfrac{\bar{V}_n}{\text{SSD}_V} & \dfrac{1}{n} + \dfrac{\bar{V}_n^2}{\text{SSD}_V} \end{bmatrix}. \tag{3.4.11}$$

To apply this approach, we have to require that $\text{SSD}_V > 0$ for each $n \geq 2$ and $\text{SSD}_V \stackrel{\text{a.s.}}{\longrightarrow} \infty$ as $n \to \infty$. This will assure that $\lim_{n\to\infty}\Sigma(\mathbf{X}^{(n)}) = 0$ in a proper metric (the largest eigenvalue).

Applying Fieller's (1940) theorem we obtain confidence intervals for $x_\gamma(\boldsymbol{\theta})$ in the following manner. Let

$$W_n = (\eta - \hat{\beta}_{0,n}) - x_\gamma(\boldsymbol{\theta})(\hat{\beta}_{1,n} + \sigma Z_\gamma). \tag{3.4.12}$$

The *conditional* distribution of W_n, *given* $\mathbf{X}^{(n)}$, is normal with mean zero and variance

$$V\{W_n \mid \mathbf{X}^{(n)}\} = \frac{\sigma^2}{\text{SSD}_V}\left[1 + x_\gamma^2(\boldsymbol{\theta})\frac{Q_n}{n} - 2x_\gamma(\boldsymbol{\theta})\bar{V}_n\right]. \tag{3.4.13}$$

Indeed, $E\{\hat{\beta}_{0,n} \mid \mathbf{X}^n\} = \beta_0$ and $E\{\hat{\beta}_{1,n} \mid \mathbf{X}^n\} = \beta_1$. It follows that the conditional distribution of W_n^2, given $\mathbf{X}^{(n)}$, is like that of $V\{W_n \mid \mathbf{X}^{(n)}\}\chi^2[1]$. Thus,

$$P\{W_n^2 \leq V\{W_n \mid \mathbf{X}^{(n)}\}\chi^2_{1-\alpha}[1] \mid \mathbf{X}^{(n)}\} = 1 - \alpha.$$

The event

$$(\eta - \hat{\beta}_{0,n})^2 + x_\gamma^2(\boldsymbol{\theta})(\hat{\beta}_{1,n} + \sigma Z_\gamma)^2 - 2x_\gamma(\boldsymbol{\theta})(\eta - \hat{\beta}_{0,n})(\hat{\beta}_{1,n} + \sigma Z_\gamma)$$
$$\leq \frac{\sigma^2}{\mathrm{SSD}_V}\left(1 + x_\gamma^2(\boldsymbol{\theta})\frac{Q_n}{n} - 2x_\gamma(\boldsymbol{\theta})\bar{V}_n\right)\chi^2_{1-\alpha}[1]$$

has probability $1 - \alpha$. Writing this as $A_n x_\gamma^2(\theta) - 2B_n x_\gamma(\boldsymbol{\theta}) + C_n \leq 0$, where

$$A_n = (\hat{\beta}_{1,n} + \sigma Z_\gamma)^2 - \frac{\sigma^2}{\mathrm{SSD}_V} \cdot \frac{Q_n}{n}\chi^2_{1-\alpha},$$
$$B_n = (\hat{\beta}_{1,n} + \sigma Z_\gamma)(\eta - \hat{\beta}_{0,n}) + \frac{\sigma^2}{\mathrm{SSD}_V}\bar{V}_n\chi^2_{1-\alpha},$$

and

$$C_n = (\eta - \hat{\beta}_{0,n})^2 - \frac{\sigma^2}{\mathrm{SSD}_V}\chi^2_{1-\alpha}. \tag{3.4.14}$$

Hence, the two real roots of the quadratic equation

$$A_n\xi^2 - 2B_n\xi + C_n = 0 \tag{3.4.15}$$

are $(1 - \alpha)$-level confidence limits for $x_\gamma(\boldsymbol{\theta})$ and where $\chi^2_{1-\alpha}$ is the $(1 - \alpha)$th quantile of the chi-squared distribution with one degree of freedom. Two real roots for Eq. (3.4.15) exist with probability $1 - \alpha$.

Let $\boldsymbol{\xi}_{n,\alpha}$ and $\bar{\boldsymbol{\xi}}_{n,\alpha}$ denote the two roots of Eq. (3.4.15). The sequence of dosages is defined as $X_1 = x^*$ and

$$X_{n+1} = \boldsymbol{\xi}_{n,\alpha}\Big]_{x^*}^{x^{**}}, \quad n \geq 1. \tag{3.4.16}$$

If for some n_0 real roots of Eq. (3.4.15) do not exist, we set $X_{n_0+1} = X_{n_0}$. By construction, $P_{\boldsymbol{\theta}}\{X_n \leq x_\gamma(\boldsymbol{\theta})\} \geq 1 - \alpha$ for all $\boldsymbol{\theta}$. That is, *the sequence* (3.4.16) *is feasible*. To secure the consistency of $\{X_n\}$, that is, $\lim_{n\to\infty} \boldsymbol{\xi}_{n,\alpha} = x_\gamma(\boldsymbol{\theta})$ in probability, it is sufficient to require that $\mathrm{SSD}_V \to \infty$ a.s. To achieve this, we modify the sequence (3.4.16) slightly. Let $I^* = \{n_j = 2^j, j = 1, 2, \cdots\}$ and fix Δ at $0 < \Delta$ but small. Then define

$$\hat{X}_n = \begin{cases} \max\{X_n - \Delta, x^*\} & \text{if } n \in I^*, \\ X_n & \text{if } n \notin I^*, \end{cases} \tag{3.4.17}$$

where $\{X_n\}$ is given by (3.4.16). The sequence $\{\hat{X}_n\}$ is feasible. Moreover, the lower confidence limits $\hat{\boldsymbol{\xi}}_{n,\alpha}$, based on $\{\hat{X}_n\}$, converge in probability to

$x_\gamma(\boldsymbol{\theta})$. The partial means $\hat{\bar{X}}_N = (1/N)\sum_{n=1}^{N} \hat{X}_n$ converge in probability to $x_\gamma(\boldsymbol{\theta})$. Thus we proved:

Theorem 3.4.2 *The sequence $\{\hat{X}_n\}$ is feasible and consistent.*

Finally we mention that the requirement of σ^2 known is not essential since after each stage one can estimate σ^2 by the usual regression estimator $\hat{\sigma}_n^2$, which has a distribution like $\sigma^2\{\chi^2[n-2]/(n-2)\}$ independently of $\hat{\beta}_{0,n}$ and $\hat{\beta}_{1,n}$. Fieller's theorem can be modified by replacing $\sigma^2\chi_{1-\alpha}^2$ with $\hat{\sigma}_n^2 \cdot F_{1-\alpha}[1, n-2]$.

3.4.2 Bayesian Adaptive Designs, σ Known

In a Bayesian framework the feasibility requirement is formulated in the following manner. Let $h(\beta_0, \beta_1)$ be a prior p.d.f. of (β_0, β_1). Let $\{X_n\}$ be a sequence of design levels. We say that $\{X_n\}$ is *Bayesian feasible* at level $1-\alpha$ if

$$P_H\{X_{n+1} \le x_\gamma(\boldsymbol{\theta}) \mid \mathcal{B}_n\} \ge 1-\alpha, \quad n = 0, 1, 2, \ldots, \tag{3.4.18}$$

where $P_H\{\cdot \mid \mathcal{B}_n\}$ denotes the posterior probability under H given $\mathcal{B}_n$. Eichhorn and Zacks (1981) investigated the properties of Bayesian designs for prior bivariate normal distributions of (β_0, β_1).

Let the prior distribution of (β_0, β_1) be a bivariate normal with mean $(\bar{\beta}_0, \bar{\beta}_1)$ and covariance matrix

$$\Sigma_0 = \begin{bmatrix} v_0 & c_0 \\ c_0 & w_0 \end{bmatrix}.$$

The posterior distribution of (β_0, β_1) after n trials given $(x_1, Y_1), \ldots, (x_n, Y_n)$ is normal with mean vector and covariance matrix having recursive formulas

$$\begin{pmatrix} \beta_0^{(n)} \\ \beta_1^{(n)} \end{pmatrix} = \begin{pmatrix} \beta_0^{(n-1)} \\ \beta_1^{(n-1)} \end{pmatrix} + \frac{Y_n - \beta_0^{(n-1)} - \beta_1^{(n-1)} x_n}{D_n} \times \begin{pmatrix} v_{n-1} + c_{n-1}x_n \\ c_{n-1} + w_{n-1}x_n \end{pmatrix} \tag{3.4.19}$$

with

$$D_n = \sigma^2 x_n^2 + v_{n-1} + 2x_n c_{n-1} + x_n^2 w_{n-1} \tag{3.4.20}$$

and

$$\Sigma_n = \Sigma_{n-1} - \frac{1}{D_n}\Sigma_{n-1}\begin{bmatrix} 1 & x_n \\ x_n & x_n^2 \end{bmatrix}\Sigma_{n-1}. \tag{3.4.21}$$

Let v_n, c_n, and w_n denote the posterior variance of β_0, covariance of β_0, β_1, and variance of β_1. Let $\boldsymbol{\xi}_{\alpha,n}$ denote a $1-\alpha$ lower credibility limit of $x_\gamma(\boldsymbol{\theta})$ given $\mathcal{B}_n$, that is,

$$P_H\left\{\frac{\eta-\beta_0}{\beta_1+\sigma Z_\gamma} \geq \boldsymbol{\xi}_{\alpha,n} \mid \mathcal{B}_n\right\} = 1-\alpha. \tag{3.4.22}$$

From the posterior distribution of $\beta_0 + \boldsymbol{\xi}_{\alpha,n} \cdot (\beta_1 + \sigma Z_\gamma)$, given $\mathcal{B}_n$, we find that $\boldsymbol{\xi}_{\alpha,n}$ is the smallest root of the equation

$$((\eta - \beta_0^{(n)}) - \xi(\beta_1^{(n)} + \sigma Z_\gamma))^2 = \chi^2_{1-2\alpha}(v_n + 2\xi c_n + \xi^2 w_n). \tag{3.4.23}$$

Equivalently, $\boldsymbol{\xi}_{\alpha,n}$ is the smallest real root of the quadratic equation

$$\xi^2 A_n^* - 2\xi B_n^* + C_n^* = 0, \tag{3.4.24}$$

where

$$\begin{aligned} A_n^* &= (\beta_1^{(n)} + \sigma Z_\gamma)^2 - \chi^2_{1-2\alpha} w_n, \\ B_n^* &= (\eta - \beta_0^{(n)})(\beta_1^{(n)} + \sigma Z_\gamma) + \chi^2_{1-2\alpha} c_n, \\ C_n^* &= (\eta - \beta_0^{(n)})^2 - \chi^2_{1-2\alpha} v_n. \end{aligned} \tag{3.4.25}$$

The adaptive design given by the sequence $\{X_n\}$, where

$$X_{n+1} = \boldsymbol{\xi}_{\alpha,n}\big]_{x^*}^{x^{**}}, \tag{3.4.26}$$

is Bayesian feasible.

Let $\mathbf{X}^{(n)} = (1, x_n)'$ and $\hat{\boldsymbol{\beta}}^{(n)} = (\beta_0^{(n)}, \beta_1^{(n)})$. Define

$$Z_n = \frac{Y_n - \hat{\boldsymbol{\beta}}^{(n-1)'}\mathbf{x}^{(n)}}{D_n^{1/2}}, \quad n = 1, 2, \ldots .$$

Let $E_H\{Z_n \mid \mathcal{F}_{n-1}\}$ denote the predictive distribution of Z_n under the prior H given $\mathcal{F}_{n-1}$. Notice that $D_n = V_H\{Y_n \mid \mathcal{F}_{n-1}\}$. Since $E_H\{Z_n \mid \mathcal{F}_{n-1}\} = 0$ a.s., we obtain from (3.4.19) that $E_H\{\hat{\boldsymbol{\beta}}^{(n)} \mid \mathcal{F}_{n-1}\} = \hat{\boldsymbol{\beta}}^{(n-1)}$ a.s. and $\{\hat{\boldsymbol{\beta}}_n, \mathcal{F}_n, n \geq 1\}$ is a martingale. Moreover, $E_H\{|Z_n| \mid \mathcal{F}_{n-1}\} = \sqrt{2/\pi}$. Thus, since all X_n are restricted to the closed interval $[x^*, x^{**}]$, (3.4.19) and (3.4.20) imply that

$$\sup_n E\{|Z_n|\mathbf{x}^{(n)'}\boldsymbol{\Sigma}_n\mathbf{x}^{(n)}\} < \infty. \tag{3.4.27}$$

Thus, the martingale convergence theorem (see Shiryaev, 1984, p. 476) implies that

$$\lim_{n\to\infty} \hat{\boldsymbol{\beta}}^{(n)} = \boldsymbol{\beta}^{(\infty)} \text{ a.s. } [H] \text{ and } \boldsymbol{\xi}_{n,\alpha} \to \xi^{(\infty)} \text{ a.s. } [H],$$

where $\hat{\boldsymbol{\beta}}^{(\infty)}$ is a random vector having a singular bivariate normal distribution concentrated on the line

$$\beta_0 + x_\gamma \beta_1 = \eta - x_\gamma \sigma Z_\gamma.$$

Eichhorn and Zacks (1981) showed that a discrete version of (3.4.26) converges a.s. to within a δ-neighborhood of $x_\gamma(\boldsymbol{\theta})$.

■ EXAMPLE 3.1

In the present example we illustrate the Bayesian adaptive procedure. Without loss of generality, assume that $\eta = 0$. The data are generated by simulation from a normal distribution $N(\beta_0+\beta_1 x, \sigma^2 x^2)$ with $\beta_0 = -10$, $\beta_1 = 3$, and $\sigma = 1$. The design levels are restricted to the interval with $x^* = 1$ and $x^{**} = 10$. For $\alpha = 0.05$ and $\gamma = 0.99$ we have $x_\gamma(\boldsymbol{\theta}) = 1.878$. We start with the prior bivariate normal distribution with mean $\beta_0^{(0)} = -15$ and $\beta_1^{(0)} = 2.75$ and covariance matrix with $v_0 = 9$, $c_0 = 0$, and $w_0 = 0.25$. In Table 3.5 we provide the values of X_n, $\beta_0^{(n)}$, $\beta_1^{(n)}$, v_n, c_n, w_n.

Table 3.5: Simulated Bayesian Design

n	X_n	$\beta_0^{(n)}$	$\beta_1^{(n)}$	v_n	c_n	w_n
1	1.380	−8.850	2.921	1.098	−0.220	0.244
2	1.464	−8.848	2.921	0.775	−0.267	0.237
3	1.530	−8.955	2.899	0.677	−0.287	0.233
4	1.596	−9.111	2.854	0.635	−0.300	0.299
5	1.588	−9.028	2.889	0.677	−0.308	0.226
10	1.736	−9.317	2.728	0.589	−0.324	0.214
15	1.788	−9.353	2.656	0.587	−0.328	0.204
20	1.816	−9.352	2.609	0.587	−0.328	0.200
25	1.802	−9.369	2.685	0.587	−0.327	0.196
30	1.830	−9.359	2.617	0.587	−0.326	0.192
35	1.824	−9.375	2.657	0.586	−0.325	0.190
40	1.820	−9.384	2.683	0.586	−0.325	0.188
45	1.844	−9.352	2.607	0.586	−0.324	0.186
50	1.847	−9.357	2.610	0.585	−0.323	0.185

Notice that after 50 stages the posterior correlation $c_n/(v_n \cdot w_n)^{1/2} = -0.982$. The posterior correlation approaches -1 as n grows. ■

3.5 STOCHASTIC APPROXIMATION

Stochastic approximations are other types of adaptive designs which approximate a solution θ of an equation $M(x) = 0$ without specifying the functional form of $M(x)$. More specifically, suppose that $Y(x)$ is a random variable such that $E\{Y(x)\} = M(x)$ and $V\{Y(x)\} = \sigma^2(x)$. More generally, if $X_1, X_2, \ldots$ is a sequence of random variables, $E\{Y(X_n) \mid X_n\} = M(X_n)$, and $V\{Y(X_n) \mid X_n\} = \sigma^2(X_n)$. We are looking for a sequence $\{X_n, n \geq 1\}$ such that $X_n \to \theta$ a.s. This is a stochastic sequence which approximates θ, where $M(\theta) = 0$.

Robbins and Monro (1951) suggested the iterative stochastic approximation

$$X_{n+1} = X_n - a_n Y(X_n), \quad n = 1, 2, \ldots, \tag{3.5.1}$$

where $\{a_n\}$ is a sequence of real numbers such that $\sum_{n=1}^{\infty} a_n = \infty$ and $\sum_{n=1}^{\infty} a_n^2 < \infty$. Generally, a_n could be a random variable depending on $(X_1, \ldots, X_n)$, $n \geq 1$. It is known that under some general conditions $X_n \to \theta$ a.s. (see Blum, 1954; Robbins and Siegmund, 1971). Also, after suitable normalization, X_n converges in distribution to $N(0, 1)$ (Sacks, 1958). In the spirit of the parametric procedures of Section 3.4, which approximate $x_\gamma(\theta)$ from below, Anbar (1977) developed a modified Robbins–Monro procedure which converges to θ from below. His iterative sequence is

$$X_{n+1} = X_n - a_n(Y(X_n) - b_n), \tag{3.5.2}$$

where a_n and b_n are measurable functions of $(X_1, \ldots, X_n)$. It is required that $\sum_{n=1}^{\infty} a_n^2 < \infty$ and $\sum_{n=1}^{\infty} |a_n b_n| < \infty$ a.s., $\sum a_n = \infty$ on the set $\{\sup_{n\geq 1} |X_n| < \infty\}$. There are also some general requirements on $M(x)$ and on $\sigma(x)$ in a neighborhood of the solution θ.

Wu (1985) considered stochastic approximation procedures for estimating the pth quantile of a tolerance distribution F. He discussed iterative sequences of the form

$$X_{n+1} = X_n - \frac{c}{n}(Y(X_n) - p), \tag{3.5.3}$$

where $Y(X_n)$ is a binary random variable with $P(Y(X) = 1 \mid X = x) = F(x)$. Following Anbar (1977), Wu used the scheme

$$X_{n+1} = X_n - \frac{1}{\hat{\beta}_n n}(Y(X_n) - p), \tag{3.5.4}$$

where

$$\hat{\beta}_n = \frac{\sum_{i=1}^{n} Y_i(X_i - \bar{X}_n)}{\sum_{i=1}^{n}(X_i - \bar{X}_n)^2}. \tag{3.5.5}$$

Wu compared these stochastic procedures to the MLE parametric procedure for the logistic tolerance distribution via simulations. For additional results, see Lai and Robbins (1979), Ljung (1977), Kushner and Clark (1978), Spall (1992), Spall and Cristion (1994), and Kushner and Yin (1997).

CHAPTER 4

ADAPTIVE METHODS FOR SAMPLING FROM FINITE POPULATIONS

4.1 BASIC THEORY

A *finite population* (F.P.) of size N is a set $\mathcal{U} = \{u_1, \ldots, u_N\}$ of well-specified units whose values $\{Y_1, \ldots, Y_N\}$ or some functions of them are subjects of a survey. Often N is either too large or too expansive for a complete survey of all units of $\mathcal{U}$, in particular if observing the value of a unit requires its destruction. Notice that a value Y of a unit u could be categorical, ordinal or scalar, unidimensional, or vector valued. Generally the objective of the survey is to draw inference on some function of $\mathbf{Y}_N = (Y_1, \ldots, Y_N)'$, denoted by $\theta(\mathbf{Y}_N)$, based on a subset $\mathbf{s} \subset \mathcal{U}$, called a *sample.* Examples of functions of interest are $\theta(\mathbf{Y}_N) = \sum_{i=1}^{N} Y_i$, which is the *population total*, or $\theta(\mathbf{Y}_N) = (1/N)\sum_{i=1}^{N}(Y_i - \overline{Y}_N)^2$, which is the *population variance.* Here $\overline{Y}_N = (1/N)\sum_{i=1}^{N} Y_i$ is the *population mean.* In these examples Y_i $(i = 1, \ldots, N)$ are real values. If Y_i are categorical, we might be interested in the frequencies of Y-values in each category or some functions of them. We call a function $\theta(\mathbf{Y}_N)$ a *population quantity.*

There are two approaches in the theory of sampling from F.P. to construct a probability structure on $\mathcal{U}$ for the purpose of statistical inference. One approach (the classical) is the *design* approach, and the other one (the modern) is the *modeling* (superpopulation) approach. In the following sections we explain these approaches and provide some basic results.

4.1.1 Design Approach

A *design space* $\mathcal{D}$ over $\mathcal{U}$ is a set of samples $\mathbf{s}_1, \mathbf{s}_2, \ldots$ which are subsets of $\mathcal{U}$. Each sample $\mathbf{s} \in \mathcal{D}$ is assigned a probability $p(\mathbf{s})$, and we require that $\sum_{\mathbf{s}\in\mathcal{D}} p(\mathbf{s}) = 1$. The design space does not have to include all possible subsets of $\mathcal{U}$. Also, the size of different samples of $\mathcal{D}$ does not have to be the same. For example, suppose that $\mathcal{U} = \{u_1, u_2, \ldots, u_{10}\}$ and $\mathcal{D} = \{\{u_1, u_2, u_{10}\}, \{u_1, u_3, u_{10}\}, \ldots, \{u_1, u_9, u_{10}\}\}$. Here we have eight samples of equal size. Suppose that $p(\mathbf{s}) = 1/8$ for each $\mathbf{s} \in \mathcal{D}$. One sample is chosen from $\mathcal{D}$ with probability $p(\mathbf{s})$. This is done with the aid of random numbers, R, which are uniformly distributed in $(0, 1)$. If $0 < R \leq 0.125$ we select the sample $\{u_1, u_2, u_{10}\}$, if $0.125 < R \leq 0.25$ we select the sample $\{u_1, u_3, u_{10}\}$, and so on. Another example of a design on $\mathcal{U}$ could be $\mathcal{D} = \{\{u_1, u_2, u_3\}, \{u_4, u_5\}, \{u_6, u_7, u_8, u_9, u_{10}\}\}$. If we denote the samples in $\mathcal{D}$ as $\mathbf{s}_1, \mathbf{s}_2, \mathbf{s}_3$ from left to right, $P(\mathbf{s})$ could be $P(\mathbf{s}_1) = 3/10$, $P(\mathbf{s}_2) = 2/10$, and $P(\mathbf{s}_3) = 5/10$. The design is specified by the pair $(\mathcal{D}, P)$.

In adaptive sampling designs, as will be shown later, one may select in a given stage sample from one design and then, according to a decision function, which is applied on the observed values of the previous samples, choose a new sample from a different design or stop sampling. In the present section we restrict the discussion to one-stage sampling designs.

Given a sample $\mathbf{s}$ chosen from $(\mathcal{D}, P)$, let $\mathbf{y}_s$ be the vector of Y-values of the units in $\mathbf{s}$. In other words, if $\mathbf{s} = \{u_{i_1}, u_{i_2}, \ldots, u_{i_n}\}$ and $\mathbf{y}_s = (Y_{i_1}, Y_{i_2}, \ldots, Y_{i_n})$ we say that $\mathbf{y}_s$ is *compatible* with $\mathbf{Y}_N$ and denote this relationship by $\mathbf{y}_s \subset \mathbf{Y}_N$. If we choose $\mathbf{s}$ from $\mathcal{D}$ according to P, then $(s, \mathbf{y}_s)$ is the *sample statistic* and $\mathbf{y}_s$ is a *random vector*. The probability distribution of $\mathbf{y}_s$ is

$$p(\mathbf{y}_s; \mathbf{Y}_N) = I\{\mathbf{y}_s \subset \mathbf{Y}_N\} P(\mathbf{s}). \tag{4.1.1}$$

The vector $\mathbf{Y}_N$ is a *parametric vector* of this sampling distribution.

In the above example of $\mathcal{D} = \{\{u_1, u_i, u_{10}\}, i = 2, \ldots, 9\}$, if $\mathbf{Y}_{10} = (1, 2, 3, \ldots, 10)$, then

$$p(\mathbf{y}_s; \mathbf{Y}_{10}) = \begin{cases} 1/8 & \text{if } \mathbf{y}_s = (1, i, 10),\ i = 2, \ldots, 9, \\ 0 & \text{otherwise.} \end{cases}$$

The *size* of a sample $\mathbf{s} \in \mathcal{D}$ is

$$n(\mathbf{s}) = \sum_{i=1}^{N} I\{u_i \in \mathbf{s}\}. \tag{4.1.2}$$

For each unit of $\mathcal{U}$ we compute its *inclusion probability*

(4.1.3)
$$\pi_i = \sum_{\mathbf{s}\in\mathcal{D}} I\{u_i \in \mathbf{s}\}P(\mathbf{s}), \quad i = 1,\ldots,N.$$

Thus, the inclusion probabilities depend on the design $(\mathcal{D}, P)$. From (4.1.2) and (4.1.3) we obtain

(4.1.4)
$$\begin{aligned}\sum_{i=1}^{N} \pi_i &= \sum_{s\in\mathcal{D}}\sum_{i=1}^{N} I\{u_i \in \mathbf{s}\}P(s) \\ &= \sum_{s\in\mathcal{D}} n(\mathbf{s})P(s).\end{aligned}$$

This is the *expected sample size* according to $(\mathcal{D}, P)$. We denote it as $E_P\{n(\mathbf{s})\}$. Similarly, from (4.1.3), $\pi_i = E_P\{I\{u_i \in \mathbf{s}\}\}$, $i = 1,\ldots,N$. Generally, if $(\mathbf{s}, \mathbf{y}_s)$ is a sample statistic and $f(\mathbf{s}, \mathbf{y}_s)$ is a given function of it, then $E_P\{f(\mathbf{s}, \mathbf{y}_s)\} = \sum_{\mathbf{s}\in\mathcal{D}} P(\mathbf{s})f(\mathbf{s}, \mathbf{y}_s)$. Generally, $f(\mathbf{s}, \mathbf{y}_s)$ may depend also on s as shown in the following example for $\mathcal{U} = \{u_1,\ldots,u_{10}\}$:

$\mathcal{D}$	$\{u_1, u_3, u_{10}\}$	$\{u_1, u_2, u_9\}$	$\{u_4, u_5, u_6, u_7, u_8\}$
P	0.3	0.2	0.5
f	$(Y_1 + Y_{10})/2$	$(Y_2 + Y_9)/2$	Y_6

In this example,

$$\begin{aligned}E_P\{f(\mathbf{s}, \mathbf{y}_s); \mathbf{Y}_{10}\} &= 0.3\frac{Y_1 + Y_{10}}{2} + 0.2\frac{Y_2 + Y_9}{2} + 0.5Y_6 \\ &= 0.15Y_1 + 0.10Y_2 + 0.5Y_6 + 0.10Y_9 + 0.15Y_{10}.\end{aligned}$$

Let $\theta(\mathbf{Y}_N)$ be a population quantity (parameter) and let $\hat{\theta}(\mathbf{s}, \mathbf{y}_s)$ be its estimator. An estimator is P *unbiased* if

(4.1.5)
$$E_P\{\hat{\theta}(s, \mathbf{y}_s); \mathbf{Y}_N\} = \theta(\mathbf{Y}_N) \quad \text{for all } \mathbf{Y}_N.$$

The *variance* of $\hat{\theta}\{\mathbf{s}, \mathbf{y}_s)$ is

(4.1.6)
$$V_P\{\hat{\theta}(s; \mathbf{y}_s)\} = E_P\{(\hat{\theta}(s, \mathbf{y}_s) - \theta(\mathbf{Y}_N))^2; \mathbf{Y}_N\}.$$

An important homogeneous linear estimator of the population total, T, is the *Horvitz–Thompson (HT) estimator*

(4.1.7)
$$\begin{aligned}\hat{T}_{\mathrm{HT}}(\mathbf{s}; \mathbf{y}_s) &= \sum_{i\in s} \frac{y_i}{\pi_i} \\ &= \sum_{i=1}^{N} I\{u_i \in \mathbf{s}\}\frac{Y_i}{\pi_i}.\end{aligned}$$

It is easy to prove that this estimator is P unbiased. The *P-variance* of the HT estimator is

$$V_P\{\hat{T}_{\mathrm{HT}}(\mathbf{s};\mathbf{y}_s)\} = \sum_{i=1}^{N} \frac{Y_i^2}{\pi_i} + \sum\sum_{i \neq j} \frac{Y_i Y_j}{\pi_i \pi_j} \pi_{ij} - T^2, \tag{4.1.8}$$

where π_{ij} is the inclusion probability of *both* u_i and u_j, that is,

$$\begin{aligned} \pi_{ij} &= \sum_{\mathbf{s} \in \mathcal{D}} P(s) I\{u_i \in \mathbf{s} \textit{ and } u_j \in \mathbf{s}\} \\ &= \sum_{\mathbf{s} \in \mathcal{D}} I\{u_i \in \mathbf{s}\} I\{u_j \in \mathbf{s}\} P(\mathbf{s}). \end{aligned} \tag{4.1.9}$$

A commonly used design is the so-called *simple random sample.* We distinguish between simple random samples *without replacement* (SRSWOR) and simple random samples *with replacement* (SRSWR). In these designs *all* possible samples are of *fixed* size, n. The SRSWOR of n units from N in $\mathcal{U}$ can be selected in a sequential manner as follows. The first unit, U_1, is chosen from $\mathcal{U}$ with equal selection probabilities $1/N$. The second unit of s, U_2, is chosen from $\mathcal{U} - U_1$ with equal probabilities $1/(N-1)$, and so on. There are $\prod_{j=0}^{n-1}(N-j)$ possible samples with equal $P(\mathbf{s}) = 1/\prod_{j=0}^{n-1}(N-j)$.

An SRSWR of size n from N units in $\mathcal{U}$ is chosen so that all the N^n possible samples are equally probable. We can choose the sample units one by one with equal probabilities $1/N$. A chosen unit is recorded and replaced in $\mathcal{U}$ and can be chosen again.

To simplify notation, an SRSWOR design of n from N will be denoted by SRS(N, n). An SRSWR design will be denoted by SRSW(N, n). The inclusion probabilities under SRS(N, n) are $\pi_i = n/N$, $i = 1, \ldots, N$, and $\pi_{ij} = n(n-1)/[N(N-1)]$ for all $i \neq j = 1, \ldots, N$. Thus, the HT estimator of T is

$$\begin{aligned} \hat{T} &= \frac{N}{n} \sum_{i \in \mathbf{s}} y_i \\ &= N\overline{y}_s, \end{aligned} \tag{4.1.10}$$

where $\overline{\mathbf{y}}_s = (1/n)\sum_{i \in s} y_i$ is the sample mean. Accordingly, $\overline{y}_s$ is an unbiased linear estimator of the population mean $\overline{Y}_N = (1/N)\sum_{i=1}^{N} Y_i$. Let

$$S_N^2 = \frac{1}{N-1} \sum_{i=1}^{N} (Y_i - \overline{Y}_N)^2$$

denote the population (adjusted) variance and

$$s_n^2 = \frac{1}{n-1} \sum_{i \in \mathbf{s}} (y_i - \overline{y}_s)^2$$

the sample variance. One can prove:

Theorem 4.1.1 *Under SRS(N, n),*

$$E_P\{s_n^2; \mathbf{Y}_N\} = S_N^2 \quad \textit{for all } \mathbf{Y}_N. \tag{4.1.11}$$

Also,

$$V_P\{\overline{y}_s; \mathbf{Y}_N\} = \frac{S_N^2}{n}\left(1 - \frac{n}{N}\right). \tag{4.1.12}$$

■

There are more complicated sampling designs, like stratified and cluster designs, which will be discussed in other sections.

4.1.2 Modeling Approach

In the modeling approach, the population vector $\mathbf{Y}_N$ is considered to be a realization of a *random vector*. If the modeling is parametric, the joint distribution of $\mathbf{Y}_N$ has to be specified up to a given parametric family. The parameter values of this distribution may or may not be known. For example, one could specify that $\log \mathbf{Y}_N = (\log Y_1, \ldots, \log Y_N)'$ has a multivariate normal distribution with mean $\boldsymbol{\mu}_N$ and covariance matrix V_N. The parameters of this model are $(\boldsymbol{\mu}_N, V_N)$.

If the parameters $(\boldsymbol{\mu}, V)$ are unknown, we may have to estimate them from the sample data. Suppose that the size of the sample $\mathbf{s}$ is n. Without loss of generality we can write $\mathbf{Y}'_N = (\mathbf{y}'_s, \mathbf{Y}'_r)$, where $\mathbf{y}_s$ is the n-dimensional subvector of the observed sample value and $\mathbf{Y}_r$ is an $(N-n)$-dimensional vector of the unobserved values of $\mathbf{Y}_N$. Let $\theta(\mathbf{Y}_N)$ be a population quantity of interest. Since $\theta(\mathbf{Y}_N)$ is a random variable, we do not estimate it but *predict* it. Suppose one can write $\theta(\mathbf{Y}_N) = \theta(\mathbf{y}_s) + \theta_{rs}(\mathbf{y}_s, \mathbf{Y}_r)$. Since $\mathbf{y}_s$ is observable, $\theta(\mathbf{y}_s)$ is *known* while $\theta_{rs}(\mathbf{y}_s, \mathbf{Y}_r)$ has to be predicted. Thus, a predictor of $\theta(\mathbf{Y}_N)$ is written as

$$\hat{\theta}_N = \theta(\mathbf{y}_s) + \hat{\theta}_{rs}(\mathbf{s}, \mathbf{y}_s). \tag{4.1.13}$$

The predictor is a function of $(\mathbf{s}, \mathbf{y}_s)$. For example, suppose that $\theta(\mathbf{Y}_N) = \sum_{i=1}^N Y_i = T$. Then, $\theta(\mathbf{y}_s) = \sum_{i\in\mathbf{s}} Y_i$ and $\theta_{rs}(\mathbf{y}_s, \mathbf{Y}_r) = \sum_{j\in r} Y_j$. Thus, to predict T we have to predict $\sum_{j\in r} Y_j$. Another example is $\sigma_N^2 = (1/N)\sum_{i=1}^N (Y_i - \overline{Y}_N)^2$. We can write

$$\sigma_N^2 = \frac{n}{N}\sigma_s^2 + \left(1 - \frac{n}{N}\right)\sigma_r^2 + \frac{n}{N}\left(1 - \frac{n}{N}\right)(\overline{y}_s - \overline{Y}_r)^2, \tag{4.1.14}$$

where

$$\sigma_s^2 = \frac{1}{n}\sum_{i\in s}(Y_i - \overline{y}_s)^2, \quad \sigma_r^2 = \frac{1}{N-n}\sum_{j\in r}(Y_j - \overline{Y}_r)^2.$$

Here $\theta(\mathbf{Y}_N) = \sigma_N^2$, $\theta(\mathbf{y}_s) = (n/N)\sigma_s^2$ and

$$\theta_{rs}(\mathbf{y}_s, \mathbf{Y}_r) = \left(1 - \frac{n}{N}\right)\sigma_r^2 + \frac{n}{N}\left(1 - \frac{n}{N}\right)(\overline{y}_s - \overline{Y}_r)^2. \tag{4.1.15}$$

The problem of predicting σ_N^2 is that of predicting $(1 - n/N)\sigma_r^2 + (n/N)(1 - n/N)\ (\overline{y}_s - \overline{Y}_r)^2$. In the following we show a few predictors of T and of σ_N^2 under several population models. Before doing specific examples we mention that a predictor $\hat{\theta}(s, \mathbf{y}_s)$ of $\theta(\mathbf{Y}_N)$ is called ψ *unbiased* if

$$E_\psi\{\hat{\theta}(s, \mathbf{y}_s) - \theta(\mathbf{Y}_N)\} = 0 \quad \text{for all } \psi. \tag{4.1.16}$$

The ψ-MSE of $(\hat{\theta}(s, \mathbf{y}_s) - \theta(\mathbf{Y}_N))$ for ψ-unbiased predictors is

$$\psi\text{-MSE}\{\hat{\theta} - \theta\} = E_\psi\{[\hat{\theta}(\mathbf{s}, \mathbf{y}_s) - \theta(\mathbf{Y}_N)]^2\}. \tag{4.1.17}$$

This is called also the prediction risk.

We present now several prediction models which are discussed at length in Bolfarine and Zacks (1992).

Prediction Model SM1

Here we assume that $E\{Y_i\} = \mu$, $i = 1, \ldots, N$, $V\{Y_i\} = \sigma^2$, $i = 1, \ldots, N$ and $\text{Cov}(Y_i, Y_j) = 0$ for all $i \neq j$. We do not assume the actual distribution. We write symbolically $\mathbf{Y}_N \sim (\mu 1_N, \sigma^2 I_N)$ where $-\infty < \mu < \infty$ is a scalar. Here $1_N' = (1, 1, \ldots, 1)$ and I_N is the identity matrix of order N.

For this model $\psi = (\mu 1_N, \sigma^2 I_N)$ and $E_\psi\{\overline{y}_s\} = E_\psi\{\overline{Y}_r\} = \mu$. Hence:

Theorem 4.1.2 *For model SM1*

$$\hat{T} = n\overline{y}_s + (N - n)\overline{y}_s = N\overline{y}_s \tag{4.1.18}$$

is a ψ-unbiased predictor of T. Moreover,

$$\psi\text{-}MSE\{\hat{T}\} = N^2\sigma^2\left(\frac{1}{n} - \frac{1}{N}\right). \tag{4.1.19}$$

A ψ-unbiased predictor of σ_N^2 is

$$\hat{\sigma}_N^2 = \frac{N-1}{N}s_n^2. \tag{4.1.20}$$

The ψ-MSE of $(\hat{\sigma}_N^2 - \sigma_N^2)$ is

$$V_\psi\{\hat{\sigma}_N^2 - \sigma_N^2\} = \left(1 - \frac{n}{N}\right)^2 V_\psi\left\{s_n^2 - \sigma_r^2 - \frac{n}{N}(\overline{y}_s - \overline{Y}_r)^2\right\}. \tag{4.1.21}$$

■

We see that the actual sample units do not play any role. For this predictive model any sample of size n will give the same result. Also here the result is independent of labels of the units in the sample. If $\mathbf{Y}_N \sim N(\mu 1_N, \sigma^2 I_N)$, then σ_s^2 is independent of σ_r^2, σ_s^2 is independent of $\overline{y}_s$, σ_r^2 is independent of $\overline{Y}_r$, and $\overline{y}_s$ is independent of $\overline{Y}_r$. Thus, in this case

$$V_\psi\{\hat{\sigma}_N^2 - \sigma_N^2\} = \frac{2\sigma^4}{n-1}\left(1 - \frac{1}{N}\right)\left(1 - \frac{n}{N}\right).$$

Prediction Model SM2

Let $\mathbf{X}_N$ be a *known* vector of covariates. The model is $\mathbf{Y}_N \sim (\beta\mathbf{X}_N, \sigma^2 \text{ diag } (\mathbf{X}_N))$, where diag$(\mathbf{X}_N)$ is a diagonal $N \times N$ matrix whose diagonal elements are $x_1, x_2, \ldots, x_N$. The vector of unknown parameters is $\boldsymbol{\psi} = (\beta, \sigma^2)$. Let $\mathbf{X}'_N = (\mathbf{X}'_s, \mathbf{X}'_r)$. From the theory of weighted least squares estimators (see Seber, 1977), the minimum variance linear unbiased estimator of β is

$$\hat{\beta}_s = \frac{\overline{y}_s}{\overline{x}_s}. \tag{4.1.22}$$

Theorem 4.1.3 *For model SM2, the best linear ψ-unbiased predictor of T is*

$$\hat{T}_R = n\overline{y}_s + (N-n)\hat{\beta}_s\overline{X}_r = \frac{\overline{y}_s}{\overline{x}_s}N\overline{X}_N. \tag{4.1.23}$$

The ψ-variance of $\hat{T}_R - T$ is

$$V_\psi\{\hat{T}_R - T\} = \sigma^2\frac{(N-n)\overline{X}_r}{n\overline{x}_s}(N\overline{X}_N). \tag{4.1.24}$$

■

According to (4.1.24), the optimal sample under SM2 is the one having the maximal value of $\overline{x}_s$. Since all values of $\mathbf{X}_N$ are known, one can choose such a sample to minimize the ψ-variance of the predictor $\hat{T}_R$. An unbiased predictor of σ_N^2 under model SM2 can be derived too.

Zacks (1969) investigated the problem of which units of the population $\mathcal{U}$ to include in the sample. In that paper it was assumed that the vector $\mathbf{Y}_N$ has a joint (prior) distribution with a specified density. This is exactly the modeling approach. Thus, the methodology of the Zacks (1969) paper can be applied to the present models SM1 and SM2. The results are the same as given above.

4.2 TWO-STAGE AND SEQUENTIAL ESTIMATION OF THE POPULATION MEAN

4.2.1 Design Approach: SRSWR

We start with simple random sampling with replacement, SRSWR. The objective is to estimate the population mean $\mu_N = \overline{Y}_N$. In a sample of size n, let X_i $(i = 1, \ldots, n)$ denote the value of the observed unit in the ith drawing. Since the sampling is with replacement, $X_1, X_2, \ldots, X_n$ are i.i.d., and their common distribution is $F_N(x) = (1/N)\sum_{i=1}^{N} I\{Y_i \le x\}$. This distribution is unknown.

Consider a fixed-width interval estimator of μ_N, $I_\delta(\overline{X}_n) = (\overline{X}_n - \delta, \overline{X}_n + \delta)$. By the central limit theorem, if n is large, then the coverage probability (CP) of $I_\delta(\overline{X}_n)$ is approximately

$$\text{CP} \cong 2\Phi\left(\frac{\delta\sqrt{n}}{\sigma_N}\right) - 1, \tag{4.2.1}$$

where σ_N^2 is the variance of F_N. Thus, if

$$n \ge \frac{\chi^2_{1-\alpha}[1]\sigma_N^2}{\delta^2}, \tag{4.2.2}$$

then the coverage probability is approximately $1-\alpha$. The problem arises when σ_N^2 is unknown. One can apply the Chow–Robbins sequential procedure (see Section 2.4) or a multistage procedure. We assume that N is very large.

The Chow–Robbins procedure is purely sequential, with an initial sample size $m \ge 2$. Let

$$S_n^2 = \frac{1}{n-1}\sum_{i=1}^{n}(X_i - \overline{X}_n)^2$$

be the sample variance based on n observations. The sequential stopping variable is

$$N(\delta) = \min\left\{n : n \ge m, n \ge \frac{\chi^2_{1-\alpha}[1]S_n^2}{\delta^2}\right\}. \tag{4.2.3}$$

Recall that S_n^2 is an unbiased estimator of σ_N^2. As mentioned in Section 2.4, Theorem 2.4.1, the Chow–Robbins sequential procedure is asymptotically consistent and efficient, as $\delta \to 0$. To illustrate the procedure when $\delta = 0.316$, we create a vector $\mathbf{Y}_N$ of $N = 10000$ random values generated from the gamma $(5, 2)$ distribution. For this random vector we have $\overline{Y}_N = 10.06617$ and $\sigma_N^2 = 50.60098$. For the above value of δ and $\alpha = 0.05$ we need a sample of minimal size $n^0 = \lfloor 3.8416 \times \sigma_N^2/\delta^2 \rfloor + 1 = 1944$. Using $m = 50$ and $N(\delta)$ of (4.2.3), in 10 simulation runs we obtained the results in Table 4.1.

Table 4.1: Simulation Estimates of $N(\delta)$, and $\overline{X}_{N(\delta)} \pm \delta$, for $\delta = 0.316$, $\alpha = 0.05$, $m = 50$

i	$N(\delta)$	$\overline{X}_{N(\delta)} - \delta$	$\overline{X}_{N(\delta)} + \delta$
1	1952	9.957	10.590
2	1795	9.666	10.299
3	1907	9.650	10.282
4	1939	9.850	10.483
5	1886	9.783	10.415
6	1872	9.702	10.335
7	2119	10.010	10.642
8	1985	9.682	10.315
9	1864	9.841	10.473
10	2106	9.738	10.370

Derived using program simcp.

The mean of these 10 stopping times is 1942.5, which is quite close to $n^0 = 1944$. Also, in all 10 cases the interval estimators covered the population mean $\overline{Y}_N$. In order to estimate the coverage probability precisely, one needs to simulate hundreds of cases. Table 4.1 is just for illustration.

A two-stage sampling procedure might often be more convenient. The procedure is:

Stage One: Draw an SRSWR of size m. Compute S_m^2 and

$$N_m = \left\lfloor \frac{\chi^2_{1-\alpha}[1] S_m^2}{\delta^2} \right\rfloor + 1. \tag{4.2.4}$$

If $N_m \leq m$, stop and estimate μ_N by $(\overline{X}_m - \delta, \overline{X}_m + \delta)$. If $N_m > m$, go to:

Stage Two: Draw an additional SRSWR of size $N_m - m$. Combine the two samples and compute $(\overline{X}_{N_m} - \delta, \overline{X}_{N_m} + \delta)$.

To evaluate the two-stage procedure, we simulated $M = 500$ cases for several values of m sampled from the above random vector $\mathbf{Y}_N$. The results are given in Table 4.2.

Table 4.2: Expected Sample Size in a Two-Stage Sampling, $\alpha = 0.05$, $\delta = 0.316$, $\mathbf{Y}_N$ as in Table 4.1

m	$E\{N_m\}$	CP
50	1973.7	0.97
100	1999.6	0.94
200	1952.8	0.95
500	1939.6	0.95

We see in Table 4.2 that the initial sample size m should be quite large.

The required sample size becomes dramatically smaller if instead of a fixed-width interval $\overline{X}_m \pm \delta$ we require that the size of the interval will be proportional to μ_N. In this case the required sample size is

$$(4.2.5) \qquad n^* = \left\lfloor \frac{\chi^2_{1-\alpha}[1]\gamma^2_N}{\lambda^2} \right\rfloor + 1,$$

where $\gamma_N = \sigma_N/\mu_N$ is the coefficient of variation and $\delta = \lambda\mu_N$. Thus, if $\mu_N = 10.066$, $\sigma_N = 7.113$, and $\lambda = 0.1$, then, for $\alpha = 0.05$, $n^* = 191.84$. This is about one-tenth of the value of n^0.

4.2.2 Design Approach: SRSWOR

In SRSWOR the random variables $X_1, \ldots, X_n$ are neither independent nor identically distributed. However, if the population size N is very large compared to the sample size n, for example, $n/N < 0.1$, properties like convergence in distribution to the normal might still approximately hold. One could test this by drawing by simulation $M = 500$ samples, without replacement, of size $n = 50$ from the population whose values are $Y_i = i$, $i = 1, \ldots, 1000$. A QQ normal plot of these 500 means shows that their distribution is approximately normal, as shown in Figure 4.1. We therefore proceed as though the sample variables are i.i.d. Notice that, as in (4.1.12), the variance of $\overline{X}_n$ is $(S^2_N/n)(1 - n/N) = S^2_N(1/n - 1/N)$. Thus, if S^2_m is the sample variance of the first-stage sample, the total sample size required in a two-stage sampling N_m is the solution of

$$\chi^2_{1-\alpha}[1]S^2_m\left(\frac{1}{N_m} - \frac{1}{N}\right) \leq \delta^2.$$

This leads to the stopping variable

$$(4.2.6) \qquad N^*_m = \min\left\{\left\lfloor N\frac{\chi^2_{1-\alpha}[1]S^2_m}{N\delta^2 + \chi^2_{1-\alpha}[1]S^2_m}\right\rfloor + 1, N\right\}.$$

Notice that if $\delta = 0$ then $N^*_m = N$. Otherwise, if $\delta > 0$ then $N^*_m < N$. Also, the second-stage sampling is an SRS$(N - m, N_m - m)$, that is, a SRSWOR from $\mathcal{U} - \mathbf{s}_1$, where $\mathbf{s}_1$ is the first-stage sample. After stopping we estimate $\overline{Y}_N$ by the average of the combined sample, that is,

$$(4.2.7) \qquad \hat{\overline{Y}}_N = \frac{m\overline{X}^{(1)}_m + (N_m - m)^+\overline{X}^{(2)}_{N_m-m}}{\max\{m, N_m\}},$$

where $\overline{X}^{(1)}_m$ is the mean of the first sample and $\overline{X}^{(2)}_{N_m-m}$ is the mean of the second sample. The conditional expectation of $\hat{\overline{Y}}_N$, given $\mathbf{X}_{s_1}$, is

$$(4.2.8) \qquad E\{\hat{\overline{Y}}_N \mid \mathbf{X}_{s_1}\} = \overline{Y}_N P\{N_m > m\} + E\{\overline{X}^{(1)}_m I\{N_m \leq m\}\}.$$

If

$$P\{N_m \leq m\} = P\left\{S_m^2 \leq \frac{Nm\delta^2}{(N-m)\chi^2_{[1-\alpha]}[1]}\right\}$$

is small, then $\hat{\bar{Y}}_N$ is approximately unbiased. For the vector $\mathbf{Y}_N$ of Section 4.2.1, on which we base the numerical examples, a simulation estimate of $P\{N_m \leq m\}$ with 1000 runs is zero.

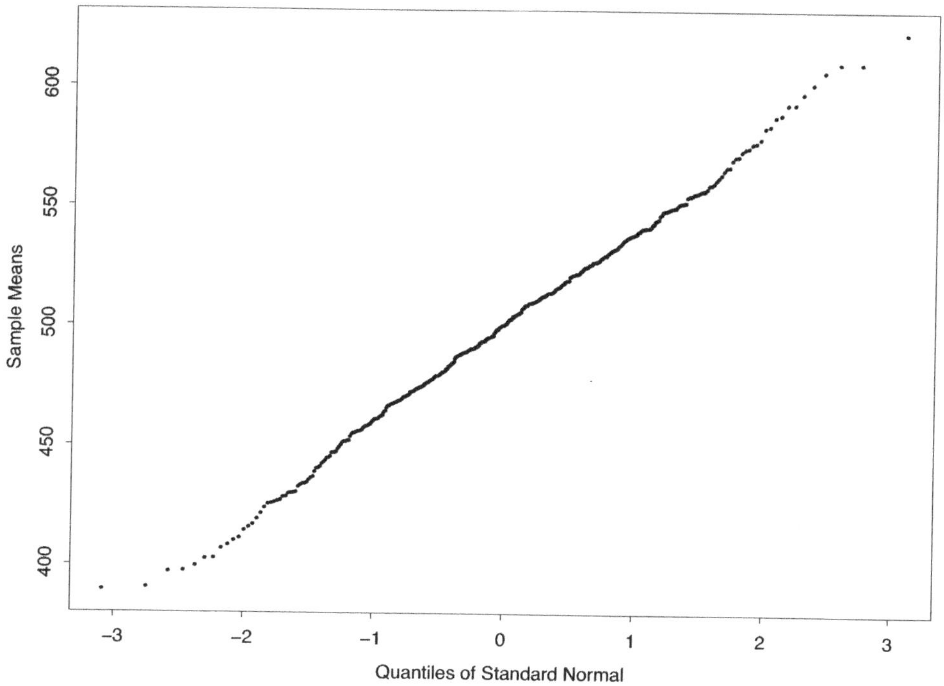

Figure 4.1 Normal QQ plot.

In Table 4.3 we present the simulation estimates of $E\{N_m^*\}$ and the CP as a function of m for the parameters of Table 4.2. We performed $M = 500$ simulation runs in each case.

Table 4.3: Simulation Estimates of $E\{N^*_m\}$ and CP for $\alpha = 0.05$ and $\delta = 0.316$, $N = 10000$

m	$E\{N^*_m\}$	CP
50	1642.70 ± 43.43	0.93 ± 0.02
100	1644.70 ± 33.91	0.96 ± 0.02
200	1635.62 ± 20.41	0.94 ± 0.02
500	1631.29 ± 13.98	0.94 ± 0.02

Derived using program simts2.

In Table 4.3 we see that, for the simulated example, the expected sample size N^*_m is approximately 16.4% of N when $\delta = 0.316$. The coverage probabilities are not significantly different from $1-\alpha = 0.95$. We see also by comparing Table 4.2 and Table 4.3 that the two-stage procedure with SRSWOR is more efficient than that with SRSWR.

An *adaptive sequential* procedure can be based on a similar stopping rule. After the initial sample of size m, we start drawing the units from $\mathcal{U}$ one by one. After each observation, we compute the sample variance of the combined sample and use the stopping variable

$$(4.2.9) \qquad N^*(\delta) = \min\left\{n : n \geq m, \ \frac{N\chi^2_{1-\alpha}[1]S^2_n}{N\delta^2 + \chi^2_{1-\alpha}[1]S^2_n} \leq n\right\}.$$

Then $M = 100$ simulation runs of this stopping rule, with the parameters of Table 4.3, for $m = 50$ gave $E\{N^*(\delta)\} = 1645.56 \pm 16.37$ and CP $= 0.94 \pm 0.02$. The sequential procedures stops on the average at about 16.5% of the population size. The coverage probability is not significantly different than 0.95. (Use function simseqwor.) It seems that the sequential procedure is not more efficient than the two-stage one.

4.2.3 Modeling Approach

In model SM1, even without assuming the actual distribution of the observed variables $Y_1, Y_2, \ldots$, the results are similar to those of the SWSWOR of Section 4.2.2. We do not estimate the r.v. $\overline{Y}_N$. We wish to find a prediction interval of fixed-width 2δ. Since $V\{\overline{Y}_n - \overline{Y}_N\} = \sigma^2(1/n - 1/N)$, we would use either the two-stage sampling procedure with N_m given by (4.2.6) or the sequential procedure with $N^*(\delta)$ given by (4.2.9).

4.3 ADAPTIVE ALLOCATION OF STRATIFIED SRS

4.3.1 Basic Theory

Stratified SRS is a design method in which the population $\mathcal{U}$ is partitioned first to k strata $\mathcal{U}_1, \ldots, \mathcal{U}_k$ such that $\bigcup_{i=1}^k \mathcal{U}_i = \mathcal{U}$ and $\mathcal{U}_i \cap \mathcal{U}_j = \emptyset$ for all $i \neq j$. If the partition is done so that each stratum is as homogeneous as possible with respect to the variable Y and the difference between means of different strata is as large as possible, then the estimation of the population mean $\overline{Y}_N$ might be substantially more precise than in SRS. More specifically, suppose that the strata sizes are N_i, $i = 1, \ldots, k$. Let $\overline{Y}_{N_i}$ be the mean of $\mathcal{U}_i$ and $S^2_{N_i}$ the variance of $\mathcal{U}_i$, $i = 1, \ldots, k$. We also let $W_i = N_i/N$, $i = 1, \ldots, k$. From each one of the k strata an SRS(N_i, n_i) is drawn independently.

Let $\overline{Y}_{s_i}$ be the mean of the sample from $\mathcal{U}_i$. An unbiased estimator of the population mean is

$$\hat{\overline{Y}}_N = \sum_{i=1}^{k} W_i \overline{Y}_{s_i}. \tag{4.3.1}$$

The P-variance of this estimator is

$$V_P\{\hat{\overline{Y}}_N\} = \sum_{i=1}^{k} W_i^2 S^2_{N_i} \left(\frac{1}{n_i} - \frac{1}{N_i}\right). \tag{4.3.2}$$

The following is the sample *allocation problem*. Given a total sample size, n, how should $n_i \geq 0$ be determined so that $\sum_{i=1}^k n_i = n$?

An allocation is called *proportional* if

$$n_i = nW_i, \quad i = 1, \ldots, k. \tag{4.3.3}$$

Under proportional allocation, we obtain from (4.3.2) that

$$V_P\{\hat{\overline{Y}}_N\} = \left(\frac{1}{n} - \frac{1}{N}\right) \sum_{i=1}^{k} W_i S^2_{N_i}. \tag{4.3.4}$$

Notice that $\sigma^2_N = [(N-1)/N] S^2_N$ can be written as

$$\sigma^2_N = \sum_{i=1}^{k} W_i \sigma^2_{N_i} + \sum_{i=1}^{k} W_i (\overline{Y}_{N_i} - \overline{Y}_N)^2 \tag{4.3.5}$$

and $V_P\{\hat{\overline{Y}}_N\}$ can be written as

$$V_P\{\hat{\overline{Y}}_N\} = \frac{1}{n}\left(1 - \frac{n-1}{N-1}\right) \sum_{i=1}^{k} W_i \sigma^2_{N_i}. \tag{4.3.6}$$

The variance of the sample mean from an unstratified SRS(N, n) is

$$V_P\{\overline{Y}_{\mathbf{s}}\} = \frac{1}{n}\left(1 - \frac{n-1}{N-1}\right) \sigma^2_N. \tag{4.3.7}$$

It follows that

$$V_P\{\overline{Y}_{\mathbf{s}}\} - V_P\{\hat{\overline{Y}}_N\} = \frac{1}{n}\left(1 - \frac{n-1}{N-1}\right)\sum_{i=1}^{k} W_i(\overline{Y}_{N_i} - \overline{Y}_N)^2. \tag{4.3.8}$$

Thus, if $\sum_{i=1}^{k} W_i(\overline{Y}_{N_i} - \overline{Y}_N)^2$ is large, the increase in precision (decrease of variance) in stratified SRS under proportional allocation could be substantial.

An *optimal allocation* can further reduce the variance of the unbiased estimator. To find this allocation, we minimize (4.3.2) under the constraint $\sum_{i=1}^{k} n_i = n$. For this, we write the Lagrangian

$$L(\underset{\sim}{n}, \lambda) = \sum_{i=1}^{k} W_i^2 \frac{S_{N_i}^2}{n_i} - \lambda\left(n - \sum_{i=1}^{k} n_i\right). \tag{4.3.9}$$

Differentiating $L(\underset{\sim}{n}, \lambda)$ with respect to n_i $(i = 1, \ldots, k)$ and λ, we obtain

$$\frac{\partial}{\partial n_i} L(\underset{\sim}{n}, \lambda) = -W_i^2 \frac{S_{N_i}^2}{n_i^2} + \lambda, \quad i = 1, \ldots, k,$$

$$\frac{\partial}{\partial \lambda} L(\underset{\sim}{n}, \lambda) = \sum_{i=1}^{k} n_i - n.$$

Setting these partial derivatives equal to zero and solving yield the optimal allocation

$$n_i^0 = n \frac{W_i S_{N_i}}{\sum_{j=1}^{k} W_j S_{N_j}}, \qquad i = 1, \ldots, k. \tag{4.3.10}$$

We see in (4.3.10) that the optimal allocation requires the knowledge of the standard deviations S_{N_i} for all strata. Also, the proportional allocation is close to optimal if S_{N_i} are almost equal in all strata.

4.3.2 Two-Stage Procedure for a Fixed-Width Interval Estimation of $\overline{\mathrm{Y}}_{\mathrm{N}}$ Under Stratified Sampling

Similar to the two-stage procedure of Section 4.2, we suggest the following two-stage procedure for stratified sampling.

Stage One: Allocate a sample of size m *proportionally* among the strata. That is, $n_i^{(1)} = W_i m$, $i = 1, \ldots, k$. Let $S^2_{n_i^{(1)}}$ $(i = 1, \ldots, k)$ be the sample unbiased estimates of $S_{N_i}^2$. Determine the size of the combined sample, N_m, as

$$(4.3.11) \qquad N_m = \left\lfloor N \frac{\chi^2_{1-\alpha}[1] \sum_{i=1}^{k} W_i S^2_{n_i^{(1)}}}{N\delta^2 + \chi^2_{1-\alpha}[1] \sum_{i=1}^{k} W_i S^2_{n_i^{(1)}}} \right\rfloor + 1.$$

If $N_m \leq m$, stop sampling and estimate $\overline{Y}_N$ by $(\overline{Y}_m \pm \delta)$, where $\overline{Y}_m = \sum_{i=1}^k W_i \overline{Y}_{n_i}$. If $N_m > m$, go to stage two.

Stage Two: Allocate the remaining sample size $N_m - m$ "optimally" among the strata as

$$(4.3.12) \qquad n_i^{(2)} = (N_m - m) \frac{W_i^{(2)} S_{n_i^{(1)}}}{\sum_{j=1}^{k} W_j^{(2)} S_{n_j^{(1)}}},$$

where $W_i^{(2)} = (N_i - n_i^{(1)})/(N - m)$, $i = 1, \ldots, k$. Estimate $\overline{Y}_N$ by $\hat{\overline{Y}}_N \pm \delta$, where

$$(4.3.13) \qquad \hat{\overline{Y}}_N = \sum_{i=1}^{k} W_i \frac{n_i^{(1)} \overline{Y}_{n_i^{(1)}} + n_i^{(2)} \overline{Y}_{n_i^{(2)}}}{n_i^{(1)} + n_i^{(2)}}.$$

$\overline{Y}_{n_i^{(2)}}$ being the means of the second-stage samples.

Theorem 4.3.1 *Under the two-stage stratified sampling given by (4.3.11) and (4.3.12), $\hat{\overline{Y}}_N$ is P unbiased, that is,*

$$E_P\{\hat{\overline{Y}}_N\} = \overline{Y}_N \quad \textit{for all } \overline{Y}_N.$$

Proof: Let $\mathcal{F}_1$ be the σ-field generated by $(\overline{Y}_{n(1)}, S^2_{n_i^{(1)}}, i = 1, \ldots, k)$. Notice that, given $n_i^{(2)}$, the second-stage sample is an SRS$(N_i - n_i^{(1)}, n_i^{(2)})$ for each stratum. Hence

$$E_P\{\overline{Y}_{n_i^{(2)}} \mid \mathcal{F}_1\} = \frac{N_i \overline{Y}_{N_i} - n_i^{(1)} \overline{Y}_{n_i^{(1)}}}{N_i - n_i^{(1)}}.$$

Hence, substituting this in (4.3.13), we get

$$E_P\{\hat{\overline{Y}}_N \mid \mathcal{F}_1\} = \sum_{i=1}^{k} W_i \overline{Y}_{n_i^{(1)}} \quad \text{a.s.}$$

Finally, since $E_P\{\overline{Y}_{n_i^{(1)}}\} = \overline{Y}_{N_i}, i = 1, \ldots, k\}$, we obtain

$$\begin{aligned} E_P\{\hat{\overline{Y}}_N\} &= \sum_{i=1}^{k} W_i \overline{Y}_{N_i} \\ &= \overline{Y}_N, \quad \text{all } \mathbf{Y}_N. \end{aligned}$$

■

The standard error of $\hat{\overline{Y}}_N$ can be estimated by bootstrapping (see Kenett and Zacks, 1998).

To illustrate this two-stage stratified allocation, we constructed a population of size $N = 1000$ with $k = 3$ strata in the following manner. We took a vector $\mathbf{Y}_{1000} \sim G(5, 2)$. The first 250 components of this vector we put in the first stratum, the next 500 components in the second stratum, and the last 250 components in the third stratum. Furthermore we added the value 10 to each component of stratum 2 and value 20 to each component of stratum 3. The parameters of this stratified population are:

i	N_i	$\overline{Y}_{N_i}$	$S^2_{N_i}$
1	250	10.20085	44.49879
2	500	20.05112	55.71654
3	250	29.96159	46.82828

We then simulated from this population $M = 100$ runs of the two-stage stratified allocation procedure (4.3.11)–(4.3.13). Also, in order to illustrate the possible higher efficiency stratification, we ran in parallel from the same population the nonstratified two-stage procedure of the previous section. The results are given in Table 4.4.

Table 4.4: Simulation Estimates of $\mathbf{E\{N^*_m\}}$ and CP for $\alpha = 0.05$, $\delta = 0.316$

	Stratified		Nonstratified	
m	$E\{N^*_m\}$	CP	$E\{N^*_m\}$	CP
100	657.32 ± 9.32	0.93 ± 0.05	784.58 ± 4.05	0.95 ± 0.04
200	659.78 ± 5.79	0.91 ± 0.06	790.66 ± 3.39	0.93 ± 0.05

Derived using programs simts2, simtsst.

The CP in all cases is not significantly different from $1 - \alpha = 0.95$. The expected sample sizes in the stratified cases are substantially smaller than in the nonstratified cases.

4.4 ADAPTIVE SEARCH FOR SPECIAL UNITS

Thompson and Seber (1996, pp. 178) discuss adaptive two-stage optimal allocation in stratified sampling. They describe a procedure for estimating the total weight of fish (biomass) in a given area of the sea. The objective is to obtain a reasonable estimator. This is different from our objective of determining the total sample size required to attain a fixed-width interval estimator of the mean $\overline{Y}_N$ with close to nominal coverage probability. The search procedure discussed here is appropriate for estimating the size or volume of a rare clustered population, like spatially clustered rare animal or plant species or some mineral. The adaptive procedure which is presented here follows that of Thompson (1990), Thompson (1992), and Thompson and Seber (1996). The location of these clusters of interest is unknown, and the objective is to discover their location by a special sampling design. First the spatial region $\mathcal{R}$ is partitioned to N units $\{U_1, \dots, U_N\}$. A random sample of n units is chosen initially from the N specified units of the region. Let Y be the value observed in a chosen unit. If Y belongs to a specified set C, we add to the sample additional units in the neighborhood. To be more specific, suppose that each unit of $\mathcal{R}$ has several neighboring units. Suppose that Y is equal to the number of rare species observed in the unit. If $Y = 0$, the result is recorded and another unit is chosen from the initial sample. On the other hand, if $Y > 0$, we add to the sample all the units in the neighborhood of the observed unit. If any of the added units has a value $Y > 0$, all its neighborhood units are added and so on, until all added units in the boundary have zero values. All the neighboring units with $Y > 0$ are called a *network*. The network plus the empty boundary units is called a *cluster*. If an initial sample unit is empty ($Y = 0$) we say that we have a network of size $m = 1$.

Let A_i ($i = 1, \dots, n$) be the set of indexes of units in R which belong to the network of the ith unit in the initial sample. Define

$$\overline{Y}_{A_i} = \sum_{j \in A_i} \frac{Y_j}{m_i}, \quad i = 1, \dots, n. \tag{4.4.1}$$

Thompson and Seber (1996) suggest the following estimator of $\mu = \overline{Y}_N$,

$$\hat{\mu} = \frac{1}{n} \sum_{i \in \mathbf{s}_1} \overline{Y}_{A_i}. \tag{4.4.2}$$

If the initial sample is an SRS(N, n), then

$$E_P\{\hat{\mu}\} = \frac{1}{N} \sum_{i=1}^{N} \overline{Y}_{A_i} = \mu \tag{4.4.3}$$

and

$$V\{\hat{\mu}\} = \frac{1}{n}\left(1 - \frac{n}{N}\right) \sigma_A^2, \tag{4.4.4}$$

where

$$\sigma_A^2 = \frac{1}{N-1} \sum_{i=1}^{N} (\overline{Y}_{A_i} - \mu)^2. \tag{4.4.5}$$

An unbiased estimator of σ_A^2 is

$$\hat{\sigma}_A^2 = \frac{1}{n-1} \sum_{i \in \mathbf{s}_1} (\overline{Y}_{A_i} - \hat{\mu})^2, \tag{4.4.6}$$

where $\mathbf{s}_1$ is the initial sample. Notice that each unit of the population (region) has a $\overline{Y}_{A_i}$ value which is either zero or the average of the Y-values in the network which intersects it.

The reader is referred to Thompson and Seber (1966) for other estimators and other search designs, which are called there "adaptive cluster designs."

4.5 ADAPTIVE ESTIMATION OF THE SIZE OF A FINITE POPULATION

The problem of estimating the size of a finite population is of interest in ecology, wild life management, fishery, and so on. There are different approaches to study this problem (see Seber, 1985). We focus attention on the *capture–recapture* method, which is performed sequentially. See on this subject the papers of Freeman (1972), Samuel (1968, 1969), Pollock and Otto (1983), and others. The present section is based on the paper of Zacks, Pereira, and Leite (1990). In the capture–recapture method one performs a sequence of trials. In each trial a random sample is drawn from the population. The number of untagged elements in the sample is recorded. All elements are then tagged and the sample is returned to the population. This method would be appropriate for estimating the number of fish in a pond. The method is sequential, and the question is how many times to repeat the procedure until a good estimate of the population size is available. A one-by-one capture–recapture (see Samuel, 1968, 1969) is applicable when one is trapping big animals.

Consider a population of unknown size N. The population is closed during the study (no migration, births, or deaths). Let M_k ($k = 1, 2, \ldots$) denote the size of the kth sample, and let U_k ($k = 1, 2, \ldots$) denote the number of untagged elements in the kth sample. Let $T_k = \sum_{i=1}^{k} U_i$. Obviously $U_1 = M_1$ and $0 \leq U_k \leq M_k$ for all $k \geq 2$. Also $N \geq \max_{1 \leq k} M_k$. Here T_k is the number of distinct elements of the population observed in the first k samples.

We assume that different samples are *conditionally independent* given $M_1, M_2, \ldots$. Let $\mathbf{D}_k = (U_1, \ldots, U_k)'$ and $\mathbf{M}_k = (M_1, \ldots, M_k)'$. The *like-*

lihood function of N given $(\mathbf{M}_k, \mathbf{D}_k)$ is

$$
\begin{aligned}
L(N; \mathbf{M}; \mathbf{D}_k) &= \prod_{i=1}^{k} \frac{\binom{N - t_{j-1}}{u_j}\binom{t_{j-1}}{M_j - u_j}}{\binom{N}{M_j}} \\
&= \frac{\prod_{j=2}^{k} \binom{t_{j-1}}{M_j - u_j}}{\prod_{j=1}^{k} u_j!} K(N; \mathbf{M}_k, t_k),
\end{aligned}
\tag{4.5.1}
$$

where the kernel of the likelihood is

$$
K(N; \mathbf{M}_k, t_k) = \begin{cases} \dfrac{N!}{(N - t_k)! \prod_{j=1}^{k} \binom{N}{M_j}}, & N \geq t_k, \\ 0, & N < t_k. \end{cases}
\tag{4.5.2}
$$

The minimal sufficient statistic for N after k samples is T_k.

Theorem 4.5.1 *Let $\{\pi(n), n \geq 0\}$ be a prior probability distribution of N. The posterior probability distribution of N is*

$$
\pi(n; M_k, T_k) = \begin{cases} \dfrac{\pi(n) K(n; \mathbf{M}_k, T_k)}{\sum_{n=T_k}^{\infty} \pi(n) K(n; \mathbf{M}_k, T_k)}, & n \geq T_k, \\ 0, & n < T_k. \end{cases}
\tag{4.5.3}
$$

■

If $M_k^* = \max_{1 \leq i \leq k} M_i$ and $M_k^* \leq t \leq \sum_{j=1}^{k} M_j$, then, as proven in Zacks, Pereira, and Leite (1990),

$$
\sum_{n=t}^{\infty} \pi(n) K(n; \mathbf{M}_k, t) < \infty.
$$

The Bayes estimator of N for the squared-error loss is the mean of the posterior distribution, and the Bayes risk is the variance of the posterior distribution. Thus, the Bayes estimator of N given $(\mathbf{M}, T_k = t)$ is

$$
B(k, t) = \sum_{n=t}^{\infty} n \pi(n; \mathbf{M}_k, t).
\tag{4.5.4}
$$

Let $R(k, t)$ denote the posterior risk given $T_k = t$. Important asymptotic results, proven in Zacks, Pereira, and Leite (1990), are:

Theorem 4.5.2 *If $\pi(n) > 0$ for all $n \geq 0$, then* *(i)* $\lim_{k\to\infty} T_k = N$ *a.s.* $[P_N]$;

(ii) $\lim_{k\to\infty} B(k, T_k) = N$ *a.s.* $[P_N]$;

(iii) $\lim_{k\to\infty} R(k, T_k) = 0$ *a.s.* $[P_N]$. ■

Thus, for prior distributions like Poisson and negative binomial, the Bayesian estimator will give the correct result if the number of samples is sufficiently large.

We continue now with the Poisson prior, that is, $\pi(n) = e^{-\lambda}\lambda^n/n!$, $n = 0, 1, \ldots$. We also assume that $M_j = M$ for all $j \geq 1$. Under these assumptions, $B(k,t)$ exists for all (k, T_k). From (4.5.2) and (4.5.3) we obtain, after some algebraic manipulation, the formula

$$B(k,t) = t + \lambda \frac{\sum_{n=0}^{\infty} \lambda^n a_n(k, t+1, M)}{\sum_{n=0}^{\infty} \lambda^n a_n(k, t, M)}, \tag{4.5.5}$$

where

$$a_n(k,t,M) = \left(n! \prod_{i=1}^{M} (n+t+1-i)^k\right)^{-1}. \tag{4.5.6}$$

Formula (4.5.6) is inconvenient for computations since the terms $a_n(k,t,M)$ decrease rapidly to zero. For example, $a_{10}(20, 50, 10) = \exp(-818.1125)$. Zacks, Pereira, and Leite (1990) have proven:

Theorem 4.5.3 *For the Poisson prior distribution and* $M_j = M$, *all* $j \geq 1$,

$$B(k,t) = t + \lambda \frac{\sum_{n=0}^{\infty} \lambda^n \frac{1}{n!} \prod_{j=1}^{M} \left(\frac{t+1-j}{n+t+2-j}\right)^k}{\sum_{n=0}^{\infty} \lambda^n \frac{1}{n!} \prod_{j=1}^{M} \left(\frac{t+1-j}{n+t+1-j}\right)^k}. \tag{4.5.7}$$

The Bayesian risk is

$$R(k,t) = [B(k,t) - t][B(k,t+1) - B(k,t)]. \tag{4.5.8}$$

■

Formula (4.5.7) can be applied also for computing $R(k,t)$.

In Table 4.5 we present values of $B(k,t)$ and $R(k,t)$ for a population of size $N = 50$ when the T_k were determined by simulation. The prior distribution is Poisson with $\lambda = 20$.

Table 4.5: Values of $\mathbf{B(k,t)}$ and $\mathbf{R(k,t)}$ for Poisson Prior with $\boldsymbol{\lambda = 20}$, $\mathbf{N = 50}$, $\mathbf{M = 1}$

k	T_k	$B(k,T_k)$	$R(k,T_k)$
3	2	19.008	19.979
13	10	20.660	15.516
40	25	30.480	7.073
70	33	35.926	3.458
100	42	44.128	2.383
150	48	48.969	1.025
300	50	50.053	0.053

In a sequential procedure the important question is that of the stopping rule. Freeman (1972) did dynamic programming to find the optimal boundary for a truncated procedure. We have used the simpler, suboptimal stopping rule

(4.5.9) $$K_\epsilon = \min\{k \geq 2 : R(k,T_k) < \epsilon\}.$$

For $N = 50$, $M = 15$, $\epsilon = 0.1$, and $\lambda = 10$, we have found empirically that the boundary for K_ϵ is

(4.5.10) $$b_m(k) = \lfloor 7.5 + 3.25k \rfloor - 1.$$

As soon as $T_k < b_m(k)$, we stop sampling.

Let $\{b_m(k), k \geq 1\}$ be a monotone increasing sequence of integer values such that $b_m(k) < km$ and $\lim_{k\to\infty} b_m(k) = \infty$. Define the corresponding stopping variable

(4.5.11) $$K(b_m) = \min\{k \geq 1 : T_k \leq b_m(k)\}.$$

We have indicated that $T_k \to N$ a.s. $[P_N]$. Thus, since $N < \infty$, $P\{K(b_m) < \infty\} = 1$. We develop the probability distribution of $K(b_m)$.

Let

(4.5.12) $$h_k^{(N,m)}(t) = P_N\{T_k = t, K(b_m) \geq k\}.$$

We determine this function recursively. Obviously $h_1^{(N,m)}(t) = I\{t = m\}$. Since $T_k = T_{k-1} + U_k$, we have, for $k \geq 2$,

(4.5.13) $$h_k^{(N,m)}(t) = \sum_{u=b_m(k-1)+1}^{(b_m(k)-1)\wedge t} h_{k-1}^{(N,m)}(u) P_N\{U_k = t-u \mid T_{k-1} = u\}.$$

Moreover,

(4.5.14) $$P_N\{U_k = t-u \mid T_{k-1} = u\} = \frac{\binom{N-u}{t-u}\binom{u}{m-t+u}}{\binom{N}{m}}.$$

Finally,

$$P_{N,m}\{K(b_m) = k\} = \sum_{j=b_m(k-1)+1}^{b_m(k)} h_k^{(N,m)}(j). \tag{4.5.15}$$

For example, for $N = 50$, $m = 15$, $\lambda = 10$, and $\epsilon = 0.1$, we get the following probability distribution of $K(b_m)$:

k	12	13	14
$P\{K(b_m) = k\}$	0.003164	0.390343	0.606488

4.6 APPLICATIONS IN SOFTWARE RELIABILITY

Software is a complex system of programs, routines, and symbolic languages that control the functioning of the hardware of a computer. A specific software is considered reliable if it performs its specified functions or tasks according to defined standards of expectation. In the present section we present statistical modeling which is connected with the process of fault detection and correction during the final testing phase. The most important questions are which modules should be tested and how long one should continue testing.

4.6.1 Sequential Stopping for Time Domain Models

Time domain models are those which specify the distribution of times between failures of the software. Suppose that the software contains N functional units which have faults and which cause failure if applied. In the testing process any detected fault is immediately corrected (rectified) and the number of faults is reduced by 1. Jelinski and Moranda (1972) assumed that the N faults are associated with N independent homogeneous Poisson processes with rate Λ. Thus, let $U_{(1)} < U_{(2)} < \cdots < U_{(N)}$ denote the N-order statistics of a sample of N i.i.d. random variables having exponential distribution with mean $\nu = 1/\Lambda$. In the present problem the sample size N is *unknown* and has to be predicted from the data.

Let $J(t) = \sum_{i=1}^{N} I\{U_{(i)} \leq t\}$, $0 < t < \infty$, be the number of failures observed up to time t. Let $W_n = \sum_{i=1}^{n} U_{(i)}$, $n = 1, 2, \ldots$. Define the stochastic process

$$W(t) = \sum_{n=0}^{N-1} I\{U_{(n)} \leq t < U_{(n+1)}\}W_n + W_N \cdot I\{t \geq U_{(N)}\}. \tag{4.6.1}$$

The likelihood function of (N, ν) at time t is

(4.6.2)

$$L(N, \nu; t, J(t), W(t)) = \frac{N!}{(N - J(t))!}\nu^{J(t)} \cdot \exp\{-\nu W(t) - \nu(N - J(t))t\}.$$

In a Bayesian framework we could assume that N and ν are priorly independent; N has a prior Poisson distribution with mean η and ν has a prior gamma distribution $G(\xi, \alpha)$. Thus, the posterior p.d.f. of (N, ν) at time t is

$$h(N, \nu \mid t, J(t), W(t)) = \frac{\eta^{N-J(t)} \nu^{\alpha+J(t)-1} \exp\{-\nu[W(t) + \xi + (N - J(t))t]\}}{\Gamma(\alpha + J(t))(N - J(t))! \sum_{m=0}^{\infty} \frac{\eta^m}{m!} [W(t) + \xi + mt]^{-(\alpha+J(t))}}, \tag{4.6.3}$$

$n \geq J(t)$, $0 < \nu < \infty$.

Let $M(t) = N - J(t)$ denote the (unknown) number of remaining faults at time t. Let $\eta(t, J(t), W(t)) = E\{M(t) \mid t, J(t), W(t)\}$. Define

$$\Psi(\eta, \lambda, x, u) = e^{-\eta} \sum_{m=0}^{\infty} \frac{\eta^m}{m!} (x + um)^{-\lambda}; \tag{4.6.4}$$

then

$$\eta(t, J(t), W(t)) = \eta \frac{\Psi(\eta, \alpha + J(t), W(t) + \xi + t, t)}{\Psi(\eta, \alpha + J(t), W(t) + \xi, t)}. \tag{4.6.5}$$

For large values of η we compute Ψ by the normal approximation,

$$\Psi(\eta, \lambda, x, t) \cong \frac{1}{\sqrt{2\pi\eta}} \int_{\eta-4\sqrt{\eta}}^{\eta+4\sqrt{\eta}} \exp\left\{-\frac{1}{2\eta}(u - \eta)^2\right\} (x + ut)^{-\lambda} \, du. \tag{4.6.6}$$

One can prove that the function $\eta(t, J(t), W(t))$ is decreasing in t in the intervals (t_i, t_{i+1}) with discontinuities at the failure points, t_i, $i \geq 1$.

Let $K[\$]$ be the cost (penalty) of finding a fault in the field (after release of the software), and let $c[\$]$ be the cost of testing per time unit. Thus, the posterior risk at time t is

$$R(t; J(t), W(t)) = ct + K\eta(t, J(t), W(t)). \tag{4.6.7}$$

The following is a reasonable stopping time:

$$T_s = \inf\{t > 0 : t = \tau^0(t)\}, \tag{4.6.8}$$

where

$$\tau^0(t) = \arg\min_{\tau \geq t} R(\tau; J(t), W(t)). \tag{4.6.9}$$

Table 4.6 demonstrates this procedure.

Table 4.6: Values of τ^0(t) for Simulated Failure Times, N = 10, $\alpha = 1$, $\xi = 1$, $\eta = 10$, K = 1, c = 0.2

t_i	$J(t_i)$	$W(t_i))$	$\eta(t_i; J(t_i), W(t_i))$	$\tau^0(t_i)$
0.0349	1	0.0349	9.5053	2.335
0.1047	2	0.1396	8.5765	8.605
0.1729	3	0.3125	7.7000	4.773
0.3500	4	0.6624	6.3593	3.650
0.5495	5	1.2120	5.2068	3.250
0.6006	6	1.8126	4.7972	3.101
1.6674	7	3.4800	2.0373	3.767
1.7586	8	5.2386	2.3297	4.159
1.8612	9	7.0998	2.4580	4.561
2.2050	10	9.3049	2.1782	4.905

Since there are only $N = 10$ faults, there will be no failure after time $t = 2.2050$. Therefore, at time $\tau^0(2.205) = 4.905$ we stop.

4.6.2 Sequential Stopping for Data Domain Models

Chernoff and Ray (1965) studied the problem of optimal stopping in rectifying sampling inspection. Let $\mathcal{U}$ be a finite population of N^* elements having proportion θ, $0 < \theta < 1$, of defective ones.

The loss due to releasing $\mathcal{U}$ with $N_\theta = \lfloor N^*\theta \rfloor$ defectives is $KN_\theta[\$]$. The cost of inspecting and rectifying n elements is $cn[\$]$. All defective elements found during an inspection are replaced by good ones (or are corrected). The risk after inspecting n elements is

$$\begin{aligned} R(\theta; n) &= (N^* - n)\theta K + cn \\ &= N_\theta K - n(\theta K - c). \end{aligned} \tag{4.6.10}$$

If $\theta K > c$, it is optimal to inspect *all* the elements of $\mathcal{U}$. The problem is that θ is unknown. Chernoff and Ray developed an approximately optimal Bayes sequential stopping rule under a beta prior distribution for θ. We show here a different approach. First, we assume that a vector of *known* covariates $\mathbf{x} = (x_1, \ldots, x_p)'$ is available for each element of $\mathcal{U}$. Also we allow different inspection costs and different penalty costs (c_i, K_i) $i = 1, \ldots, N$.

Let $Y_i = 1$ if the ith element has a fault and $Y_i = 0$ otherwise. Let $\theta(\mathbf{x}) = P\{Y = 1 \mid \mathbf{x}\}$. We apply a quantal response model (see Section 3.2) $\theta(\mathbf{x}) = F(\boldsymbol{\gamma}'\mathbf{x})$, where $(\gamma_1, \ldots, \gamma_p)$ are regression coefficients, and $F(\ )$ is a standard distribution. If $\boldsymbol{\gamma}$ is known, the risk of *not* inspecting $\mathcal{U}$ is

$$R_0 = \sum_{i=1}^{N} K_i F(\mathbf{x}_i'\boldsymbol{\gamma}). \tag{4.6.11}$$

If we inspect a sample $\mathbf{s} = (i_1, \ldots, i_n)$, the risk is

$$R_1(\mathbf{s}) = R_0 - \sum_{i \in \mathbf{s}} (K_i F(\mathbf{x}_i' \boldsymbol{\gamma}) - c_i). \tag{4.6.12}$$

Accordingly, only elements for which $F(\mathbf{x}_i' \boldsymbol{\gamma}) > c_i / K_i$ should be inspected. The problem is to devise an adaptive selection and stopping rules when $\boldsymbol{\gamma}$ is unknown.

We continue with a concrete example. Each unit has one covariate x_i, which relates to its size (number of lines of code) or complexity. We consider the model

$$\theta(x; \gamma) = e^{-\gamma/x}, \quad 0 < \gamma < \infty, \quad 0 < x < \infty. \tag{4.6.13}$$

Thus, the probability of fault is an increasing function of x. The cost structure is

$$\begin{aligned} c_i &= c x_i, \qquad & i &= 1, \ldots, N, \\ K_i &= K x_i, \qquad & i &= 1, \ldots, N. \end{aligned}$$

Thus,

$$\sum_{i \in \mathbf{s}} (K_i \theta(x_i; \gamma) - c_i) = \sum_{i \in \mathbf{s}} x_i (K e^{-\gamma/x_i} - c). \tag{4.6.14}$$

This quantity is maximized if $\mathbf{s}$ contains the n units having the *largest* x-values. The MLE of γ is the root of the equation

$$\sum_{i=1}^{n} \frac{e^{-\gamma/x_i}}{x_i(1 - e^{-\gamma/x_i})} = \sum_{i=1}^{n} \frac{Y_i}{x_i(1 - e^{-\gamma/x_i})}. \tag{4.6.15}$$

The MLE *does not* exist if $\sum_{i=1}^{N} Y_i = 0$ or if $\sum Y_i = n$. On the other hand, if $0 < \sum_{i=1}^{n} Y_i < n$, there exists a unique solution to (4.6.15) which can be obtained numerically. The Fisher information is

$$I_n(\gamma) = \sum_{i=1}^{n} \frac{e^{-\gamma/x_i}}{x_i^2(1 - e^{-\gamma/x_i})}. \tag{4.6.16}$$

Let $\hat{\gamma}_n$ be the MLE of γ after n observations. An assymptotically (large n) lower confidence limit for γ at level $1 - \alpha$ is approximately

$$\hat{\gamma}_{n,\alpha}^{(L)} = \hat{\gamma}_n - Z_{1-\alpha} \left(\frac{1}{I_n(\hat{\gamma}_n)} \right)^{1/2}. \tag{4.6.17}$$

We adopt the stopping rule

$$M^* = \min(n \geq m : K \exp\{-\hat{\gamma}_{n,\alpha}^{(L)} / x_{[n+1]}\} < c\}, \tag{4.6.18}$$

where $x_{[n+1]}$ is the largest x-value of the $N^* - n$ units not yet observed. If $M^* \geq N^*$, we stop at N^*. Notice that for (4.6.15), if $\hat{\gamma}_{n,\alpha}^{(L)} < -\min\{x_i\}\log(c/K)$, then $M^* = N^*$. To illustrate the sequential stopping rule (4.6.18), we created a population $\mathcal{U}$ with $N^* = 1000$ elements (modules) of varying number of lines of code which range from $\min\{x_i\} = 28$ to $\max\{x_i\} = 72$. For our model we considered $\gamma = 75$. For this parameter, the probability of a fault in the smallest module is $\exp\{-75/28\} = 0.0687$ and the probability of a fault in the largest module is $\exp\{-75/72\} = 0.3529$. We ran the simulation program $M = 100$ times and obtained the results in Table 4.7.

Table 4.7: Simulation Estimates of the Characteristics of (4.6.18), $\gamma = 75$, N = 1000, m = 50, c = 1, K = 3

		Quantiles of M^*		
$E\{M^*\}$	STD$\{M^*\}$	0.25	0.50	0.75
144.27	88.1061	61	121	192

Derived using programs seqsim, gmle.

The minimum and maximum of these simulation runs are 50 and 375, respectively.

4.7 SAMPLING INSPECTION SCHEMES

Sampling inspection schemes are used in industry, military, and business where large quantities of commodities are received from vendors. If the manufacturing process of a "certified" vendor is under strict statistical process control, one may not need to subject delivered material to sampling inspection. However, if the vendor has not yet established high standards of quality or for periodic auditing, sampling inspection is performed in order to test whether the items in a given lot (finite population) satisfy certain quality standards. On the basis of the observed sample a hypothesis that the proportion of nonconforming items in the lot is smaller than the accepted quality level (AQL) is tested. There are three types of sampling procedures: single samples, two-stage (double) sampling, and sequential sampling. The corresponding tests are classified to two main categories: by attributes and by continuous variables. In the spirit of the adaptive processes we confine attention in the present section to two-stage (double) and sequential sampling by attributes. For a comprehensive review of methods and theories of sampling inspection schemes, see Kenett and Zacks (1998, Chapter 9).

4.7.1 Two-Stage Sampling for Attributes

Suppose that the lot is of size N. In the first stage a random sample of size n_1 is drawn from the lot without replacement, that is, SRS(N, n_1). Let X_1 denote the number of nonconforming items in the first sample. The rules for stopping or continuing are: If $X_1 \leq c_1$, stop sampling and accept the lot. If $X_1 \geq c_2$, $c_2 > c_1+1$, stop sampling and reject the lot. If $c_1 < X_1 < c_2$, take an additional (second-stage) random sample, SRS$(N-n_1, n_2)$, of size n_2 without replacement from the units not sampled in the first stage. Let X_2 be the number of nonconforming items in the second sample. If $X_1+X_2 \leq c_3$ accept the lot, otherwise reject it. Suppose that D is the number of nonconforming items in the lot originally, and $p = D/N$. The probability of accepting such a lot is

(4.7.1)

$$\text{OC}(p) = H(c_1; D, N, n_1) + \sum_{j=c_1+1}^{c_2-1} h(j; D, N, n_1) H(c_3 - j; D - j; N - n_1, n_2),$$

where

$$h(i; M, N, n) = \frac{\binom{M}{i}\binom{N-M}{n-i}}{\binom{N}{n}}, \tag{4.7.2}$$

$i = 0, \ldots, n$, is the p.d.f. of the hypergeometric distribution and

$$H(i; M, N, n) = \sum_{j=0}^{i} h(j; M, N, n) \tag{4.7.3}$$

is the corresponding c.d.f. The function OC(p) is called the *operating characteristics* function. It gives the probability of *accepting* a lot having proportion p of nonconforming items. For example, if $N = 1000$, $n_1 = 120$, $n_2 = 240$, $c_1 = 0$, $c_2 = c_3 = 7$, we have OC$(0.01) = 0.9892$ and OC$(0.03) = 0.084$. Accordingly, if a lot with $p \leq 0.01$ is considered acceptable and one with $p \geq 0.03$ rejectable, the probability of error of Type I (producer's risk) is $\alpha = 0.07$ and the probability of error of Type II (consumer's risk) is $\beta = 0.08$. When we test the hypothesis $H_0 : p \leq p_0$ against $H_1 : p \geq p_1$, the value p_0 is the AQL and p_1 is the LTPD (limit-tolerated proportion defective). Since there are five parameters to determine, different combinations of $(n_1, n_2, c_1, c_2, c_3)$ may yield close values of α and β. It is therefore common to consider the combination $n_2 = 2n_1$, $c_2 = c_3 = 3c_1$. For this combination we should search just for n_1 and c_1. For example, if $N = 1000$, $n_1 = 200$, $n_2 = 400$, $c_1 = 3$, $c_2 = c_3 = 9$, we obtain OC$(0.01) = 0.9892$ and OC$(0.045) = 0.0114$. Here $\alpha = 0.01$ but $\beta = 0.01$. Let $\pi(p)$ be the probability that the two-stage sampling terminates after the first stage. This is

$$\pi(p) = 1 - \sum_{j=c_1+1}^{c_2-1} h(j; M, N, n). \tag{4.7.4}$$

Let N^* denote the total sample size, that is,

$$N^* = \begin{cases} n_1 & \text{if terminate after 1st stage,} \\ n_1 + n_2 & \text{otherwise.} \end{cases} \tag{4.7.5}$$

The expected total sample size is

$$\begin{aligned} E\{N^*; p) &= \pi(p)n_1 + (1 - \pi(p))(n_1 + n_2) \\ &= n_1 + n_2 \sum_{j=c_1+1}^{c_2-1} h(j; N_p, N, n). \end{aligned} \tag{4.7.6}$$

This expected total sample size is denoted also by ASN(p). For the above two-stage scheme $(200, 400, 3, 9, 9)$ the expected total sample size is ASN(0.01) = 247.9 and ASN(0.045) = 370.6. One could ask whether this two-stage sampling is more efficient than a single-stage sampling inspection by attribute. In a single sample there are two parameters, n, the sample size, and c, the test criterion. Letting X be the number of nonconforming items in an SRS(N, n) sample, we accept the lot if $X \leq c$ and reject it if $x > c$. For a given AQL, LTPD, α, and β we can determine n and c so that the Type I error probability is smaller than α and Type II error probability is smaller than β. In the present case of AQL = 0.01, LTPD = 0.045, $\alpha = \beta = 0.01$, we get that the single-stage sample should have $n = 318$ and $c = 7$.

Indeed, in such a test, if $\tilde{\alpha}$ and $\tilde{\beta}$ denote the probabilities of Type I and II errors, then

$$\tilde{\alpha} = 1 - H(7; \lfloor Np_0 \rfloor, N, n)$$

and

$$\tilde{\beta} = H(7; \lfloor Np_1 \rfloor, N, n).$$

We find that, for $N = 1000$, $p_0 = 0.01$, $p_1 = 0.045$, $n = 318$, $\tilde{\alpha} = 0.0023$, and $\tilde{\beta} = 0.0098$. On the other hand, if $n = 318$ and $c = 8$, we have $\tilde{\alpha} = 0.001$ and $\tilde{\beta} = 0.0286$. See Kenett and Zacks (1998, Chapter 9) for more details.

Comparing the two-stage procedure to the single-stage one, we find that if $p = 0.01$ the ASN is by 22% smaller than 318. On the other hand, if $p = 0.045$ the ASN is by 17% larger than 318. The indication is that if $p \leq$ AQL we should do a two-stage sampling with n_1 smaller than the required sample size of the corresponding single-stage sample. The value of c_1 can be found by a search so that $\tilde{\alpha}$ and $\tilde{\beta}$ will be smaller than the prescribed α and β.

4.7.2 Sequential Sampling for Attributes

The sequential procedure takes first an initial SRS(N, n) sample. Then, according to the Wald SPRT, it performs the likelihood ratio test and continues by drawing additional observations, one by one, until the stopping variable is attained. The stopping variable is

$$N_m = \min\left\{n : n \geq m, \log \frac{h(J_n; M_1, N, n)}{h(J_n; M_0, N, n)} \leq \log \frac{\beta}{1-\alpha} \quad \text{or} \quad \log \frac{h(J_n; M_1, N, n)}{h(J_n; M_0, N, n)} \geq \log \frac{1-\beta}{\alpha}\right\}, \tag{4.7.7}$$

where J_n is the number of nonconforming elements in a sample of size n. Also, if AQL $= p_0$ and LTPD $= p_1$, then $M_0 = [Np_0]$ and $M_1 = [Np_1]$. Here $[x]$ is the largest integer smaller or equal to x. If at the time of stopping $\log h(J_{N_m}; M_1, N, N_m) - \log h(J_{N_m}; M_0, N, N_m) \geq \log((1-\beta)/\alpha)$ the lot is rejected; otherwise the lot is accepted. For the theory of Wald SPRT see Chapter 10 and Siegmund (1985). One can immediately prove that, for the stopping variable (4.7.7), $\tilde{\alpha} + \tilde{\beta} \leq \alpha + \beta$. Table 4.8 presents simulation estimates of the characteristics of N_m based on 100 runs.

Table 4.8: Simulation Estimates of the Characteristics of $\mathbf{N_m}$, $\mathbf{N = 1000}$, $\mathbf{p_0 = 0.01}$, $\mathbf{p_1 = 0.045}$, $\boldsymbol{\alpha = \beta = 0.01}$, $\mathbf{m = 50}$

$[Np]$	$E\{N_m\}$	SE$\{N_m\}$	Quantiles		
			0.25	0.50	0.75
10	186.55	6.2337	156.5	157	203.5
45	91.47	5.4477	50	72	124.5

Derived using programs seqfpsim, seqfp2.

We see in Table 4.8 that when $p = p_0$ the expected value of N_m is considerably smaller than ASN(0.01) $= 247.9$ in the two-stage sampling with parameters $(200, 400, 3, 9, 9)$. The expected value of N_m when $p = 0.045$ is about $1/4$ of the corresponding ASN(0.045) for that two-stage sampling.

4.8 DYNAMIC BAYESIAN PREDICTION

Consider the normal regression model

$$\mathbf{Y}_N \sim N((X)\boldsymbol{\beta}, V), \tag{4.8.1}$$

where (X) is an $N \times p$ matrix of known covariates, $\boldsymbol{\beta}$ is an *unknown* vector of regression coefficients, and V is a *known* covariance matrix of $\mathbf{Y}_N$. In a Bayesian framework we assume that the prior distribution of $\boldsymbol{\beta}$ is normal, that is,

$$\boldsymbol{\beta} \sim N(\mathbf{b}, B). \tag{4.8.2}$$

Without loss of generality, assume that the sample $\mathbf{s}$ consists of the first n $(n < N)$ components of $\mathbf{Y}_N$. Thus, we partition

$$\mathbf{Y}'_N = (\mathbf{Y}'_s, \mathbf{Y}'_r),$$

where $\mathbf{Y}_r$ is the vector of the $N-n$ components of $\mathbf{Y}_N$ which are not in $\mathbf{s}$. Accordingly, partition V to

$$(V) = \left[\begin{array}{c|c} V_s & V_{sr} \\ \hline V_{rs} & V_r \end{array}\right].$$

The Bayesian predictor of $T = \mathbf{Y}'_N 1_N$ (see Bolfarine and Zacks, 1992, Chapter 3) is

$$\hat{T}_B = \mathbf{Y}'_n 1_n + 1'_{N-n}[(X)_r \hat{\boldsymbol{\beta}}_B + V_{rs}V_s^{-1}(\mathbf{Y}_s - (X)_s\hat{\boldsymbol{\beta}}_B)], \tag{4.8.3}$$

where $(X)' = ((X)'_s, (X)'_r)$ and

$$\hat{\boldsymbol{\beta}}_B = ((X)'_s V_s^{-1}(X)_s + B^{-1})^{-1}((X)'_s V_s^{-1}\mathbf{Y}_s + B^{-1}\mathbf{b}) \tag{4.8.4}$$

is the Bayesian estimator of $\boldsymbol{\beta}$. The prediction risk of $\hat{T}_B$ for the squared error loss is

(4.8.5)

$$\begin{aligned} E\{[\hat{T}_B - T]^2\} &= 1'_{N-n}[V_r - V_{rs}V_s^{-1}V_{sr}]1_{N-n} \\ &\quad + 1'_{N-n}[((X)_r - V_{rs}V_s^{-1}(X)_s)((X)'_s V_s^{-1}(X)_s + B^{-1})^{-1} \\ &\quad \cdot ((X)_r - V_{rs}V_s^{-1}(X)_s)']1_{N-n}. \end{aligned}$$

Suppose now that we have to predict T at a sequence of times. The time-related model is

$$\mathbf{Y}_t = (X)_t\boldsymbol{\beta}_t + \mathbf{e}_t, \quad t = 1, 2, \ldots, \tag{4.8.6}$$

where $\mathbf{e}_t \sim N(\mathbf{0}, V_t)$ and

$$\boldsymbol{\beta}_t = \Lambda_t \boldsymbol{\beta}_{t-1} + \mathbf{u}_t, \quad t = 1, 2, \ldots . \tag{4.8.7}$$

Furthermore $\mathbf{u}_t \sim N(\underset{\sim}{0}, \Delta_t)$; $\{\mathbf{u}_t\}$ and $\{\mathbf{e}_t\}$ are independent; V_t, Δ_t, and Λ_t are known. This model is called the *normal linear dynamic model.* In such a model we can use the data from previous time points to adaptively predict T at the present time. Let $\mathbf{y}_{ts}$ denote the sample vector at time t. The sample size is n at all t. Let $\mathcal{D}_t = (\mathcal{D}_{t-1}, \mathbf{y}_{ts})$ denote all the data up to time t and $\mathcal{D}_0$ the prior information at time $t = 0$.

Suppose that at time $t-1$

$$\boldsymbol{\beta}_{t-1} \mid \mathcal{D}_{t-1} \sim N(\mathbf{m}_{t-1}, C_{t-1}). \tag{4.8.8}$$

According to (4.8.7), before observing $\mathbf{y}_{ts}$,

$$\boldsymbol{\beta}_t \mid \mathcal{D}_{t-1} \sim N(\Lambda_t \mathbf{m}_{t-1}, R_t), \tag{4.8.9}$$

where

$$R_t = \Lambda_t C_{t-1}\Lambda'_t + \Delta_t. \tag{4.8.10}$$

After observing $\mathbf{y}_{ts}$,

$$\boldsymbol{\beta}_t \mid \mathcal{D}_t \sim N(\mathbf{m}_t, C_t). \tag{4.8.11}$$

In this equation

$$\mathbf{m}_t = (X'_{ts}V_{ts}^{-1}X_{ts} + R_t^{-1})^{-1}(X_{ts}V_{ts}^{-1}\mathbf{y}_{ts} + R_t^{-1}\Lambda_t\mathbf{m}_{t-1}) \tag{4.8.12}$$

and

$$C_t = (X'_{ts}V_{ts}^{-1}X_{ts} + R_t^{-1})^{-1}. \tag{4.8.13}$$

The dynamic Bayesian predictor of T_t is therefore

$$\hat{T}_{DBt} = n\mathbf{y}_{ts} + 1'_{N-n}[X_{tr}\mathbf{m}_t + V_{tr}V_{ts}^{-1}(\mathbf{y}_{ts} - X_{ts}\mathbf{m}_t)]. \tag{4.8.14}$$

For additional details and examples, see Bolfarine and Zacks (1992, Chapter 3). See also Section 5.7.

CHAPTER 5

ADAPTIVE PREDICTION AND FORECASTING IN TIME SERIES ANALYSIS

5.1 BASIC TOOLS OF TIME SERIES ANALYSIS

A time series (T.S.) is a sequence $\{X_t\}$, $t = 0, \pm 1, \pm 2, \ldots$, of random variables. The function $f(t) : t \rightarrow E\{X_t\}$ is called the trend of the T.S. A smooth trend can often be fitted to the T.S. data. Such a trend could be locally described by a polynomial of certain order plus a trigonometric Fourier sequence of orthogonal periodic functions. In Figure 5.1 we present a smooth trend function fitted to the DOW1941 data by the method of least squares (upper left); the residuals around the smooth trend (upper right); the scatter diagram of consecutive residuals (e_t, e_{t+1}), $t = 1, \ldots, 300$ (lower left); and the one-day-ahead forecasting of the index (lower right).

The fitted trend is

$$
\begin{aligned}
f(t) = 123.34 &+ 27.73\left(\frac{t-151}{302}\right) - 15.86\left(\frac{t-151}{302}\right)^2 \\
&- 237.90\left(\frac{t-151}{302}\right)^3 + 0.1512\cos\left(\frac{4\pi t}{302}\right) \\
&+ 1.738\sin\left(\frac{4\pi t}{302}\right) + 1.770\cos\left(\frac{8\pi t}{302}\right) \\
&- 0.208\sin\left(\frac{8\pi t}{302}\right) - 0.729\cos\left(\frac{12\pi t}{302}\right) \\
&+ 0.748\sin\left(\frac{12\pi t}{302}\right).
\end{aligned}
\tag{5.1.1}
$$

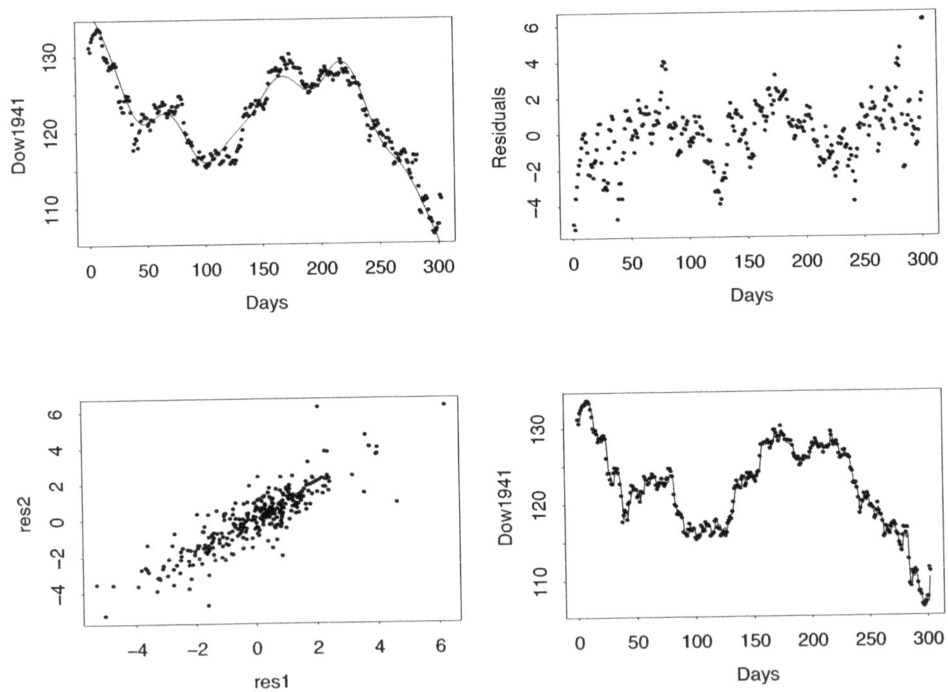

Figure 5.1

The residuals around the least squares fitted trend sum to zero. If $X_t = f(t) + U_t$, we assume that $\{U_t\}$ is a *covariance stationary* T.S. with $E\{U_t\} = 0$

for all $t = 0, \pm 1, \ldots$. A covariance stationary T.S. with $E\{U_t\} = 0$ for all t is such that

$$K(h) = \text{Cov}(U_t, U_{t+h}) = E\{U_t U_{t+h}\} \tag{5.1.2}$$

does not depend on t, $h = 0, \pm 1, \pm 2, \ldots$. Notice that $K(0) = V\{U_t\}$ is the constant variance. The simplest covariance stationary T.S. is $\{\epsilon_t\}$, where $E\{\epsilon_t\} = 0$ for all t and

$$\text{Cov}(\epsilon_t, \epsilon_{t'}) = \begin{cases} \sigma^2 & \text{if } t = t', \\ 0 & \text{if } t \neq t'. \end{cases}$$

This T.S. is called "white-noise" sequence, and we denote it by $\text{WN}(0, \sigma)^2$. A covariance stationary T.S.

$$X_t = \sum_{j=0}^{q} \beta_j \epsilon_{t-j} \tag{5.1.3}$$

is called a *moving average of order* q $(0 \leq q < \infty)$. We denote such a T.S. as $\text{MA}(q)$. The covariance function of an $\text{MA}(q)$ is

$$K(h) = \begin{cases} \sigma^2 \sum_{j=0}^{q-|h|} \beta_j \beta_{j+|h|}, & |h| = 0, \ldots, q, \\ 0, & |h| > q. \end{cases} \tag{5.1.4}$$

Notice that $K(h) = K(-h)$ for all $h = 0, \pm 1, \pm 2, \ldots$. A moving average T.S. of infinite order is

$$X_t = \sum_{j=-\infty}^{\infty} \beta_j \epsilon_{t-j}. \tag{5.1.5}$$

This random variable is defined in terms of the mean-squared limit, that is,

$$\lim_{M \to \infty} E\left\{\left[\sum_{j=-M}^{M} \beta_j \epsilon_{t-j} - X_t\right]^2\right\} = 0. \tag{5.1.6}$$

A sufficient condition for the existence of X_t is that $\sum_{j=-\infty}^{\infty} |\beta_j| < \infty$. A T.S. $\{X_t\}$ with $E\{X_t\} = 0$ for all t is called a p-order *autoregressive series* $\text{AR}(p)$ if

$$X_t + a_1 X_{t-1} + \cdots + a_p X_{t-p} = \epsilon_t, \quad \text{all } t, \tag{5.1.7}$$

where $\{\epsilon_t\}$ is a $\text{WN}(0, \sigma^2)$.

Let $\{y_t\}_{t\geq 0}$ be a sequence of real or complex variables. The z-transform of $\{y_t\}$ is defined formally as

$$Z\{y_t; z\} = \sum_{t=0}^{\infty} y_t z^{-t}, \tag{5.1.8}$$

where z is a complex number. The domain of convergence of $Z\{y_t; z\}$ is the region

$$R_c\{y\} = \{z : |z| > \limsup_{t\to\infty} |y_t|^{1/t}\}. \tag{5.1.9}$$

The z-transform is an analytic function of z within its domain of convergence. Also, if $F(z)$ is the z-transform of $\{y_t, t \geq 0\}$, then $z^{-m}F(z)$ is the z-transform of $\{y_{t-m}, t \geq 0\}$ for $z \in R_c\{y\}$. Thus, we can formally write the z-transform of the AR(p) (5.1.7) as

$$A_p(z) = 1 + a_1 z^{-1} + \cdots + a_p z^{-p} \tag{5.1.10}$$

with region of absolute convergence

$$R_c\{\mathbf{a}_p\} = \{z : |z| > 0\}, \tag{5.1.11}$$

where $\mathbf{a}_p = (1, a_1, \ldots, a_p)'$. Assume $A_p(z)$ is a polynomial of degree p in z^{-1}. The AR(p) model (5.1.7) can be written as

$$A_p(z) X_t = \epsilon_t, \quad t = 0, \pm 1, \pm 2, \ldots . \tag{5.1.12}$$

Since $|z| > 0$, we can write

$$A_p(z) = z^{-p} A_p^*(z), \tag{5.1.13}$$

where

$$A_p^*(z) = a_p + a_{p-1} z + \cdots + a_1 z^{p-1} + z^p, \tag{5.1.14}$$

$A_p^*(z)$ called the *characteristic polynomial* of the AR(p). The roots of $A_p^*(z) = 0$, $\zeta_1, \ldots, \zeta_p$, are called the *characteristic roots* of the AR(p).

Criterion for the covariance stationarity of an AR(p) T.S.: If the characteristic roots are all *within the unit disk*, then the AR(p) is covariance stationary, and one can represent the AR(p) as an infinite MA sequence

$$\begin{aligned} X_t &= \sum_{j=0}^{\infty} \beta_j z^{-j} \epsilon_t \\ &= \sum_{j=0}^{\infty} \beta_j \epsilon_{t-j}, \end{aligned} \tag{5.1.15}$$

where

$$A_p(z^{-1})^{-1} = \sum_{j=0}^{\infty} \beta_j z^{-j}. \tag{5.1.16}$$

For example, consider the AR(2)

$$X_t - X_{t-1} + 0.89X_{t-2} = \epsilon_t, \quad t = 0, \pm 1, \dots .$$

The characteristic polynomial is $A_2^*(z) = 0.89 - z + z^2$. The two characteristic roots are

$$\zeta_1 = 0.5 + 0.8i \text{ and } \zeta_2 = 0.5 - 0.8i.$$

These roots are within the unit disk. Moreover

$$\frac{1}{A_2(1/z)} = 1+\frac{1}{z}+0.11\left(\frac{1}{z}\right)^2-0.78\left(\frac{1}{z}\right)^3-0.8779\left(\frac{1}{z}\right)^4-0.1837\left(\frac{1}{z}\right)^5+\cdots .$$

Thus, this AR(2) is covariance stationary and can be represented as

$$X_t = \epsilon_t + \epsilon_{t-1} + 0.11\epsilon_{t-2} - 0.78\epsilon_{t-3} - 0.8779\epsilon_{t-4} + \cdots .$$

The covariance function $K(h)$ of a covariance stationary AR(p) can be determined by solving the *Yule–Walker equations*

$$\begin{aligned} K(h) + a_1K(h-1) + \cdots + a_pK(h-p) &= 0, \quad h > 0 \\ K(0) + a_1K(1) + \cdots + a_pK(p) &= \sigma^2. \end{aligned} \tag{5.1.17}$$

For example, for $p = 2$, the $K(h)$ for $h = 0, 1, 2$ are determined by solving

$$\begin{bmatrix} 1 & a_1 & a_2 \\ a_1 & 1+a_2 & 0 \\ a_2 & a_1 & 1 \end{bmatrix} \begin{bmatrix} K(0) \\ K(1) \\ K(2) \end{bmatrix} = \begin{bmatrix} \sigma^2 \\ 0 \\ 0 \end{bmatrix},$$

and for $h \geq 3$ we use the recursive equation

$$K(h) = -a_1K(h-1) - a_2K(h-2).$$

The correlation function is

$$\rho(h) = \frac{K(h)}{K(0)}. \tag{5.1.18}$$

A T.S. of the form

$$X_t + a_2X_{t-1} + \cdots + a_pX_t = \epsilon_t + b_1\epsilon_{t-1} + \cdots + b_q\epsilon_{t-q} \tag{5.1.19}$$

is called an autoregressive moving average ARMA(p, q). If the characteristic roots $\zeta_1, \ldots, \zeta_p$ of $A_p^*(z)$ are within the unit disk, we can write

$$\begin{aligned} X_t &= \sum_{j=0}^{\infty} \beta_j z^{-j}(1 + b_1 z^{-1} + \cdots + b_q z^{-q})\epsilon_t \\ &= \sum_{k=0}^{\infty} v_k z^{-k} \epsilon_t. \end{aligned} \tag{5.1.20}$$

The coefficients $\{v_k\}$ can be obtained by a series expansion of the *transfer function*

$$C_{p,q}(x) = \frac{B_q(x)}{A_p(x)}, \tag{5.1.21}$$

where

$$A_p(x) = 1 + a_1 x + \cdots + a_p x^p$$

and

$$B_q(x) = 1 + b_1 x + \cdots + b_q x^q.$$

The symmetric matrix of $k-1$ lag correlations,

$$R_k = \begin{bmatrix} 1 & \rho(1) & \rho(2) & \rho(3) & \cdots & \rho(k-1) \\ \rho(1) & 1 & \rho(1) & \rho(2) & \cdots & \rho(k-2) \\ \rho(2) & \rho(1) & 1 & \rho(1) & \cdots & \rho(k-3) \\ \rho(3) & \rho(2) & \rho(1) & 1 & \ddots & \vdots \\ \vdots & \vdots & \vdots & \ddots & & \\ \rho(k-1) & \rho(k-2) & \rho(k-3) & & & 1 \end{bmatrix}, \tag{5.1.22}$$

is called a *Toeplitz matrix*.

The partial autocorrelation of lag k is the correlation between $X_{t+k-1} - \hat{X}_{t+k+1}^{(k)}$ and $X_t - \sum_{j=1}^{k} \phi_j^{(k)} X_{t+j}$, where $\hat{X}_{t+k+1}^{(k)} = \sum_{j=1}^{k} \phi_j^{(k)} X_{t+k+1-j}$. The least squares vector $\boldsymbol{\phi}^{(k)}$ is the solution of the normal equations

$$R_k \boldsymbol{\phi}^{(k)} = \boldsymbol{\rho}_k, \tag{5.1.23}$$

where $\boldsymbol{\rho}_k = (\rho(1), \ldots, \rho(k))'$.

One obtains the following formula for the partial correlation of lag $k+1$:

$$\rho^*(k+1) = \frac{\rho(k+1) - \boldsymbol{\rho}_k' R_k^{-1} P_k \boldsymbol{\rho}_k}{1 - \boldsymbol{\rho}_k' R_k^{-1} \boldsymbol{\rho}_k}. \tag{5.1.24}$$

Here P_k is the permutation matrix

$$P_k = \begin{pmatrix} & & & & & 1 \\ & \ddots & & & & \\ & & 0 & & 1 & \\ & & & 1 & & \\ & & \ddots & & 0 & \\ & & & & & \ddots \\ 1 & & & & & \end{pmatrix}.$$

The partial autocorrelation function is used to determine whether a T.S. is an AR(p). One can prove that if AR(p) is covariance stationary then

(5.1.25) $$\rho^*(h) = 0 \quad \text{for } |h| > p.$$

5.2 LINEAR PREDICTORS FOR COVARIANCE STATIONARY T.S.

Let $\{X_t\}$ be a covariance stationary T.S. such that $X_t = \sum_{j=0}^{\infty} w_j \epsilon_{t-j}$ and where $\epsilon_t \sim \text{WN}(0, \sigma^2)$. Notice that $E\{X_t\} = 0$ for all t. Let $K(h)$, $h = 0, \pm 1, \pm 2, \ldots$, be the covariance function of $\{X_t\}$.

5.2.1 Optimal Linear Predictors

A linear predictor of X_{t+s} based on $\mathbf{X}_t^{(n)} = (X_t, X_{t-1}, \ldots, X_{t-n+1})'$ is

(5.2.1) $$\hat{X}_{t+s}^{(n)}(t) = \mathbf{b}_s^{(n)\prime} \mathbf{X}_t^{(n)},$$

where

$$\mathbf{b}_s^{(n)} = (b_{0,s}^{(n)}, \ldots, b_{n-1,s}^{(n)})'.$$

The PMSE of this linear predictor is given by

(5.2.2)
$$\text{PMSE}(\hat{X}_{t+s}^{(n)}(t)) = \text{Var}\{\mathbf{b}_s^{(n)\prime} \mathbf{X}_t^{(n)}\} - 2\,\text{Cov}(X_{t+s}, \mathbf{b}_s^{(n)\prime} \mathbf{X}_t^{(n)}) + V\{X_{t+s}\}.$$

Let Σ_n be the covariance matrix of $\mathbf{X}_t^{(n)}$, which is the Toeplitz matrix $\Sigma_n = K(0) R_n$, as defined in Eq. (5.1.22). The covariance of X_{t+s} and $\mathbf{X}_t^{(n)}$ is

(5.2.3) $$\boldsymbol{\gamma}_s^{(n)} = K(0) \begin{pmatrix} \rho(s) \\ \rho(s+1) \\ \vdots \\ \rho(n+s-1) \end{pmatrix}.$$

We can write the prediction MSE of $\hat{X}_{t+s}^{(n)}(t)$ as

(5.2.4) $$\begin{aligned} \text{PMSE}(\hat{X}_{t+s}^{(n)}(t)) &= \mathbf{b}_s^{(n)\prime} \Sigma_n \mathbf{b}_s^{(n)} - 2\mathbf{b}_s^{(n)\prime} \boldsymbol{\gamma}_s^{(n)} + K(0) \\ &= K(0)(\mathbf{b}_s^{(n)\prime} R_n \mathbf{b}_s^{(n)} - 2\mathbf{b}_s^{(n)} \boldsymbol{\rho}_s^{(n)} + 1), \end{aligned}$$

where $\boldsymbol{\rho}_s^{(n)} = \boldsymbol{\gamma}_s^{(n)}/K(0)$. The gradient of the PMSE with respect to (w.r.t.) $\mathbf{b}_s^{(n)}$ is

$$\nabla_b \text{PMSE} = 2\Sigma_n \mathbf{b} - 2\boldsymbol{\gamma}_s^{(n)}.$$

Thus, the optimal $\mathbf{b}$ vector is

$$\hat{\mathbf{b}}_s^{(n)} = \Sigma_n^{-1}\boldsymbol{\gamma}_s^{(n)} = R_n^{-1}\rho_s^{(n)}. \tag{5.2.5}$$

Thus, we have proven:

Theorem 5.2.1 *The optimal linear predictor based on $X_t^{(n)}$ is*

$$\hat{X}_{t+s}^{(n)}(t) = \boldsymbol{\gamma}_s^{(n)\prime}\Sigma_n^{-1}\mathbf{X}_t^{(n)} = \boldsymbol{\rho}_s^{(n)} R_n^{-1}\mathbf{X}_t^{(n)}. \tag{5.2.6}$$

■

Notice that

$$E\{\hat{X}_{t+s}^{(n)}(t)\} = 0 \tag{5.2.7}$$

and

$$\text{PMSE}\{\hat{X}_{t+s}^{(n)}(t)\} = K(0)(1 - \boldsymbol{\rho}_s^{(n)\prime} R_n^{-1}\boldsymbol{\rho}_s^{(n)}). \tag{5.2.8}$$

■ **EXAMPLE 5.1**

Let $\{X_t\}$ be a moving average smoother MAS(1) given by

$$X_t = a_{-1}\epsilon_{t-1} + a_0\epsilon_t + a_1\epsilon_{t+1}, \quad t = 0, \pm 1, \ldots,$$

where $\epsilon_t \sim \text{WN}(0, \sigma^2)$. In this case,

$$\begin{aligned}
K(0) &= \sigma^2(a_{-1}^2 + a_0^2 + a_1^2) = B_0\sigma^2, \\
K(1) &= \sigma^2(a_{-1}a_0 + a_0a_1) = B_1\sigma^2, \\
K(2) &= \sigma^2 a_{-1}a_1 = B_2\sigma^2,
\end{aligned}$$

and $K(h) = 0$ for all $|h| > 2$.

Obviously, $\boldsymbol{\gamma}_n^{(s)} = \mathbf{0}$ if $s > 2$. Thus,

$$\hat{X}_{t+s}^{(n)}(t) \equiv 0 \quad \text{for all} \quad s > 2.$$

If $s = 2$, then

$$\boldsymbol{\gamma}_2^{(n)} = \sigma^2(B_2, 0, \ldots, 0)'$$

and

$$\hat{\mathbf{b}}_2^{(n)} = \sigma^2\Sigma_n^{-1}\begin{pmatrix} B_2 \\ \mathbf{0}_{n-1} \end{pmatrix}.$$

If $s = 1$, then

$$\gamma_1^{(n)} = \sigma^2(B_1, B_2, 0, \ldots)'$$

and

$$\hat{b}_1^{(n)} = \sigma^2 \Sigma_n^{-1} \begin{pmatrix} B_1 \\ B_2 \\ 0 \end{pmatrix}.$$

Since $K(h) = 0$ for all $|h| > 2$, we construct the predictor with $n = 3$. In this case with $a_{-1} = 0.25$, $a_0 = 0.5$, $a_1 = 0.25$, $\sigma = 1$, we have

$$\Sigma_3 = \frac{1}{16} \begin{pmatrix} 6 & 4 & 1 \\ 4 & 6 & 4 \\ 1 & 4 & 6 \end{pmatrix},$$

$$\gamma_1^{(3)} = \frac{1}{16}(4, 1, 0), \quad \gamma_2^{(3)} = \frac{1}{16}(1, 0, 0)'.$$

Thus,

$$\mathbf{b}_1^{(3)} = (1.2, -0.9, 0.4)'$$

and

$$b_2^{(3)} = (0.4, -0.4, 0.2)'.$$

Finally, the best linear predictors are

$$\hat{X}_{t+1}^{(3)}(t) = 1.2X_t - 0.9X_{t-1} + 0.4X_{t-2}$$

and

$$\hat{X}_{t+2}^{(3)}(t) = 0.4X_t - 0.4X_{t-1} + 0.2X_{t-2}.$$

The PMSEs of these predictors are

$$\text{PMSE}(\hat{X}_{t+1}^{(3)}(t)) = 0.1492$$

and

$$\text{PMSE}(\hat{X}_{t+2}^{(3)}(t)) = 0.3410.$$

The predictor $\hat{X}_{t+2}^{(3)}(t)$ is obviously less accurate than $\hat{X}_{t+1}^{(3)}(t)$. In Figure 5.2 we present $\hat{X}_{t+s}(t)$ against X_t for $s = 1$ (full line) and $s = 2$ (dotted line). We see that the predictor for $s = 2$ is of no value. The correlation between X_{t+1} and $\hat{X}_{t+1}(t)$ is $r = 0.822$, which shows that the one-step ahead predictor is quite effective. ■

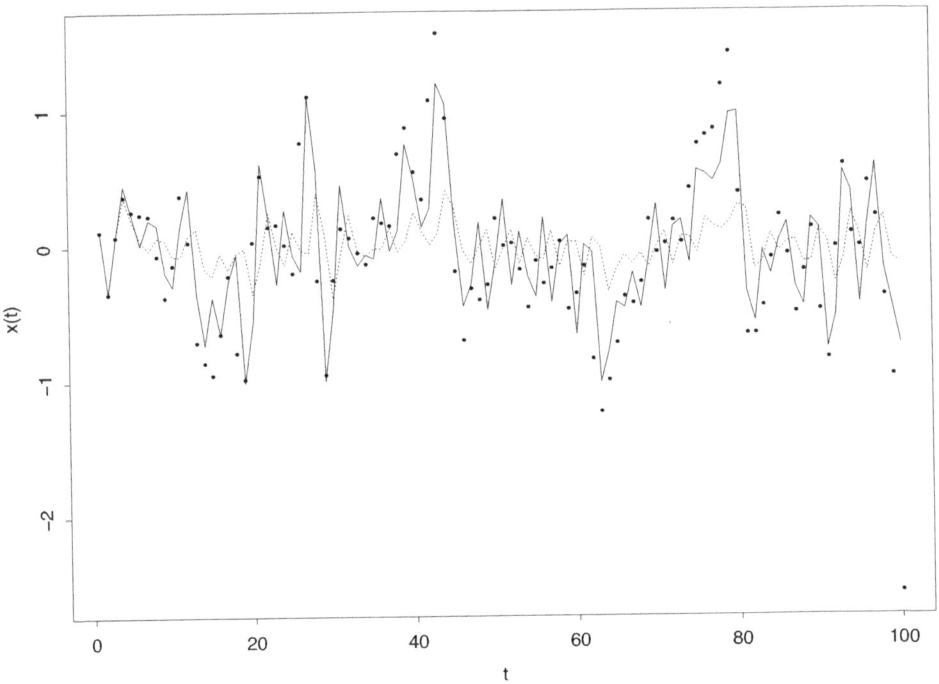

Figure 5.2. Best linear predictors, s = 1 (full line), s = 2 (dotted line).

■ EXAMPLE 5.2

Consider the AR(1) time series

$$X_t = aX_{t-1} + \epsilon_t,$$

where $\epsilon_t \sim \mathrm{WN}(0, 1)$ and $|a| < 1$. This is a covariance stationary T.S. with covariance function

$$K(h) = \frac{a^h}{1 - a^2}, \quad h = 0, \pm 1, \pm 2, \ldots .$$

We develop the formula for $\hat{X}_{t+1}^{(n)}(t)$. The covariance matrix of $\mathbf{X}_t^{(n)}$ is

$$\Sigma_n = \frac{1}{1-a^2}\begin{bmatrix} 1 & a & a^2 & \cdots & a^{n-1} \\ a & 1 & a & \cdots & a^{n-2} \\ \vdots & \vdots & \vdots & \ddots & a \\ a^{n-1} & a^{n-2} & \cdots & a & 1 \end{bmatrix}.$$

The vector $\boldsymbol{\gamma}_1^{(n)}$ is

$$\boldsymbol{\gamma}_1^{(n)} = \frac{1}{1-a^2}(a, a^2, \ldots, a^n).$$

Accordingly, the best linear predictor has coefficients

$$\mathbf{b}_1^{(n)} = \begin{bmatrix} 1 & a & \cdots & a^{n-1} \\ a & 1 & \cdots & a^{n-2} \\ \vdots & & \ddots & \vdots \\ a^{n-1} & & & 1 \end{bmatrix}^{-1} \begin{bmatrix} a \\ a^2 \\ \vdots \\ a^n \end{bmatrix} = \begin{bmatrix} a \\ 0 \\ 0 \\ \vdots \\ 0 \end{bmatrix}.$$

This result can be proven by using Cramér's method. Thus, $\hat{X}_{t+1}^{(n)}(t) = aX_t$, $t = 0, \pm 1, \ldots$. The PMSE of $\hat{X}_{t+1}^{(n)}(t)$ is

$$\begin{aligned} \text{PMSE} &= E\{(aX_t - X_{t+1})^2\} \\ &= K(0)[(1+a^2) - 2a\rho(1)] \\ &= \frac{1+a^2}{1-a^2} - \frac{2a^2}{1-a^2} = 1. \end{aligned}$$

More generally, the best predictor of X_{t+s} is $\hat{X}_{t+s}(t) = a^s X_t$. The PMSE of this optimal predictor is

$$\text{PMSE}(\hat{X}_{t+s}(t)) = \frac{1-a^{2s}}{1-a^2}.$$

Notice that also, here, the optimal predictor pulls the predictor toward the mean, zero. The PMSE grows from 1 to approximately $(1-a^2)^{-1}$ for large s. ■

5.2.2 Minimal PMSE Predictors for AR(p) T.S.

In the case of an AR(p) time series, the optimal predictor for the PMSE is the conditional expectation $E\{X_{t+s} \mid \mathbf{X}_t^{(p)}\}$, where $\mathbf{X}_t^{(p)} = (X_t, X_{t-1}, \ldots, X_{t-p+1})'$. Indeed, if $\mathbf{X}_t$ denotes the vector of all observations up to time t, $\mathbf{X}_t = (X_t, X_{t-1}, \ldots)$, then the function $\hat{P}(\mathbf{X}_t)$, which minimizes the PMSE, is $E\{X_{t+s} \mid$

$\mathbf{X}_t\}$. If we assume that the $\{\epsilon_t\}$ *are independent random variables with* $E\{\epsilon_t\} = 0$ and $V\{\epsilon_t\} = \sigma^2$, then

$$E\{\epsilon_t \mid \mathbf{X}_{t-1}\} = 0 \quad \text{for all} \quad t, \tag{5.2.9}$$

and

$$\begin{aligned} E\{X_{t+1} \mid \mathbf{X}_t\} &= E\left\{\sum_{j=1}^{p} a_j X_{t+1-j} + \epsilon_{t+1} \mid \mathbf{X}_t\right\} \\ &= a_1 X_t + a_2 X_{t-1} + \cdots + a_p X_{t-p+1} \\ &= \mathbf{a}^{(p)\prime}\mathbf{X}_t^{(p)}, \end{aligned} \tag{5.2.10}$$

where $\mathbf{a}^{(p)} = (a_1, a_2, \ldots, a_p)'$. Thus, $E\{X_{t+1} \mid \mathbf{X}_t\}$ depends only on $\mathbf{X}_t^{(p)}$. Similarly,

$$\begin{aligned} E\{X_{t+2} \mid \mathbf{X}_t\} &= E\left\{a_1 X_{t+1} + \sum_{j=2}^{p} a_j X_{t+2-j} + e_{t+2} \mid \mathbf{X}_t\right\} \\ &= \sum_{j=2}^{p} a_j X_{t+2-j} + a_1 E\{X_{t+1} \mid \mathbf{X}_t^{(p)}\} \\ &= \sum_{j=0}^{p-2} a_{j+2} X_{t-j} + a_1 \left(\sum_{j=0}^{p-1} a_{j+1} X_{t-j}\right) \\ &= \mathbf{a}_2^{(p)\prime}\mathbf{X}_t^{(p)}, \end{aligned} \tag{5.2.11}$$

where $\mathbf{a}_2^{(p)\prime} = (a_{j,2}^{(p)})$ and

$$a_{j,2} = a_1 a_{j+1} + I\{j \le p-2\} a_{j+2}, \quad j = 0, \ldots, p-1.$$

Thus, the best predictor of X_{t+2} is the linear predictor $\hat{X}_{t+2}(t) = \sum_{j=0}^{p-1} a_{j,2}^{(p)} X_{t-j}$. In a similar fashion we can show that the best predictor of X_{t+s} is a linear predictor $\mathbf{a}_s^{(p)\prime}\mathbf{X}_t^{(p)}$. A recursive formula for $\mathbf{a}_s^{(p)}$ can be determined as above.

The assumption that the $\{\epsilon_t\}$ are i.i.d. is stronger than the usual assumption that $\epsilon_t \sim \text{WN}(0, \sigma^2)$. With the weaker assumption we can get similar results by considering the best *linear* predictor.

Theorem 5.2.2 *For an AR(p)* $X_t + \alpha_1 X_{t-1} + \cdots + \alpha_p X_{t-p} = \epsilon_t$, $\hat{X}_{t+1}(t) = \sum_{i=1}^{p} a_i X_{t+1-i}$, *where* $a_i = -\alpha_i$ $(i = 1, \ldots, p)$. *Furthermore,*

$$PMSE\{\hat{X}_{t+1}(t)\} = E(X_{t+1} - \hat{X}_{t+1}(t))^2 = \sigma^2. \tag{5.2.12}$$

■

Indeed, $X_{t+1} - \sum_{i=1}^{p} a_i X_{t+1-i} = \epsilon_{t+1}$ according to the model. Hence $\text{PMSE}\{\hat{X}_{t+1}(t)\} = \sigma^2$.

■ **EXAMPLE 5.3**

Given a covariance stationary time series AR(2),

$$X_t = a_1 X_{t-1} + a_2 X_{t-2} + \epsilon_t,$$

where $\{\epsilon_t\}$ are i.i.d. $(0, \sigma^2)$. The best predictor of X_{t+2} is

$$\hat{X}^{(2)}_{t+2}(t) = (a_1^2 + a_2)X_t + a_1 a_2 X_{t-1}.$$

The PMSE of this predictor when $E\{X_t\} = 0$ for all t is

$$\begin{aligned}\text{PMSE}\{\hat{X}^{(2)}_{t+2}(t)\} = {} & K(0)[1 + a_1^2 a_2^2 + (a_1^2 + a_2)^2] + 2K(1)a_1 a_2 (a_1^2 + a_2) \\ & - 2K(2)(a_1^2 + a_2) - 2K(3) \cdot a_1 a_2.\end{aligned}$$

The covariance function $K(h)$ is determined according to the formula developed in the previous section. ■

5.2.3 Prediction with Unknown Covariance Structure

When the covariance function $K(h)$ is unknown and $E\{X_t\} = 0$, the optimal linear predictor $\hat{X}^{(n)}_{t+s}(t)$ cannot be determined. When the number of observations available up to time t is large, one can estimate the autocorrelations and substitute the estimates of the autocorrelations in Eq. (5.2.5) to have an estimate of the optimal linear coefficients $\hat{\mathbf{b}}_s^{(n)}$. What should be the value of the predictor when the sample size (number of observations) is small? How large should t be so that the estimated autocorrelations will yield good estimates of the optimal linear coefficients in $\mathbf{b}_s^{(n)}$? We illustrate the problem by example.

■ **EXAMPLE 5.4**

Consider an MA(2) T.S. given by

$$X_t = \epsilon_t + 0.5\epsilon_{t-1} + 0.25\epsilon_{t-2}, \quad t = 0, \pm 1, \ldots,$$

where $\epsilon_t \sim \text{WN}(0, 1)$. The autocorrelation function (ACF) of this T.S. is

$$\rho(h) = \begin{cases} 0.4762, & |h| = 1, \\ 0.1905, & |h| = 2, \\ 0, & |h| > 2. \end{cases}$$

In Figure 5.3(a) we present a realization of this T.S. and in Figure 5.3(b) its ACF based on $T = 100$ observations. Based on 100 observations we have the estimates $\hat{\rho}(1) = 0.5550$ and $\hat{\rho}(2) = 0.2076$ while all other autocorrelations are not significantly different from zero. Are these estimates of $\rho(1)$ and $\rho(2)$ significantly different from the true values? In the Appendix we find an SPLUS function, simul.acfma, according to which one can simulate the estimates of the autocorrelation functions of MA(q). In these simulations ϵ_t are i.i.d. $N(0,1)$.

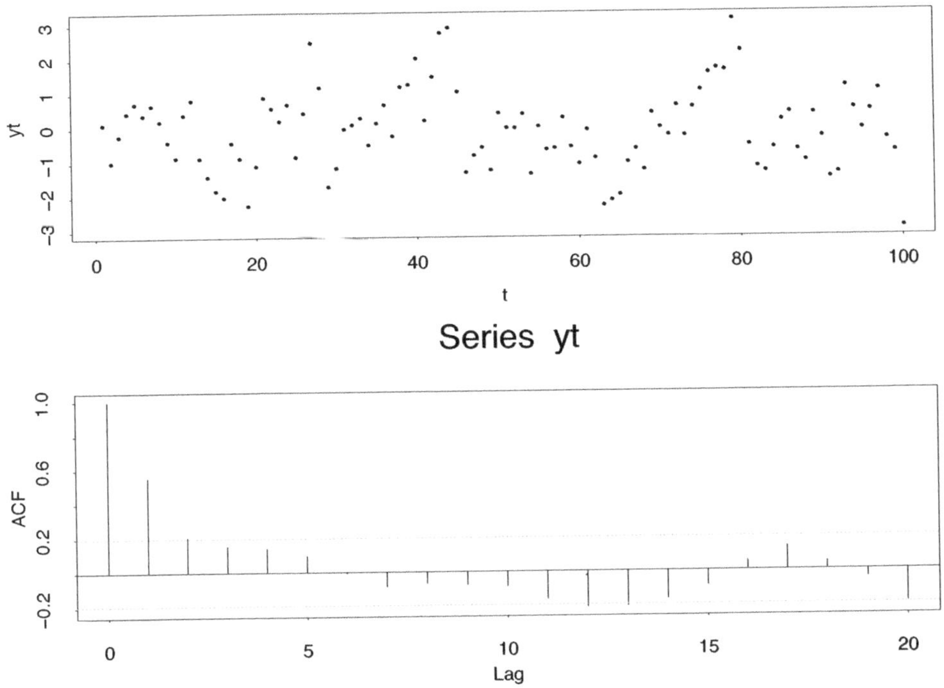

Figure 5.3: (a) A Sample of 100 MA(2) T.S. and (b) ACF of a sample of 100 MA(2) T.S.

In this function the argument ns stands for the number of simulation runs, n is for the sample size, iq is the order of the MA($\cdot$), and a is a collection set of the coefficients $a_1, \ldots, a_q$ of the MA. Such a simulation with $ns = 1000$, $n = 25, 50, 100$, $iq = 2$, and $A = (0.5, 0.25)$ gave the following results:

	$n = 25$	$n = 50$	$n = 100$	∞
$\bar{\rho}(1)$	0.3888	0.4412	0.4472	0.4762
$\bar{\rho}(2)$	0.0946	0.1335	0.1597	0.1905
STD$\{\hat{\rho}(1)\}$	0.1488	0.1226	0.0839	0
STD$\{\hat{\rho}(2)\}$	0.02111	0.01493	0.01043	0

These simulations indicate that if we have an MA(2) T.S. we need more than 100 observations to get close estimates of the correlation function. ■

Adaptive Prediction Procedure

We propose the following *adaptive procedure*:

1. After $T = 20$ observations, estimate the autocorrelation function for $h = 1, \ldots, 10$ using the SPLUS command

$$\text{ak} \leftarrow \text{acf(x, 10, plot} = \text{F)}.$$

2. Determine the best linear coefficient vector $\mathbf{b}_s^{(10)}$ for the desired s using the estimated autocorrelations and Eq. (5.2.5). For this purpose we can use the SPLUS functions toeplitz and pred1 given in the Appendix.

The result given by the function pred1 is the prediction of X_{t+1} given by $\hat{X}_{t+1}(t)$.

■ **EXAMPLE 5.5**

In the present example we compute the predicted values of $X_{21}, \ldots, X_{100}$ in a sequence of $T = 100$ values realized by the MA(2) T.S. $X_t = \epsilon_t + 0.5\epsilon_{t-1} + 0.25\epsilon_{t-2}$, $\epsilon_t \sim N(0, 1)$. The first 20 values of X_t are used for the initial estimates. In Figure 5.4 we show the results of this ad hoc prediction procedure, in comparison to the optimal linear predictor, which can be used if $\rho(h)$ is known. The predicted values were computed by using the SPLUS functions pred1 and toeplitz, which are in the Appendix. ■

5.2.4 ARIMA Forecasting

ARIMA forecasting, known also as Box–Jenkin forecasting (Box, Jenkins, and Reinsel, 1994), is an appropriate method when $\{X_t\}$ has an ARIMA(p, d, q) structure. Thus, assume that the T.S. $\{X_t\}$ has the structure

$$A_p(z^{-1})(1 - z^{-1})^d X_t = B_q(z^{-1})\epsilon_t, \tag{5.2.13}$$

$t = 0, \pm 1, \ldots$, where $\epsilon_t \sim$ i.i.d.$(0, \sigma^2)$.

Let $(B_q(z^{-1}))^{-1} = \sum_{j=0}^{\infty} \psi_j z^{-j}$. If the characteristic roots of $B_q^*(z)$ are all within the unit circle, then $\sum_{j=0}^{\infty} |\psi_j| < \infty$. Thus, the ARIMA can be expressed as an AR(∞)

$$\sum_{j=0}^{\infty} \pi_j z^{-j} X_t = \epsilon_t, \quad t = 0, \pm 1, \ldots, \tag{5.2.14}$$

where

$$\pi_j = \sum_{l=0}^{j} \psi_l c_{j-l}, \quad j = 0, 1, \ldots, \tag{5.2.15}$$

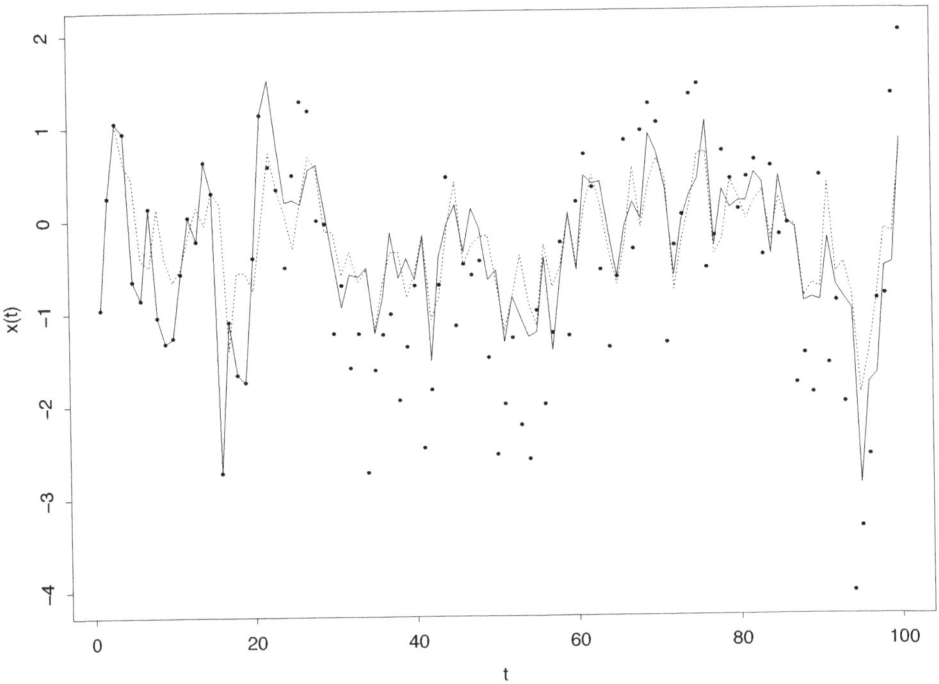

Figure 5.4: Optimal (broken line) and adaptive (solid line) predictors for MA(2), s = 1.

and

$$c_k = \sum_{i=0}^{k} (-1)^i \binom{d}{i} a_{k-i}, \quad k \geq 0.$$

Notice that if $q = 0$ then $\pi_j = 0$ for all $j > p + d$. In this case we can write

$$X_t = -\sum_{j=1}^{p+d} c_j X_{t-j} + \epsilon_t. \tag{5.2.16}$$

Consider the PMSE $E\{(\hat{X}_{t+s}(t) - X_{t+s})^2\}$ of the predictor $\hat{X}_{t+s}(t)$ of X_{t+s}. Let $\mathcal{F}_t = \sigma(X_t, X_{t-1}, \ldots)$ be the σ-field generated by the "history" of the process. The predictor which minimizes the PMSE is the conditional expectation of X_{t+s} given $\mathcal{F}_t$, that is,

$$\hat{X}^0_{t+s}(t) = E\{X_{t+s} \mid \mathcal{F}_t\}. \tag{5.2.17}$$

Thus, the optimal PMSE predictor of X_{t+1} at time t is

$$\hat{X}^0_{t+1}(t) = -\sum_{j=0}^{\infty} \pi_{j+1} X_{t-j} \tag{5.2.18}$$

since $E\{\epsilon_{t+1} \mid \mathcal{F}_t\} = 0$. For $s = 2$,

$$\hat{X}^0_{t+2}(t) = -\pi_1 E\{X_{t+1} \mid \mathcal{F}_t\} - \pi_2 X_t - \pi_3 X_{t-1} - \cdots . \tag{5.2.19}$$

Or

$$\begin{aligned} \hat{X}^0_{t+2}(t) &= -\pi_1 \left(-\sum_{j=0}^{\infty} \pi_{j+1} X_{t-j} \right) - \sum_{j=0}^{\infty} \pi_{j+2} X_{t-j} \\ &= -\sum_{j=0}^{\infty} (\pi_{j+2} - \pi_{j+1}\pi_1) X_{t-j}. \end{aligned} \tag{5.2.20}$$

Generally, for $s \geq 2$,

$$\hat{X}^0_{t+s}(t) = -\pi_1 \hat{X}^0_{t+s+1}(t) - \cdots - \pi_{s-1} \hat{X}^0_{t+1}(t) - \sum_{j=0}^{\infty} \pi_{j+s} X_{t-j}. \tag{5.2.21}$$

To apply this method one needs first to know the values of the regression coefficients $\{\pi_j\}$ and to decide how many terms to use. In the ARIMA$(p, d, 0)$ model, the number of nonzero coefficients π_j is only $p + d$.

■ EXAMPLE 5.6

Analysis of the third-order differencing of the DOW1941 data shows that we can fit to the data an ARIMA$(7, 3, 0)$ series. We use 10 nonzero π_j values given by the expansion of

$$\begin{aligned} &(1 + 1.006X + 0.906X^2 + 0.638X^3 + 0.386X^4 + 0.283X^5 \\ &\quad + 0.209X^6 + 0.157X^7)(1 - 3X + 3X^2 - X^3). \end{aligned}$$

For $s = 1$ we obtain the predictor

$$\begin{aligned} \hat{X}^0_{t+1}(t) = {} & 1.994X_t - 0.888X_{t-1} + 0.062X_{t-2} - 0.184X_{t-3} \\ & - 0.133X_{t-4} + 0.120X_{t-5} + 0.007X_{t-6} + 0.127X_{t-7} \\ & - 0.262X_{t-8} + 0.157X_{t-9}. \end{aligned}$$

In Figure 5.5 we see the predictor $\hat{X}^0_{t+1}(t)$ plotted (lines) together with the X_t values. Here PMSE $= 1.18134$. ■

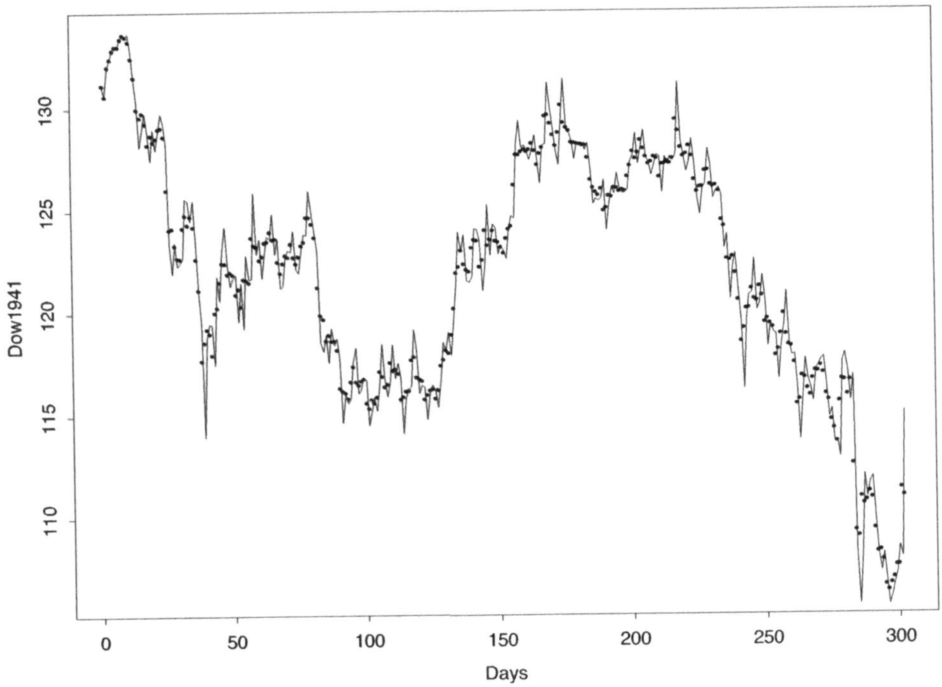

Figure 5.5: ARIMA(7,3,0) one-day-ahead predictor.

5.3 QUADRATIC LSE PREDICTORS FOR NONSTATIONARY T.S.

Generally, the time series investigated in the present section have covariance stationary residuals around an unknown trend function $f(t)$. In Section 5.1 several methods for fitting a trend function to data were mentioned. For predicting the value of X_{t+s}, $s \geq 1$, at time t, one should be able to estimate $f(t+s)$ from the data up to time t. Moreover, if the correlation structure of the residuals is known or can be estimated, one should try to reduce the prediction MSE by applying Eq. (5.2.5) for predicting the residual component. If the residuals around $f(t)$ are white noise, then the best PMSE predictor is $f(t+s)$, and it is sufficient to estimate this value of the trend. In the present section we discuss two types of predictors which fit to a neighborhood of X_t a quadratic trend by which X_{t+s} is predicted. Such methods are usually reliable only for small values of s.

For a specified n, $n \geq 5$, we fit a polynomial of degree $p = 2$ (quadratic) to the last n observations. Given this polynomial, we extrapolate to estimate

$f(t+s)$, $s \geq 1$. This approach is based on the assumption that in a close neighborhood of t, say $t-n$ to $t+n$, $f(t)$ can be approximated by

$$f_2(t) = \beta_0(t) + \beta_1(t) + \beta_2(t)t^2. \tag{5.3.1}$$

The quadratic moving LSE algorithm applies the method of ordinary least squares to estimate $\beta_0(t)$, $\beta_1(t)$, $\beta_2(t)$ on the basis of the window $\{X_{t-n+1}, \ldots, X_t\}$. With these estimates, it predicts X_{t+s} with

$$\hat{X}_{t+s}(t) = \hat{\beta}_0(t) + \hat{\beta}_1(t)(t+s) + \hat{\beta}_2(t)(t+s)^2. \tag{5.3.2}$$

After predicting $\hat{X}_{t+s}(t)$ the window of observations is moved to the right one time unit, and $\hat{X}_{t+s}(t+1)$ is predicted on the basis of the shifted window $\{X_{t-n+2}, \ldots, X_{t+1}\}$. This is called a *quadratic moving least squares estimates algorithm* (QMLSE).

In order to avoid the problem of inverting matrices which are very unbalanced for large t, we make the time shift to the time units $\{-(n-1), \ldots, 0\}$ in each cycle of the algorithm. Thus, let $\mathbf{X}_t^{(n)} = (X_t, \ldots, X_{t-n+1})'$ and define the $n \times 3$ matrix

$$A_{(n)} = \begin{bmatrix} 1 & 0 & 0 \\ \vdots & -1 & 1 \\ \vdots & \vdots & \vdots \\ 1 & -(n-1) & (n-1)^2 \end{bmatrix}.$$

Then the LSEs of $\beta_0(t)$, $\beta_1(t)$, and $\beta_2(t)$ based on a window of size n are given by

$$\hat{\boldsymbol{\beta}}^{(n)}(t) = (A'_{(n)}A_{(n)})^{-1}A'_{(n)}\mathbf{X}_t^{(n)}. \tag{5.3.3}$$

With these LSEs, the predictor is

$$\hat{X}_{t+s}^{(n)}(t) = \hat{\beta}_0^{(n)}(t) + \hat{\beta}_1^{(n)}(t) \cdot s + \hat{\beta}_2^{(n)}(t) \cdot s^2. \tag{5.3.4}$$

If, for all $j = -1, \ldots, -(n-1)$,

$$E\{X_{t+s}^{(n)}\} = \beta_0(t) + \beta_1(t)s + \beta_2(t)s^2, \tag{5.3.5}$$

then $E\{\hat{\beta}_l^{(n)}(t)\} = \beta_l(t)$, $l = 0, 1, 2$. However, if the true trend function $f(t)$ is not quadratic around t, then the LSEs (5.3.3) are biased. Assuming that in a neighborhood of t the trend is quadratic and the residuals are white noise, the variance of $\hat{X}_{t+s}^{(n)}(t)$ is given by

$$V\{\hat{X}_{t+s}^{(n)}(t)\} = \sigma^2(1, s, s^2)(A'_{(n)}A_{(n)})^{-1}\begin{pmatrix} 1 \\ s \\ s^2 \end{pmatrix}. \tag{5.3.6}$$

Using MAPLE one obtains the formula

$$
\begin{aligned}
V\{\hat{X}_{t+s}^{(n)}(t)\} = \sigma^2 \Bigg[& 3\frac{3n^2-3n+2}{n(n^2+3n+2)} + 36\frac{2n-1}{n(n^2+3n+2)}s \\
& + 36\frac{7-15n+7n^2}{n(n^2-1)(n^2-4)}s^2 \\
& + 360\frac{1}{n(n+1)(n^2-4)}s^3 \\
& + 180\frac{1}{n(n^2-1)(n^2-4)}s^4 \Bigg].
\end{aligned} \tag{5.3.7}
$$

Moreover, if $X_t = f(t) + U_t$, where $U_t \sim \text{WN}(0, \sigma^2)$, then

$$\text{PMSE}\{\hat{X}_{t+s}^{(n)}(t)\} = \sigma^2 + V\{\hat{X}_{t+s}^{(n)}(t)\}. \tag{5.3.8}$$

Thus, for $n = 10$, $\sigma^2 = 1$, and $s = 1, 2, 3$,

$$
\begin{aligned}
\text{PMSE}\{\hat{X}_{t+1}^{(10)}(t)\} &= 2.3833, \\
\text{PMSE}\{\hat{X}_{t+2}^{(10)}(t)\} &= 3.8015, \\
\text{PMSE}\{\hat{X}_{t+3}^{(10)}(t)\} &= 6.1455.
\end{aligned}
$$

If the residuals U_t are correlated, let R_n be the Toeplitz matrix determined by their correlation function. Then

$$V\{\hat{X}_{t+s}^{(n)}(t)\} = \sigma^2 \mathbf{a}_s'(A_{(n)}'A_{(n)})^{-1} \cdot A_{(n)}'R_n A_{(n)}(A_{(n)}'A_{(n)})^{-1}\mathbf{a}_s, \tag{5.3.9}$$

where $\mathbf{a}_s' = (1, s, s^2)$. The prediction MSE is, in such a case,

$$
\begin{aligned}
\text{PMSE}\{\hat{X}_{t+s}^{(n)}(t)\} = \sigma^2[& 1 + \mathbf{a}_s'(A_{(n)}'A_{(n)})^{-1}A_{(n)}'R_n A_n(A_{(n)}'A_{(n)})^{-1}\mathbf{a}_s \\
& - 2\mathbf{a}_s'(A_{(n)}'A_{(n)})^{-1}A_{(n)}'\boldsymbol{\rho}_s^{(n)}],
\end{aligned} \tag{5.3.10}
$$

where $\boldsymbol{\rho}_s^{(n)} = (\rho(s), \rho(s+1), \ldots, \rho(s+n-1))$.

The SPLUS function pred.poly computes the predicted values for a time series in an object x with window of size n according to formulas (5.3.3) and (5.3.4).

■ EXAMPLE 5.7

In Figure 5.6 we present a time series labeled DOW1941N. This time series is given by

$$X_t = f(t) + U_t, \quad t = 1, \ldots, 302,$$

where

$$f(t) = 123.3756 + 27.7297\left(\frac{t-151.0}{302}\right) - 15.8602\left(\frac{t-151.0}{302}\right)^2 - 237.8965\cdot\left(\frac{t-151.0}{302}\right)^3 \tag{5.3.11}$$

and

$$U_t = \epsilon_t + 0.5\epsilon_{t-1} + 0.25\epsilon_{t-2}, \quad t = 3, \ldots, 302, \tag{5.3.12}$$

$U_1 = \epsilon_1$, $U_2 = \epsilon_2$, where $\epsilon_t \sim \mathrm{WN}(0, 1)$.

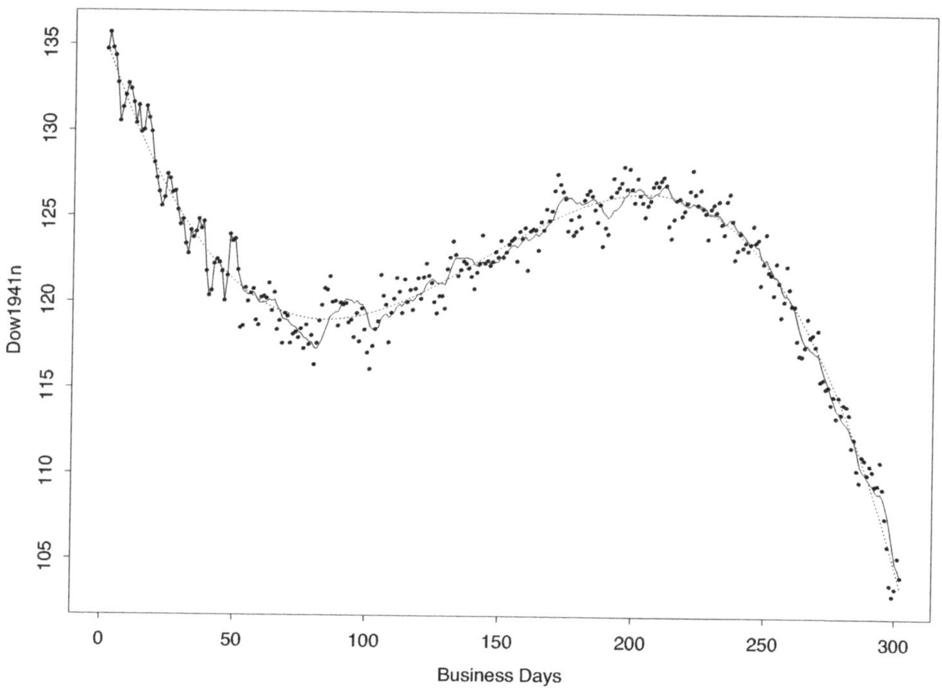

Figure 5.6: Trend estimation by quadratic moving LSE.

Applying the function pred.poly with $n = 50$ and $s = 0$, we obtain estimates of the trend by the QMLSE algorithm. The estimated trend (bold line) and the true trend (broken line) are plotted in Figure 5.6. In Figure 5.7 we plot the predicted values, computed according to the QMLSE algorithm, with $n = 50$, $s = 1$. The prediction MSE is estimated

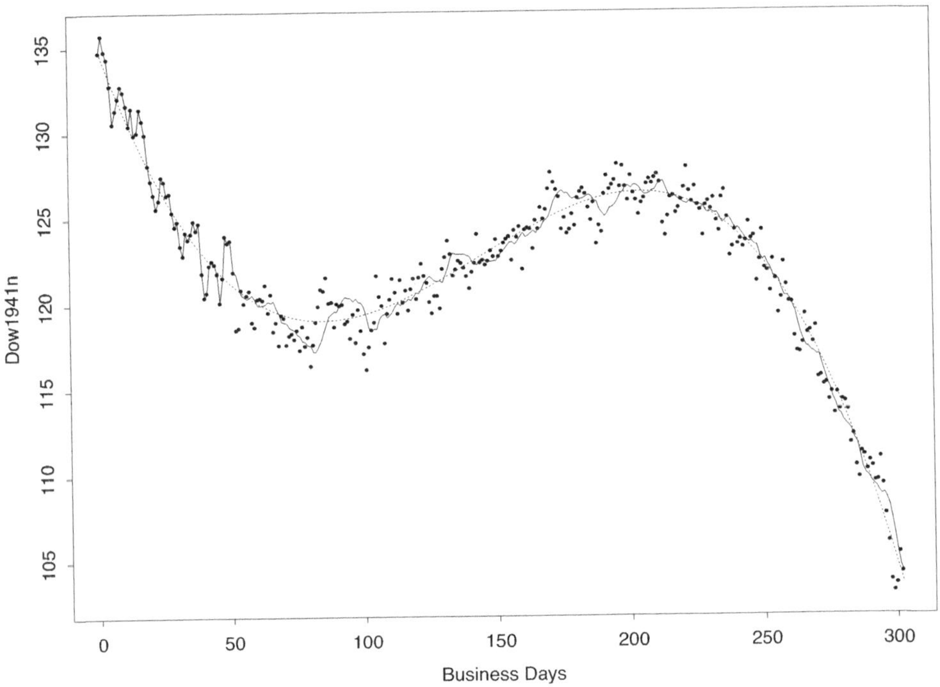

Figure 5.7: Prediction with the QMLSE algorithm, s = 1, n = 50.

as PMSE = 1.51103. The PMSE according to Eqs. (5.3.7) and (5.3.8) is 1.0877. The difference is due to the fact that $\{U_t\}$ is an MA(2) series and not a white noise. The prediction can be improved by adding a second component to the QMLSE predictor, which can be obtained by taking the linear combination $\mathbf{b}_s^{(n)\prime}\hat{\mathbf{U}}_t^{(n)}$ according to the SPLUS function pred1. The resulting predictor is shown in Figure 5.8. It has an estimated prediction MSE of PMSE = 1.0324, which is very close to the theoretical value of 1.0877. ■

5.4 MOVING AVERAGE PREDICTORS FOR NONSTATIONARY T.S.

In the present section we construct MAS(m) predictors assuming that $U_t \sim$ WN$(0, \sigma^2)$, $t = 0, \pm 1, \ldots$. These predictors, for polynomial models, are similar in structure to the QMLSE of the previous section. The difference is that we construct a window of size $2m+1$ on both sides of X_t. Thus X_{t+m+s} is

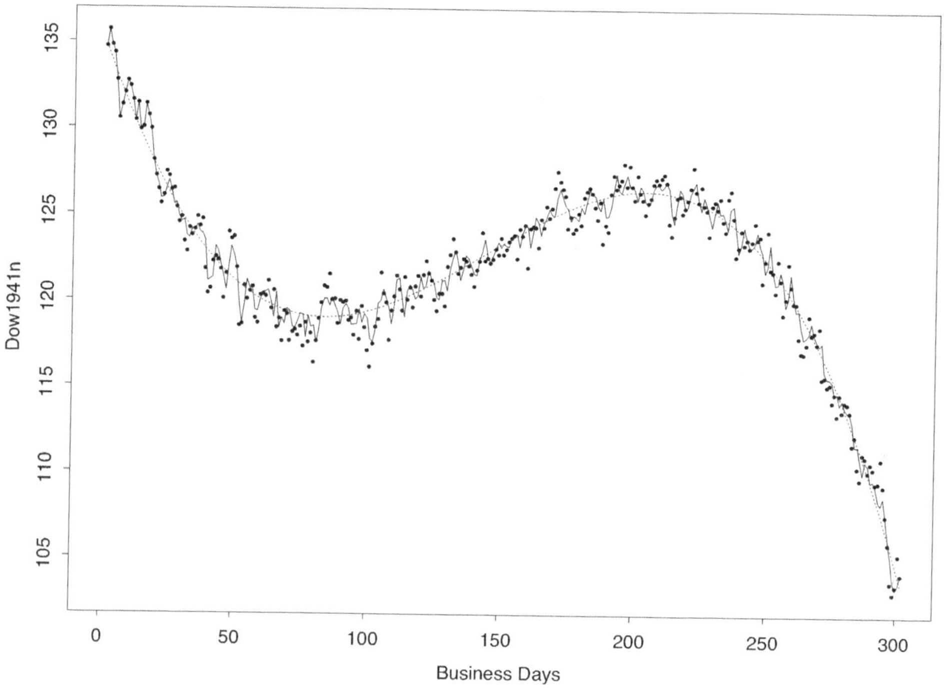

Figure 5.8: Prediction with a two-component predictor, s = 1, n = 50.

predicted on the basis of $\{X_{t-m}, \ldots, X_{t+m}\}$, $s \geq 1$. We develop here formulas for local polynomial trends. Generally, if the polynomial is of degree p, $p > 1$, and the moving window is of size $2m + 1$, we define $\mathbf{a}_{(m)} = \mathbf{a}_m^{(1)}$, where

$$\mathbf{a}_{(m)}^{(j)} = ((-m)^j, (-m+1)^j, \ldots, (-1)^j, 0, 1^j, \ldots, m^j)', \quad j = 0, 1, \ldots,$$

and construct the $(2m + 1) \times (p + 1)$ matrix

$$A_{(m)} = (1, \mathbf{a}_{(m)}, \mathbf{a}_{(m)}^{(2)}, \ldots, \mathbf{a}_{(m)}^{(p)}). \tag{5.4.1}$$

The local polynomial model is

$$\mathbf{X}_t^{(m)} = A_{(m)}\boldsymbol{\beta}(t) + \boldsymbol{\epsilon}_t^{(m)}, \tag{5.4.2}$$

where $\boldsymbol{\beta}(t) = (\beta_0(t), \ldots, \beta_p(t))'$; $\mathbf{X}_t^{(m)} = (X_{t-m}, \ldots, X_{t+m})'$ and $\boldsymbol{\epsilon}_t^{(m)} = (\epsilon_{t-m}, \ldots, \epsilon_{t+m})'$. The LSE of $\boldsymbol{\beta}(t)$ is

$$\hat{\boldsymbol{\beta}}^{(m)}(t) = (A'_{(m)}A_{(m)})^{-1}A'_{(m)}\mathbf{X}_t^{(m)}. \tag{5.4.3}$$

Notice that $\hat{\beta}_0^{(m)}(t)$ is the local polynomial LSE of $E\{X_t\}$. The predictor of X_{t+m+s} is

$$(5.4.4)\quad \hat{X}_{t+m+s}^{(m)}(t+m) = \hat{\beta}_0^{(m)}(t) + \hat{\beta}_1^{(m)}(t)(m+s) + \cdots + \hat{\beta}_p^{(m)}(t)(m+s)^p.$$

Assuming that the ϵ_t are WN$(0, \sigma^2)$, the variance of this estimator is

$$(5.4.5)\quad \begin{aligned} V\{\hat{X}_{t+m+s}^{(m)}(t+m)\} &= \sigma^2(1, (m+s), \ldots, (m+s)^p) \\ &\quad \cdot (A'_{(m)}A_{(m)})^{-1}(1, (m+s), \ldots, (m+s)^p)'. \end{aligned}$$

Furthermore, assuming that the predictor is unbiased, the prediction MSE is

$$(5.4.6)\quad \text{PMSE}\{\hat{X}_{t+m+s}^{(m)}(t+m)\} = \sigma^2 + V\{\hat{X}_{t+m+s}^{(m)}(t+m)\}.$$

In the following section explicit formulas are given for the linear case $p = 1$. Examples show that often the linear MAS predictor with $m = 3$ has smaller PMSE than MAS predictors with higher polynomial orders, $p > 1$.

5.4.1 Linear MAS Predictors

Let $S_{(m)} = A'_{(m)}A_{(m)}$. In the case of $p = 1$ we have

$$(5.4.7)\quad S_{(m)} = \begin{bmatrix} 2m+1 & 0 \\ 0 & \frac{1}{3}m(m+1)(2m+1) \end{bmatrix}.$$

Let $\hat{\mathbf{B}}^{(m)}(t) = S_{(m)}^{-1}A'_{(m)}$. Then

$$\hat{\boldsymbol{\beta}}^{(m)}(t) = \hat{\mathbf{B}}_{(m)}(t)\mathbf{X}_t^{(m)}.$$

In the case of $p = 1$, $\hat{B}_m(t)$ is a $2 \times (2m+1)$ matrix whose rows are

$$\mathbf{B}'_{(m)1} = \frac{1}{2m+1}1'_{2m+1}$$

and

$$\mathbf{B}'_{(m)2} = \frac{m(m+1)(2m+1)}{3}(-m, \ldots, -1, 0, 1, \ldots, m).$$

Theorem 5.4.1 *In the case of $p = 1$, the LSEs of $\beta_0(t)$ and $\beta_1(t)$ are*

$$(5.4.8)\quad \begin{aligned} \hat{\beta}_0^{(m)}(t) &= \frac{1}{2m+1}\sum_{j=-m}^{m} X_{t+j}, \\ \hat{\beta}_1^{(m)}(t) &= \frac{3}{m(m+1)(2m+1)}\sum_{j=1}^{m} j(X_{t+j} - X_{t-j}). \end{aligned}$$

The variance of the predictor is

$$(5.4.9)\quad V\{\hat{X}_{t+m+s}^{(m)}(t+m)\} = \sigma^2\left(\frac{1}{2m+1} + 3\frac{(m+s)^2}{(2m+1)m(m+1)}\right).$$

■

EXAMPLE 5.8

In Figure 5.9 we present the MAS linear predictor $\hat{\beta}_0^{(m)}(t) + \hat{\beta}_1^{(m)}(t) \cdot (m+s)$ for $m = 3$, $s = 1$, and $s = 2$ for the DOW1941 data. The estimated PMSE for these predictors are $\hat{\text{P}}\text{MSE}(s = 1) = 1.6681$ and $\hat{\text{P}}\text{MSE}(s = 2) = 3.5407$. The SPLUS program for computing the linear MAS(m) predictor is called mas.pred1 (see Appendix).

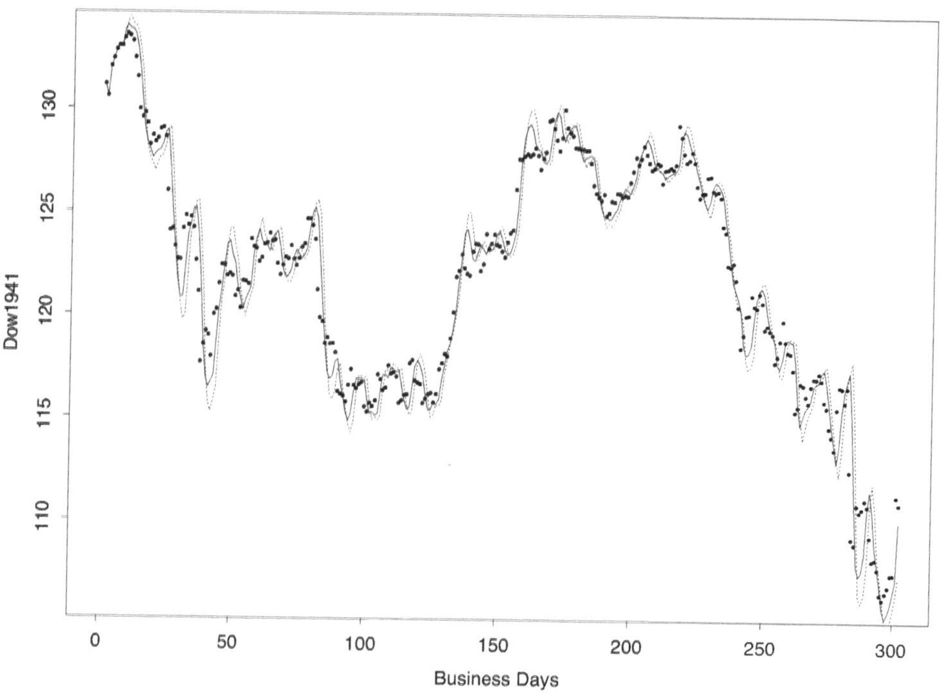

Figure 5.9: MAS linear predictor, m = 3, s = 1 (bold), s = 2 (broken).

In Figure 5.10 we show the QMLSE two-stage predictor with $n = 10$ for the DOW1941 data with $s = 1$. The estimated PMSE of this predictor is $\hat{\text{P}}\text{MSE}(s = 1) = 0.10677$. Although it is smaller than the $\hat{\text{P}}\text{MSE}$ of the linear MAS(3) predictor, it requires considerably more complicated computations. ■

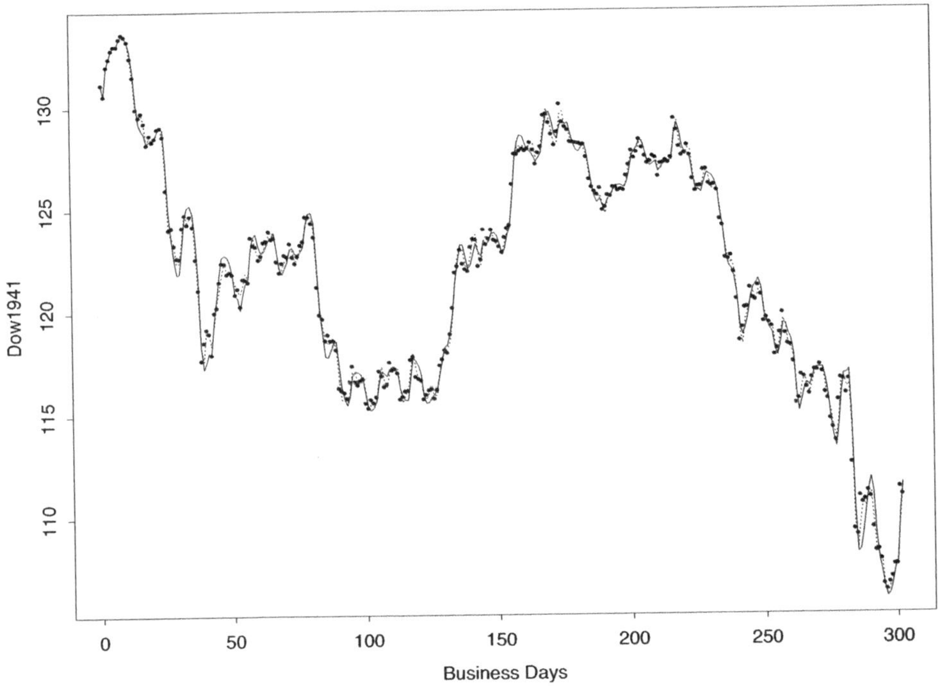

Figure 5.10: QMLSE with two-stage predictor trend (bold), s = 1 (broken).

5.5 PREDICTORS FOR GENERAL TRENDS WITH EXPONENTIAL DISCOUNTING

In the present section we present another approach to fit a trend to the data at time t by discounting past observations by a geometric factor. The computations are performed by recursive formulas, which are developed here. The exposition follows Nelson (1973).

Let

$$f(t) = \sum_{i=1}^{k} b_i Z_i(t), \tag{5.5.1}$$

where the $Z_i(t)$ are known functions. In a polynomial trend $Z_i(t) = t^{i-1}$. Let $Y_t = (X_1, \ldots, X_t)'$ and $(Z)_t$ be the matrix

$$(Z)_t = \begin{pmatrix} Z_1(1) & \cdots & Z_k(1) \\ \vdots & & \vdots \\ Z_1(t) & \cdots & Z_k(t) \end{pmatrix}.$$

The model is linear, that is,

$$\mathbf{Y}_t = (Z)_t\mathbf{b} + \boldsymbol{\epsilon}_t, \tag{5.5.2}$$

where $\boldsymbol{\epsilon}_t = (\epsilon_1, \ldots, \epsilon_t)'$ is a vector of $\mathrm{WN}(0, \sigma^2)$ random variables. The weighted LSE of $\mathbf{b}$, with a weight matrix $\mathbf{W}_t = \mathrm{diag}\{\beta^{t-j}; j = 1, \ldots, t\}$, is

$$\hat{\mathbf{b}}_t = ((Z)_t' W_t (Z)_t)^{-1} (Z)_t' W_t \mathbf{Y}_t. \tag{5.5.3}$$

The variance–covariance matrix of the LSE is

$$\mathbf{\Sigma}(\hat{\mathbf{b}}_t) = \sigma^2 ((Z)_t' W_t (Z)_t)^{-1} (Z)_t' W_t^2 (Z)_t \big((Z_t)' W_t (Z_t)\big)^{-1}. \tag{5.5.4}$$

5.5.1 Recursive Computations with Shifted Origin

For certain functions we can write

$$Z_i(t+1) = \sum_{j=1}^{k} L_{ij} Z_j(t), \quad i = 1, \ldots, k. \tag{5.5.5}$$

For example, if

$$f(t) = \sum_{i=0}^{k} b_i t^i,$$

then

$$Z_i(t) = t^i$$

$$Z_i(t+1) = (t+1)^i = \sum_{j=0}^{i} \binom{i}{j} t^j, \quad i = 0, \ldots, k.$$

Thus, if $\mathbf{Z}(t) = (1, t, t^2, \ldots, t^k)'$, then

$$\mathbf{Z}(t+1) = L\mathbf{Z}(t),$$

where L is the lower triangular matrix

$$L = \begin{pmatrix} 1 & & & & \\ 1 & 1 & & 0 & \\ 1 & 2 & 1 & & \\ \vdots & \vdots & \vdots & \ddots & \\ 1 & k & \binom{k}{2} & \cdots & 1 \end{pmatrix}.$$

Moreover, $\mathbf{Z}(t+1) = L'\mathbf{Z}(0)$. Consider the matrix

$$G_t = (Z)_t' W_t (Z)_t = \sum_{i=1}^{t} \beta^{t-i} \mathbf{Z}(i)\mathbf{Z}(i)'. \tag{5.5.6}$$

If we make a shift of the origin from 0 to t, we can write

$$G_t = \sum_{j=0}^{t-1} \beta^j \mathbf{Z}(-j)\mathbf{Z}(-j)'. \tag{5.5.7}$$

Consider the limit

$$G = \sum_{j=0}^{\infty} \beta^j \mathbf{Z}(-j)\mathbf{Z}(-j)'. \tag{5.5.8}$$

Here G is called the *steady-state matrix.* This matrix exists under certain conditions on the functions $\mathbf{Z}(t)$.

The vector $\mathbf{g}_t = (Z)_t' W_t \mathbf{Y}_t$ can be written as

$$\begin{aligned} \mathbf{g}_t &= \sum_{i=0}^{t-1} \beta^i X_{t-i} \mathbf{Z}(-i) \\ &= X_t \mathbf{Z}(0) + \beta \sum_{j=1}^{t-1} \beta^{j-1} X_{t-j} L^{-1} \mathbf{Z}(-j+1). \end{aligned} \tag{5.5.9}$$

Or,

$$\begin{aligned} \mathbf{g}_t &= X_t \mathbf{Z}(0) + \beta L^{-1} \sum_{j=0}^{t-2} \beta^j X_{t-1-j} \mathbf{Z}(-j) \\ &= X_t \mathbf{Z}(0) + \beta L^{-1} \mathbf{g}_{t-1}. \end{aligned} \tag{5.5.10}$$

Let $\hat{\mathbf{a}}(t)$ denote the LSE of $\mathbf{b}$ based on the results up to time t. Replacing G_t by the steady-state matrix, we obtain the approximation

$$\begin{aligned} \hat{\mathbf{a}}(t) &= G^{-1}\mathbf{g}_t \\ &= G^{-1}[X_t \mathbf{Z}(0) + \beta L^{-1} \mathbf{g}_{t-1}] \\ &= X_t G^{-1} \mathbf{Z}(0) + \beta G^{-1} L^{-1} G \hat{\mathbf{a}}(t-1) \\ &= X_t \mathbf{h} + H \hat{\mathbf{a}}(t-1), \end{aligned} \tag{5.5.11}$$

where

$$\mathbf{h} = G^{-1}\mathbf{Z}(0) \tag{5.5.12}$$

and

$$H = \beta G^{-1} L^{-1} G. \tag{5.5.13}$$

The vector $\mathbf{h}$ is called the *smoothing vector*. Furthermore,

$$
\begin{aligned}
L^{-1}G &= L^{-1}G(L')^{-1}L' \\
&= \sum_{j=0}^{\infty} \beta^j L^{-1}\mathbf{Z}(-j)\mathbf{Z}'(-j)(L')^{-1}L' \\
&= \sum_{j=0}^{\infty} \beta^j (L^{-1}\mathbf{Z}(-j))(L^{-1}\mathbf{Z}(-j))'L' \\
&= \sum_{j=0}^{\infty} \beta^j \mathbf{Z}(-j-1)\mathbf{Z}'(-j-1)L'.
\end{aligned} \tag{5.5.14}
$$

Letting $p = j + 1$, one obtains

$$
\begin{aligned}
L^{-1}G &= \beta^{-1} \sum_{p=1}^{\infty} \beta^p \mathbf{Z}(-p)\mathbf{Z}'(-p)L' \\
&= \beta^{-1}[G - \mathbf{Z}(0)\mathbf{Z}'(0)]L'.
\end{aligned} \tag{5.5.15}
$$

Substituting this expression, we obtain

$$
\begin{aligned}
H &= \beta G^{-1}\beta^{-1}[G - \mathbf{Z}(0)\mathbf{Z}'(0)]L' \\
&= G^{-1}[G - \mathbf{Z}(0)\mathbf{Z}'(0)]L' \\
&= [I - G^{-1}\mathbf{Z}(0)\mathbf{Z}'(0)]L' \\
&= L' - \mathbf{h}\mathbf{Z}'(0)L' \\
&= L' - \mathbf{h}(L\mathbf{Z}(0))' \\
&= L' - \mathbf{h}\mathbf{Z}'(1).
\end{aligned} \tag{5.5.16}
$$

A recursive formula for the LSE is

$$
\begin{aligned}
\hat{\mathbf{a}}(t) &= \mathbf{h}X_t + [L' - \mathbf{h}\mathbf{Z}'(1)]\hat{\mathbf{a}}(t-1) \\
&= L'\hat{\mathbf{a}}(t-1) + \mathbf{h}[X_t - \mathbf{Z}'(1)\hat{\mathbf{a}}(t-1)]
\end{aligned} \tag{5.5.17}
$$

or

$$
\hat{\mathbf{a}}(t) = L'\hat{\mathbf{a}}(t-1) + \mathbf{h}[X_t - \hat{X}_t(t-1)]. \tag{5.5.18}
$$

Finally, the predictor of X_{t+s} at time t is

$$
\hat{X}_{t+s}(t) = \mathbf{Z}'(s)\hat{\mathbf{a}}(t). \tag{5.5.19}
$$

The covariance matrix of $\hat{\mathbf{a}}(t)$ is given by

$$
\Sigma(\hat{\mathbf{a}}(t)) = \sigma^2 G^{-1} F G^{-1}, \tag{5.5.20}
$$

where

$$
F = \sum_{j=0}^{\infty} \beta^{2j}\mathbf{Z}(-j)\mathbf{Z}'(-j) \tag{5.5.21}
$$

and the variance of the predictor is

$$\begin{aligned} \mathrm{Var}\{\hat{X}_{t+s}(t)\} &= \mathrm{Var}\{\hat{\mathbf{a}}(t)'\mathbf{Z}(s)\} \\ &= \mathbf{Z}'(s)\Sigma\mathbf{Z}(s). \end{aligned} \tag{5.5.22}$$

Theorem 5.5.1 *For large values of t,*

$$E\{\hat{a}'(t)\mathbf{Z}(s)\} = \mathbf{b}'\mathbf{Z}(s)$$

and

$$\begin{aligned} PMSE(\hat{X}_{t+s}(t)) &\approx Var\{X_{t+s} - \hat{\mathbf{a}}(t)'\mathbf{Z}(s)\} \\ &= \sigma^2 + \mathbf{Z}'(s)\Sigma\mathbf{Z}(s). \end{aligned} \tag{5.5.23}$$

■

5.5.2 Linear Trend

Consider the linear model

$$X_t = b_1 + b_2 t + \epsilon_t, \quad t = 0, 1, \ldots.$$

Here $Z_1(t) = 1$ and $Z_2(t) = t$. For this case

$$L = \begin{bmatrix} 1 & 0 \\ 1 & 1 \end{bmatrix}$$

and

$$\begin{aligned} \hat{\mathbf{a}}(t) &= L'\hat{\mathbf{a}}(t-1) + \mathbf{h}e_1(t) \\ &= \begin{bmatrix} 1 & 1 \\ 0 & 1 \end{bmatrix} \begin{pmatrix} \hat{a}_1(t-1) \\ \hat{a}_2(t-1) \end{pmatrix} + \begin{pmatrix} h_1 \\ h_2 \end{pmatrix} e_1(t), \end{aligned}$$

where $e_1(t) = X_t - \hat{X}_t(t-1)$. Accordingly,

$$\hat{a}_1(t) = \hat{a}_1(t-1) + \hat{a}_2(t-1) + h_1 e_1(t) \tag{5.5.24}$$

and

$$\hat{a}_2(t) = \hat{a}_2(t-1) + h_2 e_1(t). \tag{5.5.25}$$

The matrix $\mathbf{G}(t)$ is

$$\mathbf{G}(t) = \begin{bmatrix} g_{11}(t) & g_{12}(t) \\ g_{21}(t) & g_{22}(t) \end{bmatrix},$$

where

$$g_{11}(t) = \sum_{i=0}^{t-1} \beta^i = \frac{1-\beta^t}{1-\beta}, \tag{5.5.26}$$

$$
\begin{aligned}
(5.5.27) \qquad g_{12}(t) = g_{21}(t) &= -\sum_{i=1}^{t-1} i\beta^i \\
&= -\frac{\beta(1-\beta^t - t\beta^{t-1} + t\beta^t)}{(1-\beta)^2},
\end{aligned}
$$

$$
(5.5.28) \qquad g_{22}(t) = \frac{\beta(1-\beta)}{(1-\beta)^3} - \frac{\beta^t}{(1-\beta)^3}(t^2(1-\beta)^2 + 2\beta t(1-\beta) + \beta^2).
$$

Accordingly, the steady-state matrix is

$$
(5.5.29) \qquad G = \lim_{t\to\infty} G(t) = \begin{bmatrix} \dfrac{1}{1-\beta} & -\dfrac{\beta}{(1-\beta)^2} \\ -\dfrac{\beta}{(1-\beta)^2} & \dfrac{\beta(1-\beta)}{(1-\beta)^3} \end{bmatrix}.
$$

Moreover,

$$
G^{-1} = \begin{bmatrix} 1-\beta^2 & (1-\beta)^2 \\ (1-\beta)^2 & \dfrac{(1-\beta)^3}{\beta} \end{bmatrix}.
$$

Hence, the smoothing vector is

$$
(5.5.30) \qquad \mathbf{h} = \begin{bmatrix} 1-\beta^2 & (1-\beta)^2 \\ (1-\beta)^2 & (1-\beta)^3/\beta \end{bmatrix} \begin{bmatrix} 1 \\ 0 \end{bmatrix} = \begin{bmatrix} 1-\beta^2 \\ (1-\beta)^2 \end{bmatrix},
$$

and the LSEs satisfy

$$
\begin{aligned}
(5.5.31) \qquad \hat{a}_1(t) &= \hat{a}_1(t-1) + \hat{a}_2(t-1) + (1-\beta^2)e_1(t), \\
\hat{a}_2(t) &= \hat{a}_2(t-1) + (1-\beta)^2 e_1(t).
\end{aligned}
$$

The predictors are $\hat{X}_t(t-1) = a_1(t-1) + a_2(t-1)$ and $\hat{X}_{t+1}(t) = a_1(t) + a_2(t)$. Accordingly,

$$
(5.5.32) \qquad \hat{X}_{t+1}(t) = \hat{X}_t(t-1) + \hat{a}_2(t-1) + 2(1-\beta)^2(X_t - \hat{X}_t(t-1)).
$$

Notice that $\hat{X}_t(t-1) + \hat{a}_2(t-1)$is the prediction of X_{t+1} at time $t-1$. This predictor is corrected by $2(1-\beta)^2 e_1(t)$ after X_t is observed.

5.5.3 Linear Trend with Cyclical Components

In Figure 5.11 we see the monthly demand for a seasonal commodity which has a linear trend and a cyclical variation around it. The trend function is

$$
f(t) = 50 + 0.5t + 15\cos\left(\frac{\pi t}{6}\right) - 5\sin\left(\frac{\pi t}{6}\right).
$$

The residuals around the trend function $f(t)$ are $\mathrm{WN}(0, \sigma^2)$ with $\sigma = 10$.

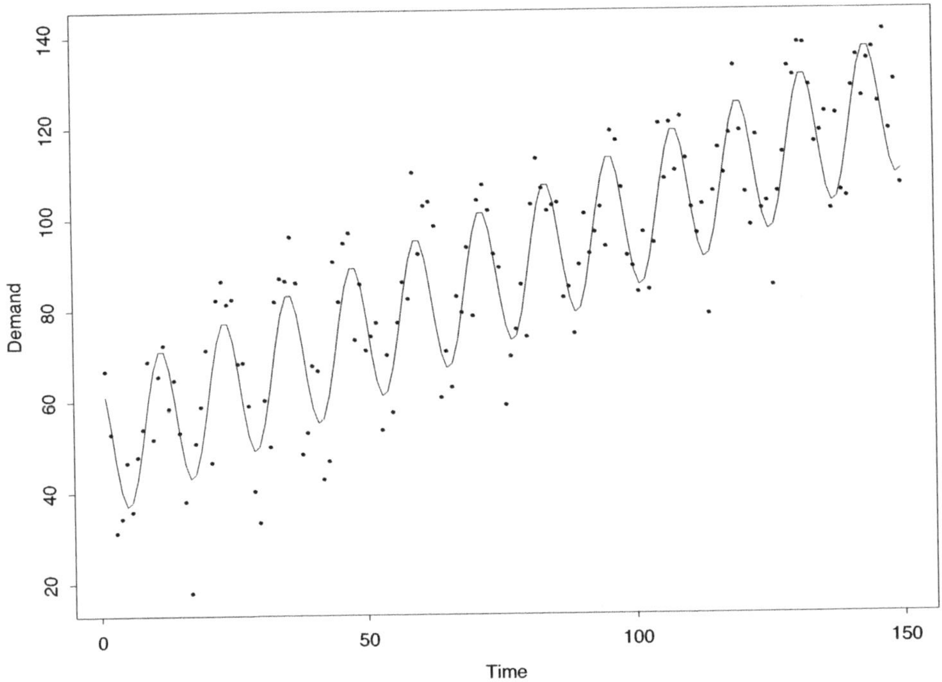

Figure 5.11: Data having linear trend with seasonal oscillations.

The model for this problem is

$$X_t = b_1 + b_2 t + b_3 \cos\left(\frac{\pi}{6}t\right) + b_4 \sin\left(\frac{\pi}{6}t\right) + e_t, \quad t = 0, \pm 1, \ldots, \tag{5.5.33}$$

where $\{e_t\}$ are $\mathrm{WN}(0, \sigma^2)$.

Let $\hat{a}_i(t)$ $(i = 1, \ldots, 4)$ be the adaptive estimators of b_i $(i = 1, \ldots, 4)$ at time t. Let $w = \pi/6$, and write

$$\mathbf{Z}(t) = (Z_1(t), \ldots, Z_4(t))',$$

where

$$\begin{aligned} Z_1(t) &= 1, \\ Z_2(t) &= t, \\ Z_3(t) &= \cos(wt), \\ Z_4(t) &= \sin(wt). \end{aligned} \tag{5.5.34}$$

Thus,

$$(5.5.35)\qquad \begin{aligned} Z_1(t+1) &= 1, \\ Z_2(t+1) &= Z_1(t) + Z_2(t), \\ Z_3(t+1) &= \cos(w)\cdot Z_3(t) - \sin(w)\cdot Z_4(t), \\ Z_4(t+1) &= \sin(w)Z_3(t) + \cos(w)Z_4(t). \end{aligned}$$

Accordingly,

$$(5.5.36)\qquad L = \begin{bmatrix} 1 & 0 & 0 & 0 \\ 1 & 1 & 0 & 0 \\ 0 & 0 & \cos w & -\sin w \\ 0 & 0 & \sin w & \cos w \end{bmatrix} = \begin{bmatrix} 1 & 0 & 0 & 0 \\ 1 & 1 & 0 & 0 \\ 0 & 0 & \frac{\sqrt{3}}{2} & -\frac{1}{2} \\ 0 & 0 & \frac{1}{2} & \frac{\sqrt{3}}{2} \end{bmatrix}.$$

The steady-state matrix is

$$G = \begin{bmatrix} G_{11} & G_{12} & \cdots & G_{14} \\ G_{21} & G_{22} & & \vdots \\ \vdots & & \ddots & \vdots \\ G_{41} & \cdots & \cdots & G_{44} \end{bmatrix},$$

where, for a discounting factor β,

$$(5.5.37)\qquad \begin{aligned} G_{11} &= \sum_{k=0}^{\infty} \beta^k = \frac{1}{1-\beta}, \\ G_{12} &= \sum_{k=0}^{\infty} \beta^k Z_1(-k) Z_2(-k) = -\sum_{k=0}^{\infty} k\beta^k = -\frac{\beta}{(1-\beta)^2}, \\ G_{13} &= \sum_{k=0}^{\infty} \beta^k Z_1(-k) Z_3(-k) = \sum_{k=0}^{\infty} \beta^k \cos(wk) \\ &= \frac{1-\beta\cos w}{1-2\beta\cos w+\beta^2}, \\ G_{14} &= -\sum_{k=0}^{\infty} \beta^k \sin(wk) \\ &= -\frac{\beta\sin(w)}{1-2\beta\cos(w)+\beta^2}; \end{aligned}$$

$$G_{21} = G_{12},$$
$$G_{22} = \sum_{k=0}^{\infty} k^2 \beta^k = \frac{\beta(1-\beta)}{(1-\beta)^3},$$
$$(5.5.38) \qquad G_{23} = -\sum_{k=0}^{\infty} k\beta^k \cos(wk) = -\frac{2\beta^2 - \beta(1+\beta^2)\cos(w)}{(1-2\beta\cos(w)+\beta^2)^2},$$
$$G_{24} = \sum_{k=0}^{\infty} k\beta^k \sin(wk) = \frac{\beta(1-\beta^2)\sin(w)}{(1-2\beta\cos(w)+\beta^2)^2};$$

$$G_{31} = G_{13},$$
$$G_{32} = G_{23},$$
$$(5.5.39) \qquad G_{33} = \sum_{k=0}^{\infty} \beta^k \cos^2(wk) = \frac{1+\beta+\beta(\beta-3)\cos^2(w)}{(1-\beta)(1+\beta(2+\beta)-4\cos^2(w))},$$
$$G_{34} = -\sum_{k=0}^{\infty} \beta^k \cos(wk)\sin(wk) = -\frac{\beta\sin(w)\cos(w)}{1+\beta^2+2\beta-4\beta\cos^2(w)};$$

$$(5.5.40) \qquad G_{44} = \sum_{k=0}^{\infty} \beta^k \sin^2(wk) = \frac{\beta(1+\beta)(1-\cos^2(w))}{(1-\beta)(1+\beta^2+2\beta-4\beta\cos^2(w))}.$$

The matrix G for $\beta = 0.95$ and $w = \pi/6$ is

$$G = \begin{bmatrix} 20 & -380 & 0.68965 & -1.84788 \\ \bullet & 14,820 & -3.62868 & 0.70090 \\ \bullet & \bullet & 10.27559 & -0.43188 \\ \bullet & \bullet & \bullet & 9.7244 \end{bmatrix}$$

The smoothing vector is then

$$\mathbf{h} = G^{-1}\mathbf{Z}(0) = (0.0960, 0.0025, 0.0927, 0.0222)'.$$

The predictor $\hat{X}_t(t-1) = \hat{\mathbf{a}}(t-1)'\mathbf{Z}(1)$. Let $e_1(t) = X_t - (\hat{\mathbf{a}}(t-1))'\mathbf{Z}(1)$, where $\mathbf{Z}'(1) = (1, 1, \sqrt{3/2}, \frac{1}{2})$. Then from the equation $\hat{\mathbf{a}}(t) = L'\hat{\mathbf{a}}(t-1) + e_1(t)\mathbf{h}$ we get

$$\begin{aligned} \hat{a}_1(t) &= \hat{a}_1(t-1) + \hat{a}_2(t-1) + 0.0960e_1(t), \\ \hat{a}_2(t) &= \hat{a}_2(t-1) + 0.0025e_1(t), \\ \hat{a}_3(t) &= \frac{1}{2}\sqrt{3}\,\hat{a}_3(t-1) + \frac{1}{2}\hat{a}_4(t-1) + 0.0927e_1(t), \\ \hat{a}_4(t) &= -\frac{1}{2}\hat{a}_3(t-1) + \frac{1}{2}\sqrt{3}\,\hat{a}_4(t-1) + 0.0222e_1(t). \end{aligned} \tag{5.5.41}$$

The formula of $G_{11}, \ldots, G_{44}$ given above can be obtained by using MAPLE.

The first f data points are used to obtain initial estimate of a_1, a_2, a_3, a_4 by the method of LSE. All other values of $\hat{a}_i(t)$, $t \geq 1$, $i = 1, \ldots, 4$, are computed according to (5.5.41). The one-month-ahead predictor ($s = 1$) is

$$\hat{X}_{t+1}(t) = \hat{a}_1(t) + \hat{a}_2(t) + \frac{1}{2}\sqrt{3}\,\hat{a}_3(t) + \frac{1}{2}\hat{a}_4(t).$$

Generally, an s-months-ahead predictor is

$$\hat{X}_{t+s}(t) = \hat{a}_1(t) + \hat{a}_2(t)\cdot s + \hat{a}_3(t)\cdot \cos\left(\frac{\pi s}{6}\right) + \hat{a}_4(t)\cdot \sin\left(\frac{\pi s}{6}\right).$$

In Figure 5.12 we see the effect of the length of the initial period f. The predictor with $f = 18$ seems to be close to the true trend $f(t)$, with estimated PMSE of 144.51. The variance around the trend $f(t)$ is $\sigma^2 = 100$. We see that the prediction $\hat{X}_{t+1}(t)$ improves as t grows.

5.6 DYNAMIC LINEAR MODELS

In the present section we consider *dynamic linear models* (DLMs) of the form

$$\mathbf{X}_t = A_t\boldsymbol{\theta}_t + \boldsymbol{\epsilon}_t \tag{5.6.1}$$

and

$$\boldsymbol{\theta}_t = G_t\boldsymbol{\theta}_{t-1} + \boldsymbol{\eta}_t, \tag{5.6.2}$$

where $\boldsymbol{\theta}_t$ is a vector of size $p \times 1$, $\mathbf{X}_t$ is a vector of size $q \times 1$, $\{\boldsymbol{\epsilon}_t\}$ is a sequence of *independent* q-dimensional random vectors and $\{\boldsymbol{\eta}_t\}$ is a sequence of independent p-dimensional random vectors, $\{\boldsymbol{\epsilon}_t\}$ are mutually independent of $\{\boldsymbol{\eta}_t\}$, and A_t and G_t are known (nonrandom) matrices of sizes $q \times p$ and $p \times p$, respectively. We will further assume that, for each t, $\boldsymbol{\epsilon}_t \sim N(\mathbf{0}, V_t)$ and $\boldsymbol{\eta}_t \sim N(\mathbf{0}, W_t)$. Many different dynamic models can be formulated in these terms. For example, T.S. with polynomial trends, having coefficients which change at random from one observation epoch to another, can be modeled as

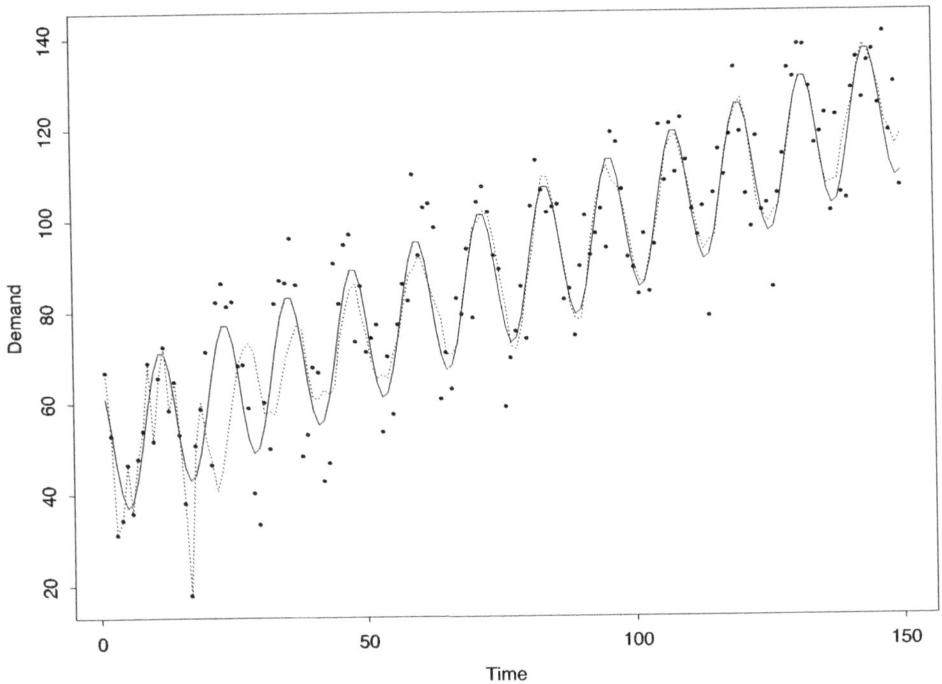

Figure 5.12: Seasonal demand data with trend (bold) and predictor, s = 1 (broken).

above, with $q = 1$, $\mathbf{A}_t = (1, t, \ldots, t^p)$, $\boldsymbol{\theta}_t = \boldsymbol{\theta}_{t-1} + \boldsymbol{\eta}_t$. The covariance matrix W_t governs the extent of possible changes in $\boldsymbol{\theta}_t$. If some components of $\boldsymbol{\theta}_t$ are fixed we can set the corresponding covariances with that component equal to zero.

The AR(p) model can be written in a DLM form with $A_t = (1, \mathbf{0}'_{p-1})$, $\boldsymbol{\theta}_t = (X_t, \ldots, X_{t-p+1})'$,

$$G_t = \begin{bmatrix} \phi_1 & \phi_2 & & & \phi_p \\ & & \ddots & & \\ 1 & 0 & & & 0 \\ & 1 & 0 & & \vdots \\ & & \ddots & \ddots & 0 \\ 0 & & & 1 & 0 \end{bmatrix},$$

and $\boldsymbol{\eta}_t' = (\epsilon_t, 0, \ldots, 0)$, where $\{\epsilon_t\}$ is a sequence of uncorrelated $(0, \sigma^2)$ random variables. For this AR(p) model, we set $V = 0$ and

$$W = \begin{bmatrix} \sigma^2 & \mathbf{0}' \\ \mathbf{0} & 0 \end{bmatrix}.$$

In the simple case where $p = 1$, $q = 1$, $A_t = 1$, and $G_t = 1$, we obtain the DLM

$$\begin{aligned} X_t &= \theta_t + \epsilon_t, \\ \theta_t &= \theta_{t-1} + \eta_t, \quad t = 0, 1, \ldots . \end{aligned} \tag{5.6.3}$$

We will call this model the *normal random walk model.* In Figure 5.13 we illustrate this normal random walk model with $\theta_0 \equiv 0$, ϵ_t i.i.d. $N(0, .09)$ and η_t i.i.d. $N(0, 1.0)$. Let ϵ_t represent the observational errors and η_t are errors imposed on the dynamics of the process mean, represented by θ_t.

5.6.1 Recursive Computations for the Normal Random Walk DLM, Constant Variances

In the present model X_t are observable random variables while θ_t are unobservable. We will develop here recursive formulas for the estimation of θ_t and the prediction of X_{t+1} given the data up to time t. Generally, if the *conditional* distribution of X given θ is $N(\theta, v)$ and if θ has a normal distribution, that is, $\theta \sim N(\tau, w)$, then the vector (X, θ) has a bivariate normal distribution

$$\begin{pmatrix} X \\ \theta \end{pmatrix} \sim N\left(\begin{bmatrix} \tau \\ \tau \end{bmatrix}, \begin{bmatrix} v + w & w \\ w & w \end{bmatrix} \right). \tag{5.6.4}$$

Thus, from normal distribution theory, the *conditional* distribution of θ, given X, is *normal* with mean

$$E\{\theta \mid X\} = \tau + \frac{w}{v + w}(X - \tau), \tag{5.6.5}$$

and

$$\begin{aligned} V\{\theta \mid X) &= w - \frac{w^2}{w + v} = w\left(1 - \frac{w}{w + v}\right) \\ &= \frac{wv}{w + v} = \left(\frac{1}{v} + \frac{1}{w}\right)^{-1}. \end{aligned} \tag{5.6.6}$$

In Bayesian terms, the distribution of θ is called a *prior distribution*, and the conditional distribution of θ, given X, is called the *posterior distribution.* We return now to the DLM, with constant variances v and w. Let $\mathbf{X}_t = (X_1, \ldots, X_t)'$. By induction we can prove that the *posterior* distribution of

θ_t given $\mathbf{X}_t$ is normal. Let m_t and c_t denote the mean and variance of the posterior distribution of θ_t given $\mathbf{X}_t$, that is,

$$\theta_t \mid \mathbf{X}_t \sim N(m_t, c_t). \tag{5.6.7}$$

Before observing X_{t+1}, the predictive distribution of X_{t+1} given $\mathbf{X}_t$ is *normal* with mean $E\{X_{t+1} \mid \mathbf{X}_t\} = E\{E\{X_{t+1} \mid \theta_t\} \mid \mathbf{X}_t\} = m_t$ and variance $c_t + w + v$. Thus, the best predictor of X_{t+1} for minimizing the PMSE is

$$\hat{X}_{t+1}(t) = E\{X_{t+1} \mid \mathbf{X}_t\} = m_t. \tag{5.6.8}$$

The corresponding PMSE is

$$\text{PMSE}\{\hat{X}_{t+1}(t)\} = c_t + w + v. \tag{5.6.9}$$

After observing X_{t+1} we compute the posterior distribution of θ_{t+1} given $\mathbf{X}_{t+1}$ in the following manner. The conditional distribution of θ_{t+1} given $\mathbf{X}_t$, namely, the $N(m_t, c_t + w)$, is used as the prior distribution. Then, the posterior distribution of θ_{t+1} given $\mathbf{X}_{t+1}$ is *normal* with mean

$$m_{t+1} = m_t + \frac{c_t + w}{c_t + w + v}(X_{t+1} - m_t) \tag{5.6.10}$$

and variance

$$c_{t+1} = \frac{(c_t + w)}{c_t + v + w} v. \tag{5.6.11}$$

Using these recursive equations, starting from some initial values (m_0, c_0), we can compute (m_t, c_t) and $\hat{X}_{t+1}(t)$ for all t. In Figure 5.13 we present the predictor $\hat{X}_{t+1}(t) = m_t$, where $m_1 = X_1$, $m_t = 0.6224 m_{t-1} + 0.3776 X_t$.

If we let $\alpha_t = (c_t + w)/(c_t + w + v)$, we can write

$$m_{t+1} = (1 - \alpha_t) m_t + \alpha_t X_{t+1}. \tag{5.6.12}$$

This recursive equation is similar to that of an exponential smoothing

$$S_{t+1} = (1 - \alpha^*) S_t + \alpha^* X_{t+1}. \tag{5.6.13}$$

Theorem 5.6.1 *In the normal random walk model* $\lim_{t\to\infty} c_t = c^*$ *and* $\lim_{t\to\infty} \alpha_t = \alpha^*$, *where*

$$c^* = \frac{w}{2}\left(\left(1 + 4\frac{v}{w}\right)^{1/2} - 1\right). \tag{5.6.14}$$

Proof: Write

$$\begin{aligned} \frac{1}{c_t} - \frac{1}{c_{t-1}} &= \frac{1}{c_{t-1} + w} - \frac{1}{c_{t-2} + w} \\ &= \frac{c_{t-1} \cdot c_{t-2}}{(c_{t-1} + w)(c_{t-2} + w)} \left(\frac{1}{c_{t-1}} - \frac{1}{c_{t-2}}\right). \end{aligned} \tag{5.6.15}$$

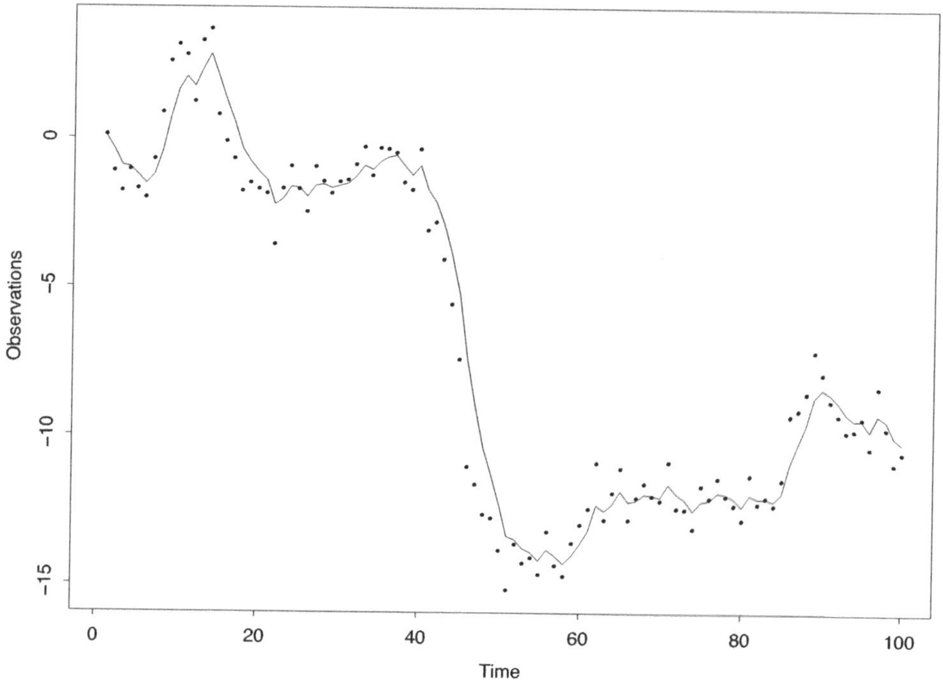

Figure 5.13: Normal random walk with a bayesian predictor.

Let

(5.6.16) $$k_t = \frac{c_t \cdot c_{t-1}}{(c_{t-1}+w)(c_t+w)}, \quad t = 1, 2.$$

Obviously, $0 < k_t < 1$ for all $t = 1, 2, \ldots$ and

(5.6.17) $$\frac{1}{c_t} - \frac{1}{c_{t-1}} = \left(\prod_{j=1}^{t-1} k_j\right)\left(\frac{1}{c_1} - \frac{1}{c_0}\right), \quad t = 2, 3, \ldots .$$

Thus, if $c_1 > c_0$, then $c_t > c_{t-1}$ for all t, and if $c_1 < c_0$, then $c_t < c_{t-1}$ for all t. Moreover, $0 < c_t < v$ for all t. It follows that $c_t \to c^*$ as $t \to \infty$. It is immediate to show that c^* is given by (5.6.14). ■

We have seen that the Bayes predictor of X_{t+1} at time t is $\hat{X}_{t+1}(t) = m_t$. The s-step-ahead predictor is

(5.6.18) $$\begin{aligned}\hat{X}_{t+s}(t) &= E\{X_{t+s} \mid \mathbf{X}_t\} \\ &= E\{\theta_{t+s} + e_{t+s} \mid \mathbf{X}_t\} = m_t.\end{aligned}$$

The conditional variance of X_{t+s} given $\mathbf{X}_t$ is

$$\begin{aligned} V\{X_{t+s} \mid \mathbf{X}_t\} &= E\{V\{X_{t+s} \mid \theta_{t+s}\} \mid \mathbf{X}_t\} \\ &\quad + V\{E\{X_{t+s} \mid \theta_{t+s}\} \mid \mathbf{X}_t\} \\ &= v + V\left\{\theta_t + \sum_{j=1}^{s} \eta_{t+j} \mid \mathbf{X}_t\right\} \\ &= c_t + sw + v. \end{aligned} \tag{5.6.19}$$

This is independent of $\mathbf{X}_t$. Hence

$$E\{V\{X_{t+s} \mid \mathbf{X}_t\}\} = c_t + sw + v \tag{5.6.20}$$

and

$$E\{m_t - X_{t+s}\} = 0.$$

Thus

$$\begin{aligned} \text{PMSE}\{\hat{X}_{t+s}(t)\} &= V\{m_t - X_{t+s}\} \\ &= c_t + sw + v. \end{aligned} \tag{5.6.21}$$

5.6.2 Incorporating External Information

Suppose that the first-order DLM model is under consideration, but an external information is available that a shift Z is going to occur in the mean θ_t, just before a given epoch t_0. Suppose that the magnitude of the shift is not known, but there is reason to believe that Z is normally distributed with mean ζ and variance τ^2. Moreover, Z is independent of all other random variables. The DLM is accordingly

$$\begin{aligned} X_t &= \theta_t + e_t, \\ \theta_t &= \theta_{t-1} + I\{t = t_0\}Z + \eta_t. \end{aligned} \tag{5.6.22}$$

The recursive equations for the determination of m_t and C_t remain as before for $t \neq t_0$. For $t = t_0$, the prior for θ is changed from $N(m_{t_0-1}, c_{t_0-1} + w)$ to $N(m_{t_0-1} + \zeta, c_{t_0-1} + w + \tau^2)$. Thus,

$$m_{t_0} = m_{t_0-1} + \zeta + \frac{c_{t_0-1} + w + \tau^2}{c_{t_0-1} + w + \tau^2 + v}(X_{t_0} - m_{t_0-1} - \zeta) \tag{5.6.23}$$

and

$$c_{t_0} = \frac{c_{t_0-1} + w + \tau^2}{c_{t_0-1} + w + \tau^2 + v} v. \tag{5.6.24}$$

This type of analysis when extraneous information is incorporated into the recursive equations is called *intervention analysis*.

■ EXAMPLE 5.9

In the present example we consider a T.S. of size $n = 50$,

$$X_t = \theta_t + e_t,$$

where

$$\theta_t = \begin{cases} 10 & \text{if } 1 \le t \le 25, \\ 15 & \text{if } 26 \le t \le 50, \end{cases}$$

and where $\{e_t\}$ are i.i.d. $N(0,1)$. Assume $t_0 = 26$ is a *change point.* Suppose that the epoch of change t_0 is *known* but the magnitude of change is not known with certainty. If we model the magnitude of change to be $Z \sim N(5,1)$, then we can use the above intervention analysis to adjust for the change. In Figure 5.14 we present the DLM predictor $\hat{X}_{t+1}(t) = m_t$ with and without intervention. The DLM parameters are $m_0 = 10$, $c_0 = 0$, $w = v = 1$, $\tau^2 = 1$, and $\zeta = 5$. We see that the intervention adjustment is very effective. Without intervention the DLM predictor adjusts itself completely only after five epochs. ■

The one-dimensional DLM discussed in this section can be computed with the SPLUS function dlm1.int (see Appendix).

5.6.3 General DLM with Applications

We consider here the general DLM

$$\text{(5.6.25)} \quad \begin{aligned} \mathbf{X}_t &= A_t\boldsymbol{\theta}_t + \mathbf{e}_t, \quad t = 1,2,\ldots, \\ \boldsymbol{\theta}_t &= G_t\boldsymbol{\theta}_{t-1} + \boldsymbol{\eta}_t, \quad t = 1,2,\ldots, \end{aligned}$$

where the matrices A_t and G_t may depend on the time t, $\{\mathbf{e}_t\}$ is a sequence of i.i.d. normal vectors $N(\mathbf{0}, V_t)$, and $\{\boldsymbol{\eta}_t\}$ are i.i.d. $N(\mathbf{0}, W_t)$. Moreover the $\{\mathbf{e}_t\}$ are mutually independent of $\{\boldsymbol{\eta}_t\}$. Let $\mathcal{D}_t = \{\mathcal{D}_{t-1}, \mathbf{X}_t\}$, $t \ge 2$, with $\mathcal{D}_1 = \{\mathbf{X}_1\}$ denote the available data after t time epochs. Let $\boldsymbol{\theta}_0 \sim N(\mathbf{m}_0, C_0)$ be the distribution of the initial value of $\boldsymbol{\theta}$. The recursive algorithm changes the parameters (m_t, C_t) and predicts X_{t+1}, in the following manner:

(i) Given $\mathcal{D}_t$, the predictor of $\mathbf{X}_{t+1}$ is $\hat{\mathbf{X}}_{t+1}(t) = A_{t+1}G_{t+1}\mathbf{m}_t$, $t = 0, 1, \ldots$.

(ii) The prediction MSE is given by

$$\text{(5.6.26)} \quad \begin{aligned} \text{PMSE}\{\hat{X}_{t+1}(t)\} &= E\{||\hat{\mathbf{X}}_{t+1}(t) - \mathbf{X}_{t+1}||^2\} \\ &= \text{tr}\{R_{t+1}\}, \end{aligned}$$

where

$$\text{(5.6.27)} \quad R_{t+1} = V_{t+1} + A_{t+1}(G_{t+1}C_tG'_{t+1} + W_{t+1})A'_{t+1'}$$

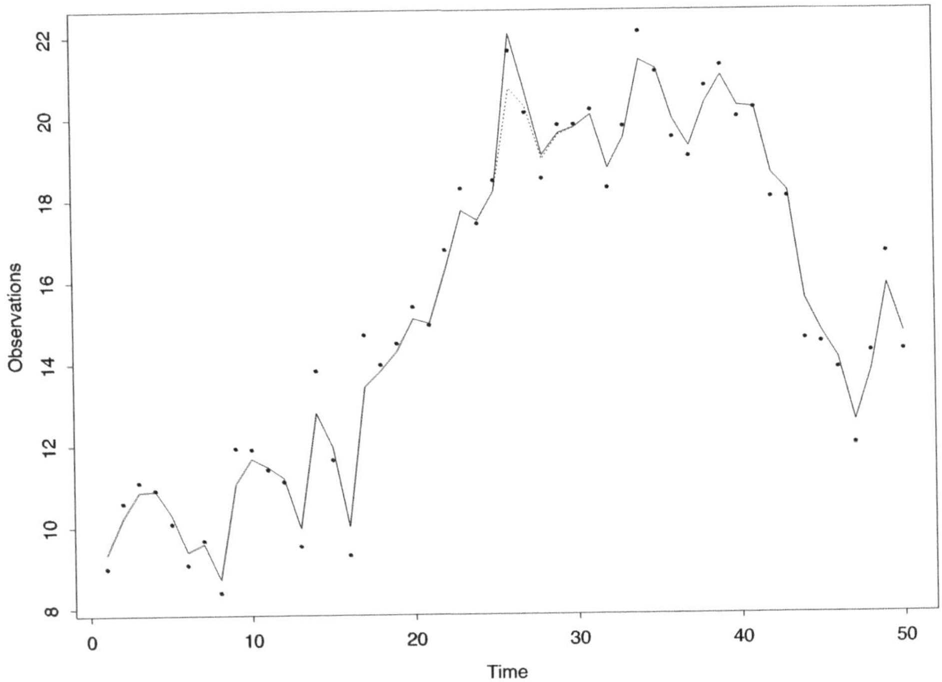

Figure 5.14: DLM prediction with and without intervention (broken line).

and $\text{tr}\{\cdot\}$ is the trace of the matrix in the curly brackets.

(iii) The prior distribution for $\boldsymbol{\theta}_{t+1}$, given $\mathcal{D}_t$, is normal $N(G_{t+1}\mathbf{m}_t, G_{t+1}C_tG_{t+1}+W_{t+1})$.

(iv) The posterior distribution of $\boldsymbol{\theta}_{t+1}$, given $\mathcal{D}_{t+1}$, is normal with mean

(5.6.28)

$$\mathbf{m}_{t+1} = G_{t+1}\mathbf{m}_t + (G_{t+1}C_tG'_{t+1} + W_{t+1})A'_{t+1} \cdot R^{-1}_{t+1}(\mathbf{X}_{t+1} - A_{t+1}G_{t+1}\mathbf{m}_t)$$

and covariance matrix

(5.6.29)

$$C_{t+1} = (G_{t+1}C_tG'_{t+1} + W_{t+1}) - (G_{t+1}C_tG'_{t+1} + W_{t+1})A'_{t+1}R^{-1}_{t+1}A_{t+1} \cdot (G_{t+1}C_tG'_{t+1} + W_{t+1}).$$

Here $\mathbf{m}_t$ is the Bayes estimator of the current position of the evolution process, $\boldsymbol{\theta}_t$, for the squared error loss. This estimator is called the *Kalman filter*, which is often written as

$$\mathbf{m}_t = G_t\mathbf{m}_{t-1} + K_t(\mathbf{X}_t - A_tG_t\mathbf{m}_{t-1}), \tag{5.6.30}$$

where

$$K_t = (G_tC_{t-1}G_t' + W_t)A_t'R_t^{-1}. \tag{5.6.31}$$

The Kalman filter can be obtained also from a more general approach of the minimum MSE linear recursive estimator of $\boldsymbol{\theta}_t$. This will be shown in Section 5.7. We now show a few applications.

5.6.3.1 DLM with Linear Growth Consider a linear growth model in which $X_t = \theta_0 + \theta_1 t + e_t$ with θ_0 and θ_1 random. This model can be formulated as a DLM with

$$X_t = \mathbf{a}_t'\boldsymbol{\theta}_t + e_t, \quad t = 1, 2, \ldots,$$
$$\boldsymbol{\theta}_t = \boldsymbol{\theta}_{t-1} + \boldsymbol{\eta}_t, \quad t = 1, 2, \ldots,$$

with $\mathbf{a}_t' = (1, t)$. Assume $\boldsymbol{\theta}_t' = (\theta_{0,t}, \theta_{1,t})$. This is a special case of the general model discussed above with $A_t = \mathbf{a}_t'$ and $G_t = I$. Let $\mathbf{m}_t$ and C_t be the posterior mean and posterior covariance matrix of $\boldsymbol{\theta}_t$ given $\mathcal{D}_t$. We obtain in the present case the recursive formulas

$$\mathbf{m}_t = \mathbf{m}_{t-1} + \frac{1}{r_t}(X_t - \mathbf{a}_t'\mathbf{m}_{t-1})(C_{t-1} + W)\mathbf{a}_t, \tag{5.6.32}$$

where

$$r_t = v + \mathbf{a}_t'(C_{t-1} + W)\mathbf{a}_t \tag{5.6.33}$$

and

$$C_t = C_{t-1} + W - \frac{1}{r_t}(C_{t-1} + W)\mathbf{a}_t\mathbf{a}_t' \cdot (C_{t-1} + W), \tag{5.6.34}$$

where v is the constant variance of e_t and W is a constant covariance matrix of $\boldsymbol{\eta}_t$. The predictor of X_{t+1} at time t is $\hat{X}_{t+1}(t) = \mathbf{a}_{t+1}'\mathbf{m}_t$.

The SPLUS function dlm.lg computes the predicted values according to a linear growth DLM. (See Appendix.)

EXAMPLE 5.10

In Figure 5.15 we illustrate the predictor $\hat{X}_{t+1}(t)$ for the sales data of a commodity in 4 years. A linear regression analysis of these data yields the linear trend $\hat{f}(t) = 285.68 + 10.1984t$. We therefore start with

$$\mathbf{m}_0 = \begin{pmatrix} 285.68 \\ 10.20 \end{pmatrix} \quad \text{and} \quad C_0 = 0.$$

The variance around this regression line is $\hat{\sigma}^2 = 2977.7$. We set $v = \hat{\sigma}^2$. For the covariance matrix W we use the variance–covariance matrix of the LSE, namely,

$$W = \begin{bmatrix} 256.063 & -7.920 \\ -7.920 & 0.323 \end{bmatrix}.$$

■

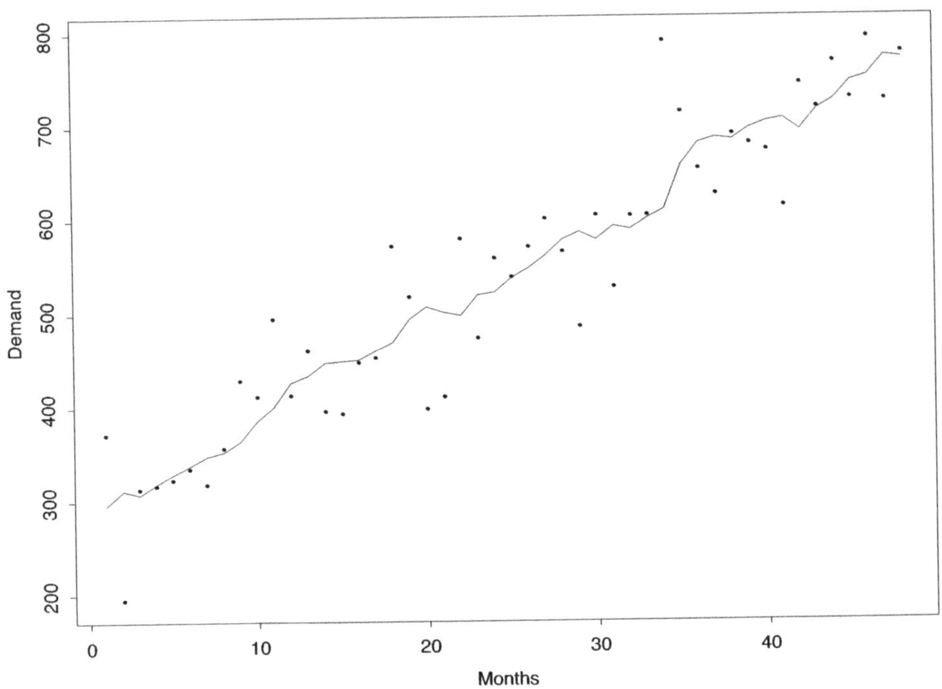

Figure 5.15: Prediction by DLM growth model.

■ EXAMPLE 5.11

In Figure 5.16 we show the DLM growth predictor for the DOW1941 data. For these recursive calculations for $\mathbf{m}_0$ we used the LSE of a regression line based on the first 50 days. For W we used the variance–covariance matrix of these LSEs. The variance around the regression line is v. These are $\mathbf{m}_0' = (134.234, -0.3115)$, $v = 3.8698$, and

$$W = \begin{pmatrix} 0.3191 & -0.0095 \\ -0.0095 & 0.0004 \end{pmatrix}.$$

We started with $C_0 = 0$. We see that the recursive procedure adjusts rapidly for the changes in the growth coefficients $\boldsymbol{\theta}_t$ and yields reasonable predictors despite the many changes in the trend of this T.S. ■

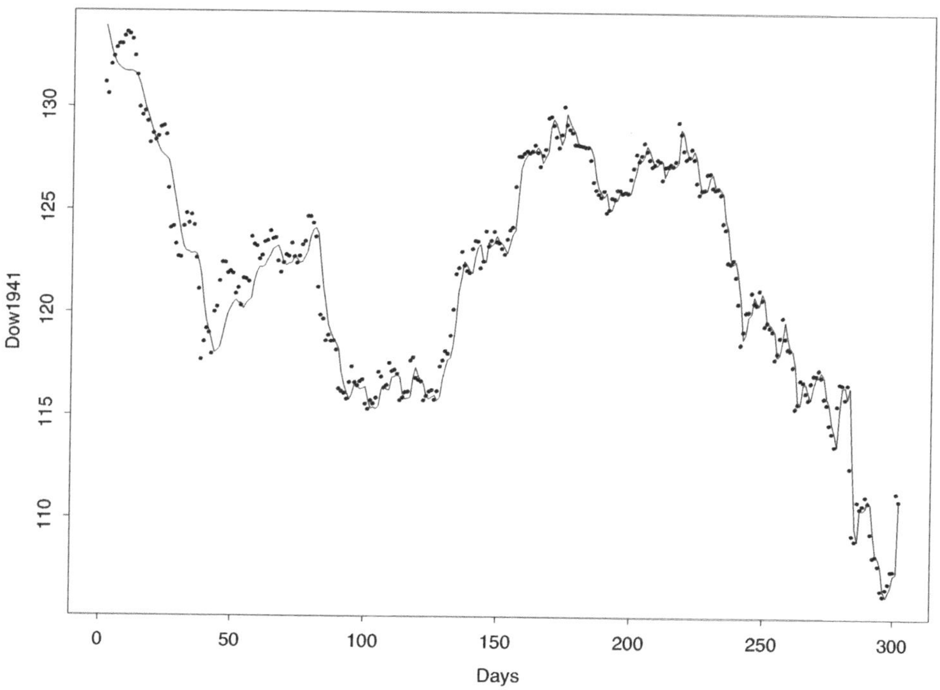

Figure 5.16: Daily Dow Jones 1941 with DLM growth predictor.

5.6.3.2 DLM with Linear Regression Suppose that a T.S. $\{Y_t\}$ is of interest. Assume k concurrent T.S. $\{X_{t,i}\}$, $i = 1, \ldots, k$, are available which are correlated with $\{Y_t\}$. The relationship between Y_t and $X_{t,i}$ is linear, that is,

$$Y_t = \beta_0 + \beta_1 X_{t,1} + \cdots + \beta_k X_{t,k} + e_t, \tag{5.6.35}$$

$t = 1, 2, \ldots$. The DLM also allows random variations in the values of the regression coefficients from one time epoch to another. Thus, the DLM with k regressors is

$$\begin{aligned} Y_t &= \mathbf{X}_t' \boldsymbol{\beta}_t + e_t \quad t = 1, 2, \ldots, \\ \boldsymbol{\beta}_t &= \boldsymbol{\beta}_{t-1} + \boldsymbol{\eta}_t, \end{aligned} \tag{5.6.36}$$

where $\mathbf{X}_t' = (1, X_{t,1}, \ldots, X_{t,k})$, $\boldsymbol{\beta}_t' = (\beta_{t,0}, \ldots, \boldsymbol{\beta}_{t,k})$. The $\{e_t\}$ are i.i.d. $N(0, v)$, the $\boldsymbol{\eta}_t$ are i.i.d. $N(\mathbf{0}, W)$; the $\{e_t\}$ and $\{\boldsymbol{\eta}_t\}$ are independent. This DLM is a special case of the general DLM with $A_t = \mathbf{X}_t'$ and $G_t = I$. The posterior distribution of $\boldsymbol{\beta}_t$ given $\mathcal{D}_t$ is $N(\mathbf{m}_t, C_t)$, and a predictor of Y_{t+1} at time t is $\hat{Y}_{t+1}(t) = \mathbf{X}_{t+1}' \mathbf{m}_t$. As before, $\mathbf{m}_t$ and C_t are determined recursively by the equations

$$\mathbf{m}_t = \mathbf{m}_{t-1} + \frac{1}{r_t}(Y_t - \mathbf{X}_t' \cdot \mathbf{m}_{t-1})(C_{t-1} + W)\mathbf{X}_t \tag{5.6.37}$$

and

$$C_t = (C_{t-1} + W) - \frac{1}{r_t}(C_{t-1} + W)\mathbf{X}_t \mathbf{X}_t'(C_{t-1} + W), \tag{5.6.38}$$

where

$$r_t = v + \mathbf{X}_t'(C_{t-1} + W)\mathbf{X}_t.$$

We present a few examples.

■ EXAMPLE 5.12

In the present example we use the monthly series of monetary international exchange rates for the years 1975–1977. We wish to predict month by month the exchange rate of the U.S. dollar Y, using as predictors the rates of exchange, relative to the U.S. dollar, of the Canadian dollar, X_1; the franc, X_2; the mark, X_3; the yen, X_4; and the lira, X_5. The following is a regression analysis of Y on X_1 to X_5 as well as a summary of the regression analysis as obtained from SPLUS.

	Value	Std. Error	t Value	Pr(> |t|)
(Intercept)	−0.2271	0.1426	−1.5922	0.1218
X_1	0.5053	0.0493	10.2541	0.0000
X_2	0.0669	0.0247	2.7117	0.0110
X_3	0.1193	0.0174	6.8515	0.0000
X_4	0.0002	0.0001	2.9747	0.0057
X_5	−0.0001	0.0001	−1.0293	0.3115

Residual standard error: 0.02602 on 30 degrees of freedom. Multiple R^2: 0.9903.

Correlation of Coefficients:

0.4854				
−0.4741	−0.7027			
−0.2017	−0.1321	−0.3982		
0.1406	0.0022	−0.1632	−0.4025	
−0.6136	−0.0065	−0.3607	0.5345	0.0262

We see first that the intercept is not significant and neither is the slope coefficient of X_5. We consider therefore a regression prediction using the variables $X_1, \ldots, X_4$ as predictors. The prediction is done by the DLMREG algorithm. If we take as initial parameters $C_0 = 0$, $V = 0.0001$, W to be the variance covariance matrix of $(\hat{\beta}_0, \hat{\beta}_1, \ldots, \hat{\beta}_4)$, and $M_0 = (-0.3172, 0.5050, 0.0002, 0.0578, 0.1289)$, we obtain the monthly predictions shown in Figure 5.17. Excluding the first month, the predictions are very close to the actual values of Y. The estimated PMSE is 0.000504. The values of $(\hat{\beta}_0, \ldots, \hat{\beta}_4)$ and W are, however, not available at the beginning. If we have similar estimates from previous years we should use them. In Figure 5.18 we show the sensitivity of the procedure to the choice of W and M_0.

The "default1" initial parameters are $C_0 = 0$, $W = I$, and $M_0 = (-0.3172, 0.5050, 0.0002,\ 0.0578)$. In the default1 case we "know" the good initial M_0. The resulting predictor is seen in Figure 5.18. The estimated PMSE is 0.000691. The "default2" initial parameters are $C_0 = 0$, $W = I$, and $M_0 = (\bar{Y}_4, 0, 0, 0, 0)'$, where $\bar{Y}_4 = (Y_1 + Y_2 + Y_3 + Y_4)/4$. The resulting predictor is unsatisfactory with estimated PMSE of 0.006158. ■

5.6.4 DLM for ARMA(p,q) T.S.

The ARMA(p, q) model was discussed in Section 5.1. In this model, for a T.S. stationary around a mean zero, we can write

$$X_t = \sum_{j=1}^{p} a_j X_{t-j} + \sum_{j=0}^{q} b_j \epsilon_{t-j},$$

where $b_0 = 1$, $a_p \neq 0$, and $b_q \neq 0$. We formulate this T.S. model as a DLM with constant matrices A, G, V, W. Let $n = \max(1 + q, p)$. If $p < n$, let $a_{p+1} = \cdots = a_n = 0$. If, on the other hand, $q < n - 1$, let $b_{q+1} = \cdots = b_{n-1} = 0$. Define $A = (1, 0, \ldots, 0)$,

$$G = \begin{bmatrix} a_1 & a_2 & \cdots & a_n \\ 1 & & & 0 \\ & & \ddots & \vdots \\ 0 & & 1 & 0 \end{bmatrix}, \tag{5.6.39}$$

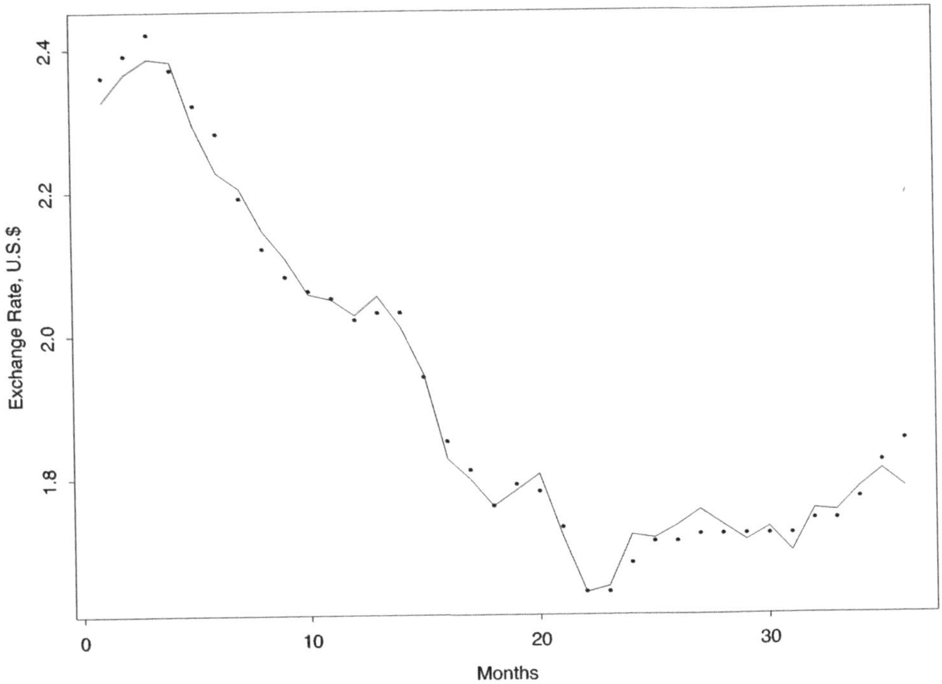

Figure 5.17: Prediction of U.S.$ exchange rate by DLMREG.

$\mathbf{h}' = (1, b_1, \ldots, b_{n-1})$. Furthermore, let $\boldsymbol{\theta}_t' = (X_t, X_{t-1}, \ldots, X_{t-n+1})$ and $\boldsymbol{\eta}_t' = (\mathbf{h}'\epsilon_t, 0, \ldots, 0)$, where $\boldsymbol{\epsilon}_t' = (\epsilon_t, \epsilon_{t-1}, \ldots, \epsilon_{t-n+1})$. Then, we can write the ARMA(p, q) T.S. as $\{Y_t\}$, where

$$\begin{aligned} Y_t &= A\boldsymbol{\theta}_t, \\ \boldsymbol{\theta}_t &= G\boldsymbol{\theta}_{t-1} + \boldsymbol{\eta}_t, \end{aligned}$$

with $V = 0$ and $W = (W_{ij}; i, j = 1, \ldots, n)$, where

$$W_{ij} = \begin{cases} \sigma^2 \left(1 + \sum_{j=1}^{n-1} b_j^2\right) & \text{if } i = 1, j = 1, \\ 0 & \text{otherwise.} \end{cases} \tag{5.6.40}$$

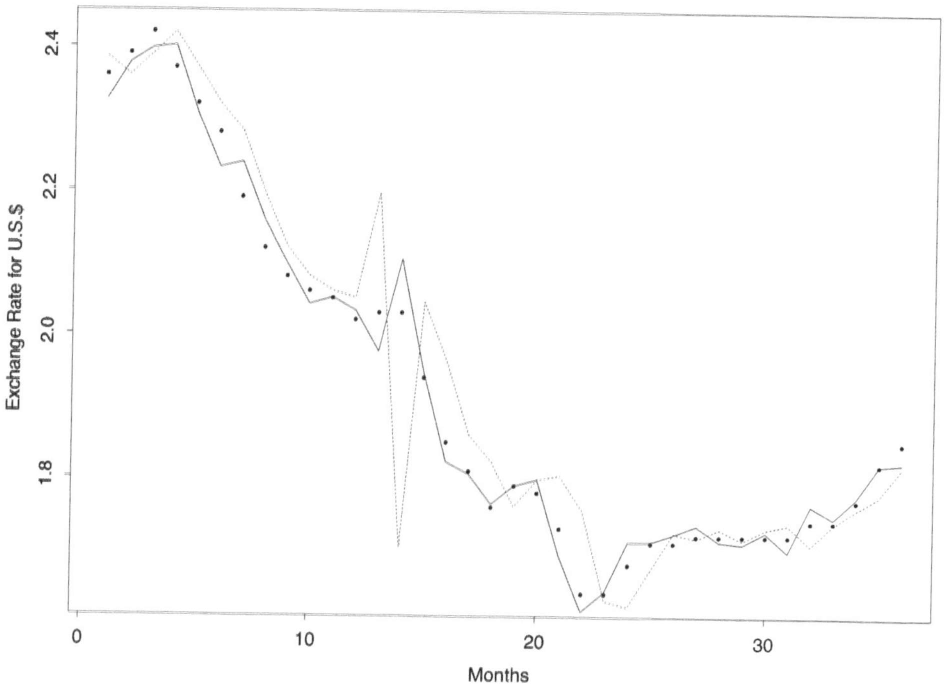

Figure 5.18: Sensitivity of DLMREG to initial parameters: default1 (bold), default2 (broken).

The recursive formulas for $\mathbf{m}_t$ and C_t become, in this case,
(5.6.41)

$$\mathbf{m}_t = \begin{bmatrix} \sum_{i=1}^{n} a_i m_{t-1,i} \\ m_{t-1,1} \\ \vdots \\ m_{t-1,n-1} \end{bmatrix} + \frac{1}{r_t}\left(Y_t - \sum_{i=1}^{n} a_i m_{t-1,i}\right)(GC_{t-1}G' + W)(1, \mathbf{0}')',$$

where $r_t = W_{11} + \mathbf{a}'C_{t-1}\mathbf{a}$ and $\mathbf{a}' = (a_1, \ldots, a_n)$. After some algebraic manipulations we obtain

$$\mathbf{m}_t = \begin{pmatrix} \mathbf{a}'\mathbf{m}_{t-1} \\ \mathbf{m}^*_{t-1} \end{pmatrix} + (Y_t - \mathbf{a}'\mathbf{m}_{t-1}) \begin{pmatrix} 1 \\ \frac{1}{r_t} C^*_{t-1}\mathbf{a} \end{pmatrix}, \tag{5.6.42}$$

where $\mathbf{m}_{t-1}^*$ and C_{t-1}^* are obtained from $\mathbf{m}_{t-1}$ and C_{t-1} by deleting the first element and the last row, respectively. The recursive equation for C_t is

$$C_t = (GC_{t-1}G' + W) - \frac{1}{r_t}\begin{bmatrix} r_t^2 & \mathbf{a}'C_{t-1}^* \\ C_{t-1}^*\mathbf{a} & C_{t-1}^*\mathbf{a}\mathbf{a}'C_{t-1}^{*\prime} \end{bmatrix}. \tag{5.6.43}$$

We start with $\mathbf{m}_0' = (X_p, X_{p-1}, \ldots, X_1)'$ and $C_0 = K_X(0) \cdot \text{toeplitz}([1, \rho_x(1), \ldots, \rho_x(n - 1)])$. Finally, the predictor of X_{t+1} at time t is

$$\begin{aligned} \hat{X}_{t+1}(t) &= E\{Y_{t+1} \mid \mathcal{D}_t\} \\ &= AG\mathbf{m}_t \\ &= \mathbf{a}'\mathbf{X}_t. \end{aligned} \tag{5.6.44}$$

Indeed $\mathcal{D}_t = \{Y_1, Y_2, \ldots, Y_t\}$ and $\mathbf{m}_t = E\{\boldsymbol{\theta}_t \mid \mathcal{D}_t\} = E\{\mathbf{X}_t \mid \mathcal{D}_t\} = \mathbf{X}_t$. This result was obtained before. The PMSE of this predictor is, according to Eq. (5.6.26),

$$\begin{aligned} \text{PMSE}\{\hat{X}_{t+1}(t)\} &= r_{t+1} \\ &= W_{11} + \mathbf{a}'C_t\mathbf{a}. \end{aligned} \tag{5.6.45}$$

■ EXAMPLE 5.13

Consider the stationary ARMA(3, 2) time series given by

$$X_t = 0.5X_{t-1} + 0.3X_{t-2} + 0.1X_{t-3} + \epsilon_t + .3\epsilon_{t-1} + .5\epsilon_{t-2}, \quad t = 4, 5, \ldots,$$

in which $\{\epsilon_t\}$ is a sequence of i.i.d. $N(0, 1)$ random variables. The initial random variables are $X_1 = N(10, 1)$, $X_2 = X_1 + N(0, 1)$, and $X_3 = X_2 + N(0, 1)$. Here $\mathbf{a} = (0.5, 0.3, 0.1)$, $b_1 = 0.3$, $b_2 = 0.5$; $A = (1, 0, 0)$. The matrix G is

$$G = \begin{bmatrix} 0.5 & 0.3 & 0.1 \\ 1 & 0 & 0 \\ 0 & 1 & 0 \end{bmatrix},$$

$V = 0$, and

$$W = \begin{bmatrix} 1.34 & 0 & 0 \\ 0 & 0 & 0 \\ 0 & 0 & 0 \end{bmatrix}.$$

We start the algorithm with $\mathbf{m}_0 = (X_3, X_2, X_1)$. The characteristic roots of

$$m^3 - 0.5m^2 - 0.3m - 0.1 = 0$$

are 0.9352, $-0.2176 + 0.2441i$, $-0.2716 - 0.2441i$. These roots belong to the unit disk. Therefore, $K_X(h)$, $|h| = 0, 1, 2, \ldots$, are obtained by solving the Yule–Walker equations (5.1.17), namely,

$$\begin{bmatrix} 1 & -0.5 & -0.3 & -0.1 \\ -0.5 & 0.7 & -0.1 & 0 \\ -0.3 & -0.6 & 0 & 1 \\ -0.1 & -0.3 & -0.5 & 1 \end{bmatrix} \begin{bmatrix} K_x(0) \\ K_x(1) \\ K_x(2) \\ K_x(3) \end{bmatrix} = \begin{bmatrix} 1.34 \\ 0.45 \\ 0.5 \\ 0 \end{bmatrix}.$$

The solution is $K_x(0) = 7.69$, $K_x(1) = 7.1495$, $K_x(2) = 7.0967$, $K_x(3) = 6.4622$. Thus, we start the algorithm with the covariance matrix

$$C_0 = \begin{bmatrix} 7.6900 & 7.1495 & 7.0967 \\ 7.1495 & 7.6900 & 7.1495 \\ 7.0967 & 7.1495 & 7.6900 \end{bmatrix}.$$

In Figure 5.19, we present this T.S. with the predictor $\hat{X}_{t+1}(t)$. For each t we also calculated the prediction interval (XL_t, XU_t), where the lower and upper limits XL_t and XU_t are given by $\hat{X}_{t+1}(t) \pm 2\sqrt{r_t}$. We see in Figure 5.19, that all the 96 points are inside the prediction region. The values of r_t for $t = 4, \ldots, 10$ are as follows:

t	4	5	6	7	8	9	10
r_t	7.312	2.601	1.979	1.834	1.794	1.783	1.780

All values of $r_t = 1.779$ for $t > 10$. ■

5.7 ASYMPTOTIC BEHAVIOR OF DLM

In the present section we discuss the asymptotic behavior of the covariance matrix C_t in a constant DLM (A, G, V, W) as $t \to \infty$. We introduce first the *spectral norm* of matrices. Let A be an $n \times m$ matrix. The spectral norm of A, denoted $||A||$, is defined as

$$||A|| = \sup_{|X|=1} ||A\mathbf{X}||, \tag{5.7.1}$$

where $||A\mathbf{X}||$ is the Euclidean norm of $A\mathbf{X}$, that is, $(\mathbf{X}'A'A\mathbf{X})^{1/2}$. Thus, to find $||A||^2$, we have to maximize $\mathbf{X}'A'A\mathbf{X}$ with respect to vectors of length 1. Writing the Lagrangian

$$L(\mathbf{X}; \lambda) = \mathbf{X}'A'A\mathbf{X} + \lambda(1 - \mathbf{X}'\mathbf{X}), \tag{5.7.2}$$

we find that the maximizing vector, $\mathbf{X}^0$, should satisfy the equation

$$(A'A)\mathbf{X}^0 = \lambda\mathbf{X}^0. \tag{5.7.3}$$

That is, $\mathbf{X}^0$ is a normalized eigenvector of $A'A$ having eigenvalue λ. Accordingly, $||A||^2$ is the *largest eigenvalue of* $A'A$.

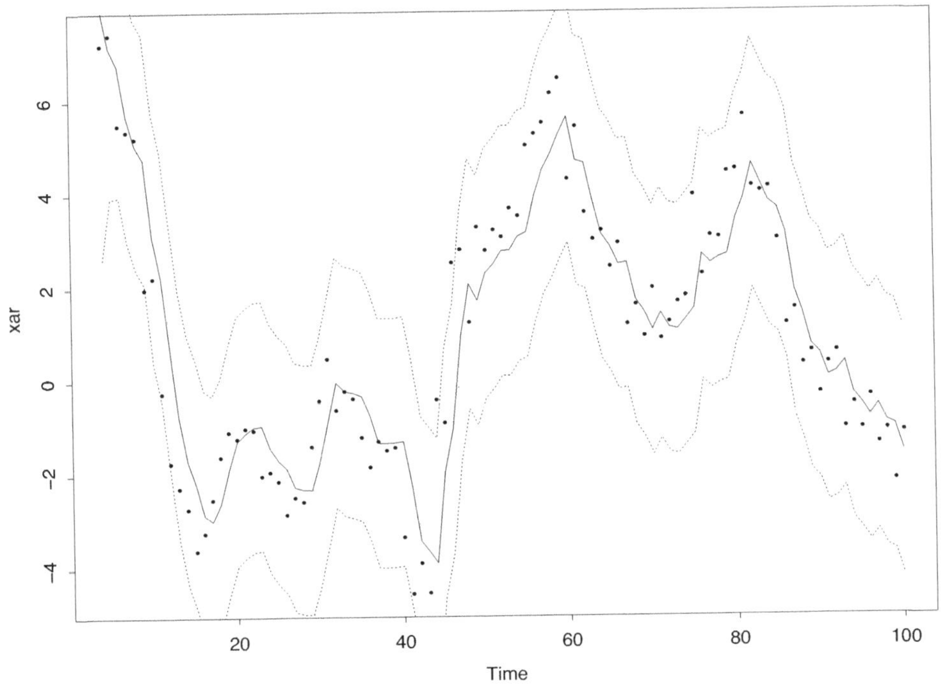

Figure 5.19: ARMA(3,2) T.S. and DLMARMA predictor.

Notice that the spectral norm, $||A||$, satisfies

$$||AB|| \leq ||A|| \cdot ||B||. \tag{5.7.4}$$

The distance between A and B is $||A - B||$. A squared matrix A is called *stable* if all its eigenvalues are *within* the unit disk. The following theorem provides a uniform bound for stable matrices.

Theorem 5.7.1 *Let $\mathcal{P}$ be a compact subset of the $n \times n$ matrices such that, if $A \in \mathcal{P}$, then all the eigenvalues of A are in the disk $\{z : |z| \leq 1 - \epsilon\}$ for some $\epsilon > 0$. Then, for any λ, $1 - \epsilon < \lambda < 1$, there exists a constant c, $0 < c < \infty$, such that (s.t.)*

$$||A^k|| \leq c\lambda^k \quad \textit{for all} \quad A \in \mathcal{P},\ k \in \mathbb{Z}^+.$$

Proof: Let $0 < 1 - \epsilon < \bar{\lambda} < \lambda < 1$.

(i) Take any $A \in \mathcal{P}$. We show that there exists a $c_A > 0$ s.t.

$$||A^k|| \leq c_A \cdot \bar{\lambda}^k, \quad k = 1, 2, \ldots .$$

Indeed, according to Jordan's decomposition of A, there exists a nonsingular matrix M s.t.

$$A = M^{-1}JM,$$

where

$$J = \begin{bmatrix} J_1 & & & & \\ & \ddots & & 0 & \\ & & J_2 & & \\ & 0 & & \ddots & \\ & & & & J_d \end{bmatrix}$$

and

$$J_i = \begin{pmatrix} \lambda_i & \delta & & 0 \\ & \ddots & \ddots & \\ & 0 & \ddots & \delta \\ & & & \lambda_i \end{pmatrix}, \quad i = 1, \ldots, d, \quad \delta = 0, 1.$$

Here λ_i is an eigenvalue of A. Thus, $A^k = M^{-1}J^kM$ and there exists a $c_1 > 0$ so that

$$||A^k|| \leq c_1 \max_{1 \leq i \leq d} ||J_i^k||.$$

Write $J_i = \lambda_i I + S_i$, where

$$S_i = \begin{pmatrix} 0 & \delta_i & 0 & \\ & \ddots & \ddots & \\ 0 & & 0 & \delta_i \end{pmatrix}, \quad \delta_i = 0, 1.$$

If $\delta_i = 0$, then $J_i^k = \lambda_i^k I$ and $||J_i^k|| \leq \bar{\lambda}^k$, since $|\lambda_i| \leq 1 - \epsilon$. If $\delta_i = 1$, then there exists a $c_2 > 0$ such that

$$||S_i^k|| \leq c_2(\bar{\lambda} - (1 - \epsilon))^k.$$

Indeed $||S_i|| = 0$ since $|S_i - \lambda I| = (-\lambda)^{r_i}$, where r_i is the dimension of δ_i. Thus, $0 \leq ||S_i^k|| \leq (||S_i||)^k = 0$. Now,

$$J_i^k = \sum_{l=0}^{k} \binom{k}{l} (\lambda_i)^l (S_i)^{k-l}.$$

Hence,

$$\begin{aligned} ||J_i^k|| &\leq \sum_{l=0}^{k} \binom{k}{l} |\lambda_i|^l ||S_i||^{k-l} \\ &\leq c_2 \sum_{l=0}^{k} \binom{k}{l} |\lambda_i|^l (\bar{\lambda} - (1 - \epsilon))^{k-l} \\ &\leq c_2((1 - \epsilon) + \bar{\lambda} - (1 - \epsilon))^k = c_2 \bar{\lambda}^k. \end{aligned}$$

Set $c_A = c_1 c_2$. Then $||A||^k \le c_A \bar{\lambda}^k$.

(ii) Let A be a fixed matrix in $\mathcal{P}$ and let $\tilde{A}$ be such that

$$||\tilde{A} - A|| < \lambda - \bar{\lambda}.$$

If $B = \tilde{A} - A$, then $\tilde{A} = A + B$. Then

$$\begin{aligned} ||\tilde{A}^k|| &= \left|\left|\sum_{l=0}^{k} \binom{k}{l} A^l B^{k-l}\right|\right| \\ &\le \sum_{l=0}^{k} \binom{k}{l} ||A^l||\ ||B^{k-l}|| \\ &\le c_A \sum_{l=0}^{k} \binom{k}{l} \bar{\lambda}^l (\lambda - \bar{\lambda})^{k-l} \\ &= c_A \lambda^k. \end{aligned}$$

(iii) Since $\mathcal{P}$ is compact, there exists a finite number of elements $A_1, \ldots, A_p$ such that

$$P \subset \bigcup_{i=1}^{p} \{\tilde{A} : ||\tilde{A} - A_i|| < (\lambda - \bar{\lambda})\}.$$

Set $c = \max_{1 \le i \le p} c_{A_i}$. Then, for any $A \in \mathcal{P}$, $||A^k|| \le c\lambda^k$.

■

Consider a DLM $\{A, G, V, W\}$. Let $\boldsymbol{\theta}_t$ be a random vector starting at $\boldsymbol{\theta}_0$. From the state equation $\boldsymbol{\theta}_t = G\boldsymbol{\theta}_{t-1} + \boldsymbol{\eta}_t$ we obtain that

$$\boldsymbol{\theta}_t = G^t \boldsymbol{\theta}_0 + \sum_{j=0}^{t-1} G^j \boldsymbol{\eta}_{t-j}. \tag{5.7.5}$$

Let $\boldsymbol{\mu}_t$ denote the expected value of $\boldsymbol{\theta}_t$ and let D_t denote the covariance matrix of $\boldsymbol{\theta}_t$. Notice the difference between $\boldsymbol{\mu}_t$ and $\mathbf{m}_t$, D_t and C_t. Since $\{\boldsymbol{\eta}_t\}$ are i.i.d. vectors, with $E\{\boldsymbol{\eta}_t\} = \mathbf{0}$ and covariance matrix W,

$$\boldsymbol{\mu}_t = G^t \boldsymbol{\mu}_0 \tag{5.7.6}$$

and

$$D_t = G^t D_0 (G^t)' + \sum_{j=0}^{t-1} G^j W (G^j)'. \tag{5.7.7}$$

Assume that G is a *stable* matrix. According to the previous theorem, there exists a $0 < c < \infty$ and a $0 < \lambda < 1$ such that $||G^t|| \le c\lambda^t \to 0$. Thus,

$$|\boldsymbol{\mu}_t| = ||G^t||\ |\boldsymbol{\mu}_0| \to 0 \quad \text{as } t \to \infty.$$

Also, if $||D_0|| < \infty$,

$$||G^t D_0(G^t)'|| \leq c^2 ||D_0|| \lambda^{2t} \to 0,$$

and if $||W|| < \infty$, then

$$\left|\left|\sum_{j=0}^{\infty} G^j W (G^j)'\right|\right| \leq c^2 \sum_{j=0}^{\infty} ||W|| \lambda^{2j} = \frac{c^2}{1-\lambda^2} ||W|| < \infty.$$

Thus $\boldsymbol{\mu}_t \to \mathbf{0}$ and

$$D_t \to D_\infty = \sum_{j=0}^{\infty} G^j W (G^j)'. \tag{5.7.8}$$

Thus, the random position of the process is distributed asymptotically around zero with finite covariance matrix D_∞ when the evolution (transition) matrix G is stable.

Notice that D_t is obtained recursively by the equation

$$D_t = G D_{t-1} G' + W. \tag{5.7.9}$$

When G is stable, then D_∞ satisfies the matrix equation (called the Liapounov equation)

$$D = GDG' + W. \tag{5.7.10}$$

The observed process $\{\mathbf{X}_t\}$ is distributed around $\boldsymbol{\theta}_t$ according to the observation equation

$$\mathbf{X}_t = A\boldsymbol{\theta}_t + \mathbf{e}_t.$$

Let $\boldsymbol{\xi}_t = E\{\mathbf{X}_t\}$ and Σ_t be the covariance matrix of $\mathbf{X}_t$. Moreover, let $K(t, t-j)$ denote the covariance matrix of $\mathbf{X}_t$ and $\mathbf{X}_{t-j}$.

From the previous results we have, for stable G,

$$\boldsymbol{\xi}_t = AG^t \boldsymbol{\mu}_0 \to \mathbf{0} \quad \text{as} \quad t \to \infty \tag{5.7.11}$$

and

$$\Sigma_t = A\left(G^t D_0 (G^t)' + \sum_{j=0}^{t-1} G^j W (G^j)'\right)A' + V. \tag{5.7.12}$$

Thus,

$$\Sigma_t \to A D_\infty A' + V \quad \text{as } t \to \infty. \tag{5.7.13}$$

The covariance of $\mathbf{X}_t$ and $\mathbf{X}_{t-j}$ is

$$
\begin{aligned}
K(t,t-j) &= E\{K(t,t-j \mid \boldsymbol{\theta}_{t-j})\} \\
&\quad + K(E\{X_t \mid \boldsymbol{\theta}_{t-j}\}, E\{X_{t-j} \mid \boldsymbol{\theta}_{t-j}\}) \\
&= AG^j D_{t-j} A',
\end{aligned} \tag{5.7.14}
$$

since $K(t,t-j) \mid \boldsymbol{\theta}_{t-j}) = 0$. Thus, for a stable matrix G, $K(t,t-j) \to AG^j D_\infty A'$ as $t \to \infty$. Moreover, when both $t, j \to \infty$, $K(t,t-j) \to 0$. Finally, if $C_t \to C^*$ as $t \to \infty$, then C^* should satisfy the equation

$$
\begin{aligned}
C^* &= (GC^*G' + W) - (GC^*B' + WA') \\
&\quad \cdot (V + BC^*B' + AWA')^{-1}(BC^*G' + AW),
\end{aligned} \tag{5.7.15}
$$

where $B = AG$. This equation is known as the *Ricatti algebraic equation.* It is known (see Davis and Vinter, 1985) that if there exist an $m \times n$ matrix F such that $G - B'F$ is stable, then C^* exists and is nonnegative definite. Moreover, C^* can be obtained from the recursive equation

$$
\begin{aligned}
C_{t+1} &= (GC_tG' + W) - (GC_tB' + WA') \\
&\quad \cdot (V + AWA' + BC_tB')^{-1} \cdot (BC_tG' + AW)
\end{aligned} \tag{5.7.16}
$$

starting with C_0.

■ **EXAMPLE 5.14**

In Example 5.13 we have seen the DLMARMA(3,2) model. The matrix

$$
G = \begin{bmatrix} 0.5 & 0.3 & 0.1 \\ 1 & 0 & 0 \\ 0 & 1 & 0 \end{bmatrix}
$$

has eigenvalues

$$
\lambda_1 = 0.9352, \quad \lambda_2 = -0.2176 + 0.2441i, \quad \lambda_3 = \bar{\lambda}_2.
$$

Thus, $|\lambda_i| < 0.94$ for all $i = 1, 2, 3$. The matrix G is stable. We see in Figure 5.19 that the process, starting at $X_1 \approx 11$, decreases fast to the zero level. Moreover, $D_\infty = \sum_{j=0}^{\infty} G^j W (G^j)'$. In the present case W is singular and is given by

$$
W = \begin{bmatrix} 1.34 & 0 & 0 \\ 0 & 0 & 0 \\ 0 & 0 & 0 \end{bmatrix}.
$$

Let $H^j = G^j W^{1/2}$. Then $D_\infty = \sum_{j=0}^{\infty} H^j (H^j)'$. Numerical evaluation yields

$$
D_\infty \cong \begin{bmatrix} 4.9231 & 4.0769 & 3.9231 \\ 4.0769 & 4.9231 & 4.0769 \\ 3.9231 & 4.0769 & 4.9231 \end{bmatrix}
$$

with eigenvalues $(12.9748, 1.000, 0.7944)$. In the present example, after 100 iterations we obtain

$$C_{100} = \begin{bmatrix} 1.0832 & 0.2103 & 0.1597 \\ 0.2103 & 0.8411 & 0.0884 \\ 0.1597 & 0.0884 & 0.7797 \end{bmatrix}.$$

The matrix $C_t \to C^*$ since $G - G'\mathbf{a}'\mathbf{a}$ has eigenvalues 0.5214, $-0.1882 + 0.2555i$, $-0.1882 - 0.2555i$. ■

We conclude the section with the remark that the stability condition for the evolution matrix G is a necessary condition for the asymptotic finiteness of the norm of the covariance matrix of $\boldsymbol{\theta}_t$. For example, the matrix $G = I$ is not stable, and the variance–covariance matrix of $\boldsymbol{\theta}_t$ is $D_t = tW$. Assume $||D_t|| \to \infty$ as $t \to \infty$. This is the case in the random walk DLM. The posterior covariance matrix C_t may still converge to a limit. For example, if $\{A, G, V, W\} = \{I_3, I_3, I_3, I_3\}$, $D_\infty = \infty$, but since $I - \mu I$ is stable, for any $0 < \mu < 1$, $C_t \to C^*$ as $t \to \infty$. In the present case $C^* = 0.618 I_3$.

5.8 LINEAR CONTROL OF DLM

5.8.1 Deterministic Linear Control

The present section follows Chapter 6 of Davis and Vinter (1985).

We consider here the control of the linear system

$$\mathbf{X}_{k+1} = A(k)\mathbf{X}_k + B(k)\mathbf{u}_k, \quad k = 0, 1, \ldots, N \tag{5.8.1}$$

with a given initial condition $\mathbf{x}_0$. This is called a *finite-horizon* system. We have to choose $\mathbf{u} = (u_0, \ldots, u_{N-1})$ to minimize

$$J_N(\mathbf{u}) = \sum_{k=0}^{N-1} ||D(k)\mathbf{x}_k + F(k)\mathbf{u}_k||^2 + \mathbf{x}'_N Q \mathbf{x}_N. \tag{5.8.2}$$

Here Q is a nonnegative definite symmetric matrix; $F'(k)F(k)$ are positive definite. The dimension of D is $p \times n$, and that of F is $p \times m$, $p > m$. We will study also what happens when $N \to \infty$. Consider the *dynamic programming* (DP) formulation. Let $V_j(\mathbf{x})$ be the minimum cost if at stage j we start at $\mathbf{x}_j = \mathbf{x}$. The DP equation (DPE) is

$$V_j(\mathbf{x}) = \min_{\mathbf{v} \in \mathbb{R}^m} [||D(j)\mathbf{x} + F(j)\mathbf{v}||^2 + V_{j+1}(A(j)\mathbf{x} + B(j)\mathbf{v})] \tag{5.8.3}$$

for all $\mathbf{x}$. The *principle of optimality* says that if $\{\mathbf{x}^*_k, \mathbf{u}^*_k\}$ is an optimal sequence over the last $N - j$ stages, that is,

$$V_l(\mathbf{x}^*_l) = \sum_{k=l}^{N-1} ||D(k)\mathbf{x}^*_k + F(k)\mathbf{u}^*_k||^2 + \mathbf{x}^{*\prime}_N Q \mathbf{x}_N, \tag{5.8.4}$$

where $l = j+1, \ldots, N-1$, and

(5.8.5)
$$V_j(\mathbf{x}^*) = ||D_j(j)\mathbf{x}^* + F(j)\mathbf{u}_j^*||^2 + V_{j+1}(A(j)\mathbf{x}^* + B(j)\mathbf{u}_j^*), \quad j = 0, 1, \ldots, N-1,$$

where $V_n(\mathbf{x}) = \mathbf{x}'Q\mathbf{x}$, then $\{\mathbf{x}_j^*, \mathbf{u}_j^*\}$, $j = 1, \ldots, N$, is optimal.

Let $V_j(\mathbf{x}) = \mathbf{x}'S_j\mathbf{x}$, $j = 0, 1, 2, \ldots$. Let $H_j(\mathbf{u})$ denote the (Hamiltonian) on the r.h.s. of the DPE, namely,

$$H_j(\mathbf{u}) = ||D_j\mathbf{x} + F_j\mathbf{u}||^2 + (A_j\mathbf{x} + B_j\mathbf{u})'S_{j+1}(A_j\mathbf{x} + B_j\mathbf{u}). \tag{5.8.6}$$

Hence,

$$\frac{\partial}{\partial \mathbf{u}} H_j(\mathbf{u}) = 2F_j'(D_j\mathbf{x} + F_j\mathbf{u}) + 2B_j'S_{j+1}(A_j\mathbf{x} + B_j\mathbf{u}).$$

Setting this to zero and solving, we obtain

$$\mathbf{u}^0(\mathbf{x}) = -M_j\mathbf{x}, \tag{5.8.7}$$

where

$$M_j = (F_j'F_j + B_j'S_{j+1}B_j)^{-1}(F_j'D_j + B_j'S_{j+1}A_j). \tag{5.8.8}$$

We require that $F_j'F_j$ is positive definite for each $j = 0, 1, \ldots, N-1$, which implies that $(F_j'F_j + B_j'S_{j+1}B_j)$ is nonsingular.

Substituting $\mathbf{u}^0(\mathbf{x})$ in the DPE we obtain

$$\begin{aligned} S_j = {} & (D_j - F_jM_j)'(D_j - F_jM_j) \\ & + (A_j - B_jM_j)'S_{j+1}(A_j - B_jM_j), \quad j = 0, 1, \ldots, N-1, \end{aligned} \tag{5.8.9}$$

where $S_N = Q$. This is a *recursive Ricatti equation.* By induction we prove that S_j are symmetric, nonnegative definite for all j. Thus, the optimal solution can be obtained by determining recursively the matrices S_j, M_j, and $\mathbf{u}_j^0 = -M_j\mathbf{x}_j^*$, where $\mathbf{x}_j^* = A_{j-1}\mathbf{x}_{j-1}^* + B_{j-1}\mathbf{u}_{j-1}^0, \ldots$. The SPLUS function rec.ricatti computes the solution S to the algebraic Ricatti equation (see Appendix).

In the infinite-horizon case, $N = \infty$, we assume that the system and the cost are time invariant. Thus, the total quadratic cost is

$$J_\infty(\mathbf{u}) = \sum_{k=0}^{\infty} ||D\mathbf{x}_k + F\mathbf{u}_k||^2 < \infty, \tag{5.8.10}$$

and the system evolution is

$$\mathbf{x}_{k+1} = A\mathbf{x}_k + B\mathbf{u}_k. \tag{5.8.11}$$

The problem makes sense as long as there is at least one control sequence $\mathbf{u}$ for which $J_\infty(\mathbf{u}) < \infty$.

A sufficient condition for this is that the pair (A, B) is *stabilizable*, that is, there exists an $m \times n$ matrix M such that $A - BM$ is *stable* (all eigenvalues are within the open unit disk). The DPE for the infinite-horizon case is

$$V(\mathbf{x}) = \inf_{\mathbf{u} \in \mathbb{R}^m} [||D\mathbf{x} + F\mathbf{u}||^2 + V(A\mathbf{x} + B\mathbf{u})]. \tag{5.8.12}$$

We say that $\mathbf{u}' = -M\mathbf{x}$ is *stabilizable control* if $\mathbf{x}_k = (A - BM)\mathbf{x}_{k-1}$, $k = 1, 2, \ldots$, and $||x_k|| \to 0$ as $k \to \infty$. We assume that $V(\mathbf{0}) = 0$. Let $V(\mathbf{x}) = \mathbf{x}'S\mathbf{x}$, where S is symmetric nonnegative definite. Assume also that $V(\mathbf{x})$ is continuous and $V(\mathbf{x}) \to 0$ as $||x|| \to 0$. The r.h.s. of the DPE is

$$H(\mathbf{u}) = ||D\mathbf{x} + F\mathbf{u}||^2 + (A\mathbf{x} + B\mathbf{u})'S(A\mathbf{x} + B\mathbf{u}). \tag{5.8.13}$$

The gradient of $H(u)$ is

$$\frac{\partial}{\partial \mathbf{u}} H(\mathbf{u}) = 2F'(D\mathbf{x} + F\mathbf{u}) + 2B'S(A\mathbf{x} + B\mathbf{u}).$$

Hence, the optimal control is

$$\mathbf{u}^0 = -M\mathbf{x}, \tag{5.8.14}$$

where

$$M = (F'F + B'SB)^{-1}(F'D + B'SA). \tag{5.8.15}$$

Substituting $\mathbf{u}^0$ in the DPE we obtain that S should satisfy

$$S = D'D + A'SA - (A'SB + D'F)(F'F + B'SB)^{-1} \cdot (B'SA + F'D). \tag{5.8.16}$$

This is the *algebraic Ricatti equation.* Notice that if $\mathbf{x}_0 = \mathbf{x}$ and $\{\mathbf{x}_k^*, \mathbf{u}_k^*\}_{k=1}^{\infty}$ is a controlled sequence, in which $\mathbf{u}_k^* = -M\mathbf{x}_k^*$, then

$$\begin{aligned} \mathbf{x}_{k+1}^* &= A\mathbf{x}_k^* + B\mathbf{u}_k^* \\ &= (A - BM)\mathbf{x}_k^* = (A - BM)^k \mathbf{x}. \end{aligned} \tag{5.8.17}$$

It follows that

$$\begin{aligned} J_N(\mathbf{u}^0) &= \sum_{k=0}^{N-1} ||D\mathbf{x}_k^* + F\mathbf{u}_k^*||^2 + \mathbf{x}_N^{*\prime} Q \mathbf{x}_N \\ &= \sum_{k=0}^{N-1} ||(D - FM)(A - BM)^k \mathbf{x}||^2 \\ &\quad + \mathbf{x}'((A - BM)^N)'Q(A - BM)^N \mathbf{x}. \end{aligned} \tag{5.8.18}$$

If $A - BM$ is stable, then there exists a λ, $0 < \lambda < 1$, $c > 0$, s.t.

$$||(A - BM)^j|| \le c\lambda^j \quad \forall j = 1, 2, \ldots .$$

Thus, if $\mathbf{x}'\mathbf{x} = r^2$, then

$$\mathbf{x}'((A-BM)^N)'Q(A-BM)^N\mathbf{x} \leq r^2||Q||c^2\lambda^{2N} \to 0 \text{ as } N \to \infty,$$

$$\lim_{N\to\infty} \sum_{k=0}^{N-1} ||(D-FM)(A-BM)^k\mathbf{x}||^2 \leq c^2r^2||D-FM|| \sum_{k=0}^{\infty} \lambda^{2k} < \infty.$$

Accordingly,

$$J_\infty(\mathbf{u}^0) = \sum_{k=0}^{\infty} ||(D-FM)(A-BM)^k\mathbf{x}||^2. \tag{5.8.19}$$

5.8.2 Stochastic Linear Control

Consider the stochastic linear evolution model

$$\mathbf{x}_{k+1} = A(k)\mathbf{x}_k + B(k)\mathbf{u}_k + C(k)\mathbf{e}_k, \quad k = 0, 1, \ldots . \tag{5.8.20}$$

We assume that the r.v.s $\mathbf{e}_1, \mathbf{e}_2, \ldots$ are *independent* $V[\mathbf{e}_k] = I$, $k = 0, 1, \ldots$, and $\mathbf{x}_0$ is a random vector,

$$E[\mathbf{x}_0] = \mathbf{m}_0, \quad V[\mathbf{x}_0] = P_0.$$

Also, $\mathbf{x}_0$ is independent of $\{\mathbf{e}_1, \mathbf{e}_2, \ldots\}$. We suppose that $\mathbf{x}_k$ can be observed directly. The objective is to minimize

$$J_N(\mathbf{u}) = E\left\{ \sum_{k=0}^{N-1} ||D(k)\mathbf{x}_k + F(k)\mathbf{u}_k||^2 + \mathbf{x}_N'Q\mathbf{x}_N \right\}, \tag{5.8.21}$$

where $Q = Q'$, $Q \geq 0$.

The DPE becomes

$$W_j(\mathbf{x}) = \min_{\mathbf{v}}[||D(j)\mathbf{x} + F(j)\mathbf{v}||^2 + E\{W_{j+1}(A(j)\mathbf{x} + B(j)\mathbf{v} + C(j)\mathbf{e})\}]. \tag{5.8.22}$$

If the horizon is finite (N say), then $W_N(\mathbf{x}) = \mathbf{x}'Q\mathbf{x}$. The solution is given by

$$W_k(\mathbf{x}) = \mathbf{x}'S_k\mathbf{x} + \alpha_k, \tag{5.8.23}$$

where S_k is the recursive solution to the discrete algebraic Ricatti equation with $S_N = Q$. For a fixed k, the conditional expectation of $W_{k+1}(\mathbf{x})$ given $\mathbf{x}$ is

$$\begin{aligned} E_{k|x}\{&W_{k+1}(A(k)\mathbf{x} + B(k)\mathbf{u} + C(k)\mathbf{e})\} \\ &= (A(k)\mathbf{x} + B(k)\mathbf{u})'S_{k+1}(A(k)\mathbf{x} + B(k)\mathbf{u}) \\ &\quad + E\{\mathbf{e}'C'(k)S_{k+1}C(k)\mathbf{e}\} + \alpha_{k+1} \\ &= (A(k)\mathbf{x} + B(k)\mathbf{u})'S_{k+1}(A(k)\mathbf{x} + B(k)\mathbf{u}) \\ &\quad + \mathrm{tr}\{C'(k)S_{k+1}C(k)\} + \alpha_{k+1}. \end{aligned} \tag{5.8.24}$$

Since the last two terms on the r.h.s. of Eq. (5.8.24) do not depend on $\mathbf{u}$, $\mathbf{u}_k^0 = -M(k)\mathbf{x}_k$. Moreover, by backwards induction, starting with $\alpha_N = 0$, we obtain

$$\alpha_k = \sum_{j=k}^{N-1} \mathrm{tr}\{\mathbf{C}'(j)S_{j+1}\mathbf{C}(j)\}, \quad k = 0, 1, 2, \ldots, N-1. \tag{5.8.25}$$

Finally,

$$\begin{aligned} E\{W_0(\mathbf{x}_0)\} &= E(\mathbf{x}_0 S_0 \mathbf{x}\} \\ &= \mathbf{m}_0' S_0 \mathbf{m}_0 + \mathrm{tr.}\{S_0 P_0\}. \end{aligned}$$

Thus, by repeated application of Eq. (5.8.20) we obtain, *for the stochastic linear control,* $\mathbf{u}_k^0 = -M(k)\mathbf{x}_k$. *The minimal cost is*

$$J_N(\mathbf{u}^0) = \mathbf{m}_0' S_0 \mathbf{m}_0 + \mathrm{tr}\{S_0 P_0\} + \sum_{i=0}^{N-1} \mathrm{tr}\{C'(i)S_{i+1}C(i)\}. \tag{5.8.26}$$

The important feature is that the matrices S_k, $k = 0, 1, \ldots$, and $M(k)$ do not depend on the $C(k)$ matrices of the noise.

The above shows that $\lim_{N\to\infty} J_N(\mathbf{u}^0) = \infty$. In order to make it finite, we need to introduce a discount factor, $0 < \rho < 1$, and a discounted total cost

$$J_N(\mathbf{u}; \rho) = E\left\{\sum_{k=0}^{N-1} \rho^k ||D\mathbf{x}_k + F\mathbf{u}_k||^2 + \rho^N \mathbf{x}_N' Q \mathbf{x}_N\right\}. \tag{5.8.27}$$

We define

$$\mathbf{x}_k^\rho = \rho^{k/2}\mathbf{x}_k, \quad A^\rho = \rho^{1/2}A, B^\rho, F^\rho, D^\rho, C^\rho;$$

the problem is then reduced to the previous one, and the optimal control is $\mathbf{u}_k^\rho = -M^\rho(k)\mathbf{x}_k^\rho$, $k = 0, 1, \ldots$,

$$\begin{aligned} J_N(\mathbf{u}^0; \rho) &= \mathbf{m}_0' S_0^\rho \mathbf{m}_0 + \mathrm{tr}\{S_0^\rho P_0\} \\ &\quad + \sum_{k=0}^{N-1} \rho^{k+1}\mathrm{tr}\{C'(k)S^\rho(k+1)C(k)\}, \end{aligned} \tag{5.8.28}$$

and

$$\lim_{N\to\infty} J_N(\mathbf{u}^0; \rho) = \mathbf{m}_0' S_0^\rho \mathbf{m}_0 + \mathrm{tr}\{S^\rho P_0\} + \frac{\rho}{1-\rho}\mathrm{tr}\{C' S^\rho C\}. \tag{5.8.29}$$

Notice that if (A, B) is stabilizable then (A^ρ, B^ρ) is stabilizable for any $0 < \rho \leq 1$. We say that (H, A) is *detectable* if there exists a matrix M such that $(A + MH)$ is *stable.*

If either one of the conditions

(i) (A, B) is stabilizable,

(ii) $(\hat{D}, \hat{A})$ is detectable, where

$$\hat{A} = A - B(F'F)^{-1}F'D,$$
$$\hat{D} = [I - F(F'F)^{-1}F']D,$$

then we must take $\rho < \rho_0$, where ρ_0 is such that (A^ρ, B^ρ) is stabilizable and $(\hat{D}, \hat{A}^\rho)$ is detectable. Generally, $\rho_0 < 1$.

If $C(k)$ is not constant, similar results apply as long as

$$\sum_{k=0}^{\infty} \rho^{k+1} \mathrm{tr}[C'(k) S^\rho C(k)] < \infty.$$

■ EXAMPLE 5.15

In Example 5.14 we have shown a DLMARMA algorithm. In the present example we illustrate a controlled AR(3) process. The uncontrolled time series is

$$X_t + 0.5X_{t-1} + 0.3X_{t-2} + 0.1X_{t-3} + \epsilon_t, \quad t = 1, 2, \ldots,$$

where $\epsilon_t \sim \mathrm{WN}(0, 1)$. The objective in the present control problem is to keep the process as close as possible to the level zero. Let $\mathbf{X}_t = (X_t, X_{t-1}, X_{t-2})'$, $t = 1, 2, \ldots$. As before, the evolution matrix is

$$G = \begin{bmatrix} 0.5 & 0.3 & 0.1 \\ 1 & 0 & 0 \\ 0 & 1 & 0 \end{bmatrix}.$$

Let

$$B = C = \begin{bmatrix} 1 & 0 & 0 \\ 0 & 0 & 0 \\ 0 & 0 & 0 \end{bmatrix}$$

and $\boldsymbol{\epsilon}_t = (\epsilon_t, \epsilon_{t-1}, \epsilon_{t-2})$. Then the controlled process is

$$\mathbf{X}_t = G\mathbf{X}_{t-1} + B\mathbf{u}_t + C\boldsymbol{\epsilon}_t, \quad t = 1, 2, \ldots.$$

We consider the cost function (5.7.14) with $D = F = I_3$.

Applying the rec.ricatti SPLUS function, we obtain after $n = 100$ iterations that $S \cong 0$. Thus $M = I$, and the optimal control vector is

$$\mathbf{u}_t^0 = -\mathbf{x}_t.$$

Thus, the optimally controlled sequence is given by the first element of each vector

$$\mathbf{Y}_t = (G - B)\mathbf{x}_t + C\mathbf{e}_t.$$

In Figure 5.20 we plot the uncontrolled AR(3) (points) against the optimally controlled AR(3) (lines). We see the extent of improvement attained by controlling the time series. This technique could be applicable in statistical process control when consecutive observations are correlated. ■

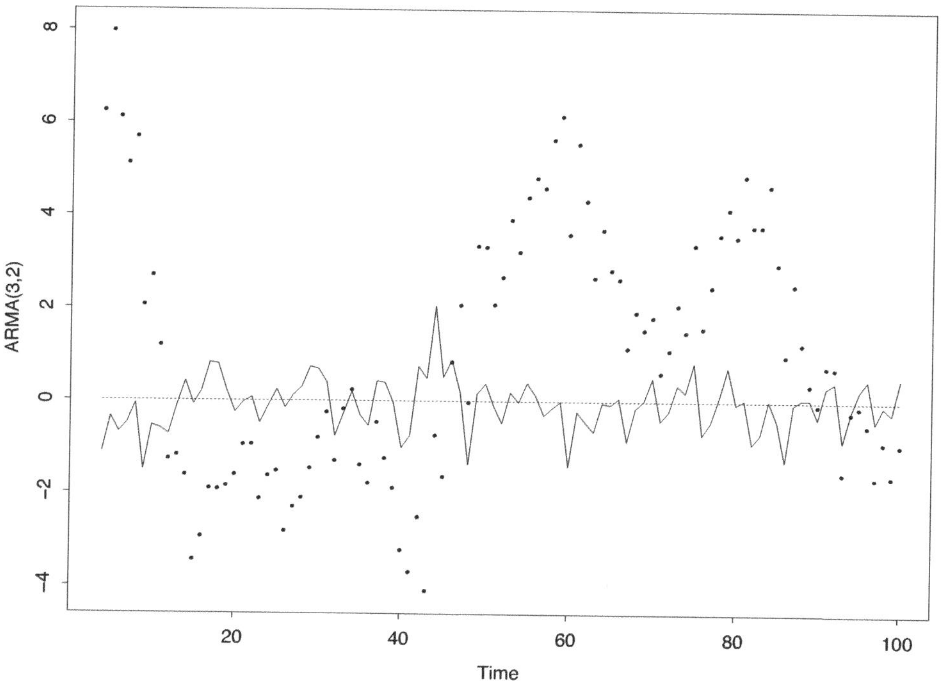

Figure 5.20: Optimally controlled AR(3) process.

CHAPTER 6

ADAPTIVE SEARCH OF AN MTD IN CANCER PHASE I CLINICAL TRIALS

6.1 UP-AND-DOWN ADAPTIVE DESIGNS

Up-and-down (UD) designs were first suggested by Anderson, McCarthy, and Tukey (1946), Dixon and Mood (1948), Dixon (1965), Tsutakawa (1967), and more. The common feature to these designs is the following. The response of each subject to a given dose, x , is binary: either a DLT response or not. Starting with a low "safe" dose, rules are given for escalating or de-escalating the dosage for the next trial. The dose at which the trial ends is estimated as the MTD. The following are some UD procedures:

1. UD1: The patients are treated in groups of size $n = 3$ (cohort groups). All patients in the same cohort receive the same dose. If no DLT is observed in a given dose, x_1, the next cohort receives the next higher dose, x_2. Otherwise, if only one patient exhibits a DLT, the next cohort remains at the same dose, x_1. If the next cohort does not exhibit any DLT, the dose is then escalated to x_2. If there are one or more DLT among the next cohort, the trial is terminated, and the estimate of the

Stage-Wise Adaptive Designs. By Shelemyahu Zacks

MTD is x_1. In UD1 there is an immediate escalation, one repeat of the same dose, or termination.

2. UD2: Treat patients in cohorts of size $n = 3$. If no DLT is observed, escalate the dose. If more than one patient manifests DLT, de-escalate the dose. Otherwise, remain at the same dose. Terminate the trial when a specified number of patients, N, have been observed.

3. UD3: Treat the patients one at a time. If DLT is manifested, de-escalate the dose. Otherwise, if at two consecutive trials no DLT is shown, escalate the dose. Terminate after a specified number of patients, N, have been treated.

4. UD4: Escalate continuously until the first DLT. Then, implement UD3.

Durham and Flournoy (1995) considered UD designs with randomization. They called these biased coin designs (BCDs). Two such designs were considered:

5. BCD1: Patients are treated one at a time. At a dose x, let $0 < b(x) < 1$ be a randomization probability. If there is *no* DLT at x, escalate with probability $b(x)$ and stay at x with probability $1 - b(x)$. If there is DLT at x, de-escalate the dose.

6. BCD2: Patients are treated one at a time. If *no* DLT at a dose x, escalate. If there is DLT, stay at x with probability $b(x)$ and de-escalate with probability $1 - b(x)$.

Let

$$Q(x) = P\{\text{DLT} \mid \text{dose} = x\}. \tag{6.1.1}$$

To evaluate the characteristics of the various UD procedures, we should assign the dosages values of $Q(x)$. We adopt here the logistic model employed by Durham and Flournoy (1995), namely,

$$Q(x) = \frac{\exp\{-3.569 + 0.549x\}}{1 + \exp\{-3.569 + 0.549x\}}. \tag{6.1.2}$$

We consider a set of six dosages with the associated values of $Q(x)$:

x	2.5	4.5	5.24	5.76	6.5	7.25
$Q(x)$	0.1	0.25	0.33	0.4	0.5	0.6

For a target of $Q(x) \leq \gamma = 1/3$, the MTD is 5.24. Suppose that in all procedures other than UD1 there are $N = 24$ patients in the trial. We estimate by $M = 1000$ simulation runs, in each case, the bias of the estimators of the MTD, the MSE of these estimators, and the proportion of cases where $x >$ MTD. This is denoted by POD. We repeat it for each one of the four UD designs and for the BCD1 design. In the BCD designs, $b(x) = Q(x)/(1-Q(x))$. All procedures start at the lowest dose of $x = 2.5$. In Table 6.1 we present the results of these simulations.

Table 6.1: Bias, MSE, and Proportion of Overdose Cases, MTD = 5.24, $\gamma = 1/3$, N = 24

Procedure	Bias	MSE	POD
UD1	−0.355	1.0428	0.231
UD2	−0.238	0.9083	0.304
UD3	−0.193	1.6821	0.366
UD4	−0.243	1.6838	0.369
BCD1	0.088	2.1858	0.462

Derived using program ud1-ud4, Bcd.

From the results of this simulation we conclude that UD1 and UD2 are the better UD procedures. It is interesting to note that while all the above UD procedures, excluding UD1, employ a fixed number $N = 24$ of patients, the number of patients treated by UD1 is random. The median number of patients in UD1 of the 1000 replicas is $N_{0.5} = 12$. We develop now the exact operating characteristics of UD1 and UD2. Starting with UD1, suppose that there are K dosages. Let ψ_j $(j = 1, \ldots, K)$ denote the conditional probability that the trial terminates at dose x_j given that it has not terminated before. Let $q_j = Q(x_j)$. We have then

$$\begin{aligned}\psi_j &= b(1;3,q_j)(1-b(0;3,q_j)) + b(2;3,q_j) + b(3;3,q_j) \\ &= 1 - b(0;3,q_j)(1+b(1;3,q_j)),\end{aligned} \tag{6.1.3}$$

$j = 1, \ldots, K-1$, and $\psi_K = 1$. Here $b(i;3,q_j)$, $i = 0, 1, \ldots, 3$, is the binomial p.d.f., namely,

$$b(i;3,q_j) = \binom{3}{i} q_j^i (1-q_j)^{3-i}. \tag{6.1.4}$$

Let P_j $(j = 1, \ldots, K)$ denote the probability of terminating at x_j. In other words, $P_j = P\{\hat{\text{MTD}} = x_j\}$. We have

$$P_j = \begin{cases} \psi_1, & j \le 1, \\ \psi_j \prod_{i=1}^{j-1}(1-\psi_i), & j = 2, \ldots, K-1, \\ \prod_{i=1}^{K-1}(1-\psi_i), & j = K. \end{cases} \tag{6.1.5}$$

Notice that $\sum_{j=1}^{K} P_j = 1$. Accordingly, the expected value of the estimator of the MTD is

$$E\{\hat{\text{MTD}}\} = \sum_{j=1}^{K} x_j P_j. \tag{6.1.6}$$

Let γ denote the tolerated probability of DLT. The MTD is then $Q^{-1}(\gamma)$. The bias of the estimator is

$$\text{Bias}(\hat{\text{MTD}}) = \sum_{j=1}^{K} x_j P_j - Q^{-1}(\gamma), \tag{6.1.7}$$

and its MSE is

$$\text{MSE}\{\hat{\text{MTD}}\} = \sum_{j=1}^{K} P_j (x_j - Q^{-1}(\gamma))^2. \tag{6.1.8}$$

We assume here that if the procedure gets to the largest dose x_K, only one application is allowed.

The conditional probability that at x_j the process terminates after the first repeat is

$$\psi_j^{(1)} = 1 - b(0; 3, q_j) - b(1; 3, q_j). \tag{6.1.9}$$

Let

$$\psi_j^{(2)} = b(1; 3, q_j)(1 - b(0; 3, q_j)) \tag{6.1.10}$$

denote the conditional probability at x_j that termination is after the second repeat. The expected total number of treated patients, N, is

$$E\{N\} = \sum_{j=1}^{K} P_j \sum_{i=1}^{j} \frac{3\psi_i^{(1)} + 6\psi_i^{(2)}}{\psi_i}. \tag{6.1.11}$$

The probability that UD1 applies dosages above the MTD is

$$\text{POD} = \sum_{j=1}^{K} I\{x_j > Q^{-1}(\gamma)\} P_j. \tag{6.1.12}$$

In Table 6.2 we give the exact values of the characteristics of UD1 computed for the case which was simulated before.

Table 6.2: Exact Values of the Characteristics of UD1, $\gamma = 1/3$, MTD = 5.24

Bias	MSE	$E\{N\}$	POD
−0.339	1.0940	13.417	0.23615

Also, the distribution of the estimator $\hat{\text{MTD}}$ in this example is:

$\hat{\text{MTD}}$	2.5	4.5	5.24	5.76	6.5	7.25
P	0.0938	0.3626	0.3074	0.1631	0.0605	0.0126

Notice that the probability that a dose will be above 5.76 is $P = 0.0731$. The dose 5.76 is the MTD for $\gamma = 0.4$, which is close to $\gamma = 0.33$.

The UD2 procedure can be evaluated as a Markov chain with K states. The process is a "birth-and-death" one.

From a state x_i the process moves to x_{i+1} with probability $p_i = b(0; 3, Q(x_i))$; it moves back to x_{i-1} with probability $s_i = 1 - b(0; 3, Q(x_i)) - b(1; 3, Q(x_i))$ and stays in the same state with probability $r_i = b(1; 3, Q(x_i))$. As before, let $q_i = Q(x_i)$. Then the matrix of transition probabilities is

$$P = \begin{bmatrix} (r_1+s_1) & p_1 & 0 & \cdots & \cdots & \cdots & 0 \\ s_2 & r_2 & p_2 & 0 & \cdots & \cdots & 0 \\ & s_3 & r_3 & p_3 & \cdots & \cdots & 0 \\ & & \ddots & \ddots & \ddots & & \\ & & & \ddots & \ddots & \ddots & p_{K-1} \\ 0 & & & & 0 & s_K & (r_K + p_K) \end{bmatrix}. \tag{6.1.13}$$

This Markov chain is irreducible, positive recurrent (see Kao, 1997, p. 169). If we treat $N = 3 \cdot m$ patients, the probability distribution of the final states is

$$\mathbf{P}'_m = \mathbf{P}'_0 P^m, \tag{6.1.14}$$

where $\mathbf{P}'_0 = (1, 0, 0, \ldots, 0)$. In other words, $\mathbf{P}'_m$ is the first row of the matrix P^m. For the data of the previous example with $N = 24$ we have

$$\mathbf{P}'_8 = (0.05566, 0.24012, 0.34844, 0.25111, 0.09032, 0.01435).$$

In Table 6.3 we present the characteristics of UD2 computed exactly.

Table 6.3: Characteristics of UD2, $\gamma = 1/3$, MTD = 5.24

Bias	MSE	N	POD
−0.057	0.81866	24	0.3558

Comparing Tables 6.2 and 6.3 we conclude that UD2, with $N = 24$, has considerably smaller bias than UD1; its MSE is slightly smaller. UD1 however requires on the average about one-half the number of patients, and its POD is smaller.

Several important studies have been published recently concerning UD designs for cancer Phase I clinical studies, in particular on the estimation of the MTD. The reader is referred to Stylianou, Proschan, and Flournoy (2003); Ivanova, Montazar-Haghighi, Mohanty, and Durham (2003); and in particular the article of Ng, Mohanty, and Balakrishnan (2007). In this paper, the authors study, in addition to the BCD rule mentioned before, also a k-in-a-row (KROW) rule, the Naroyana rule (NAR), and the CRM rule, which is discussed in the next section. The KROW is appropriate only if $\gamma = 1 - (1/2)^k$, $k \geq 1$, which is at least 0.5. This is generally too large. The NAR rule was introduced for $\gamma = 0.5$.

In our previous discussion we applied as an estimator of the MTD the last dosage used in the design. This is obviously a nonparametric estimator. Stylianou and Flournoy (2002) introduced an empirical mean estimator (EME), which is the average of the last $(N - r)$ dosages used. Another type of nonparametric estimator is the *isotonic regression* estimator suggested by Stylianou and Flournoy (2002). Suppose that h out of the K dosages were used in a trial. Let $\hat{Q}_j = X_j/n_j$, $j = 1, \ldots, h$, where X_j is the number of patients exhibiting DLT and n_j is the number of patients subjected to dosage d_j. For $i = 1, \ldots, h$, define $\hat{Q}_j^* = \hat{Q}_{j-1}I\{\hat{Q}_j \leq \hat{Q}_{j-1}\} + \hat{Q}_j I\{\hat{Q}_j > \hat{Q}_{j-1}\}$. Notice that $\hat{Q}_0 \equiv 0$ and $\hat{Q}_1^* \leq \hat{Q}_2^* \leq \cdots \leq \hat{Q}_h^*$. Let m be such that $\hat{Q}_m^* \leq \gamma \leq \hat{Q}_{m+1}^*$. The isotonic linear estimator of the MTD is

$$\hat{\text{MTD}}_{\text{LI}} = d_m + \frac{\Gamma - \hat{Q}_m^*}{Q_{m+1}^* - \hat{Q}_m^*}(d_{m+1} - d_m) \tag{6.1.15}$$

if $\hat{Q}_{m+1}^* > \hat{Q}_m^*$ and $\hat{\text{MTD}}_{\text{LI}} = d_m$ if $\hat{Q}_m^* = \hat{Q}_{m+1}^*$. Another type of isotonic estimator is given by a *logistic-type* interpolation. Recall that, for $0 < p < 1$, $\text{logit}(p) = \log[p/(1-p)]$. Accordingly,

$$\hat{\text{MTD}}_{\log I} = d_m + \frac{\text{logit}(\gamma) - \text{logit}(\hat{Q}_m^*)}{\text{logit}(\hat{Q}_{m+1}^*) - \text{logit}(\hat{Q}_m^*)} \cdot (d_{m+1} - d_m). \tag{6.1.16}$$

In case $\gamma > \hat{Q}_h^*$ the estimator is d_h, and if $\gamma < \hat{Q}_1^*$ the estimator is d_1. The MLEs of the type studied in Chapter 3 were also studied in the above-mentioned papers, with likelihood based on the logistic distribution. According to the numerical results of Ng, Mohanty, and Balakrishnan (2007), the isotonic and the MLEs of the MTD have smaller MSE than the estimators based on the last dosage.

6.2 BAYESIAN ADAPTIVE SEARCH: THE CONTINUOUS REASSESSMENT METHOD

The CRM has been applied by many researchers. This method is based on modeling a tolerance distribution in order to have a likelihood function. After observing k patients an estimator of the MTD is obtained as a function of the previous results. The application of the treatment is done one by one and the dosage for the next patient is the last estimator of the MTD or a function of it. In the present section we focus attention on Bayesian procedures. MLE estimation can follow the procedures of Chapter 3. CRM methods were investigated by O'Quigley, Pepe, and Fisher (1990), Storer (1989), Eichhorn and Zacks (1973), Tsutakawa (1980), Gastonis and Greenhouse (1992), Babb, Rogatko, and Zacks (1998), and Zacks, Rogatko, and Babb (1998). In particular see the article of Babb and Rogatko (2003) on Bayesian methods in cancer Phase I clinical trials (CPICT).

There are different formulation of the tolerance distributions in the literature. Let $F(z)$ be a c.d.f. in standard form. The relationship between a dose x and the response binary variable $Y(x)$ is given by

$$P\{Y(x) = 1 \mid x\} = F(\beta_0 + \beta_1 x), \tag{6.2.1}$$

where $\beta_1 > 0$. Recall that $Y(x) = 1$ if the response is DLT and $Y(x) = 0$ otherwise. The MTD is the dosage for which the probability of DLT is γ. Thus, the MTD is a function of $F(\cdot)$, β_0, and β_1 and is given by

$$x_\gamma = \frac{F^{-1}(\gamma) - \beta_0}{\beta_1}. \tag{6.2.2}$$

The model (6.1.2) was such a model in which $Q(x) = F(-3.569 + 0.549x)$, and $F(z)$ is the logistic distribution $F(z) = e^z/(1+e^z)$, $-\infty < z < \infty$.

In Section 3.3 we presented the Bayesian procedure for the adaptive estimation of the design point maximizing the Fisher information. Here we wish to estimate at each stage the MTD, x_γ. We will, for the sake of presentation, use the two-parameter logistic tolerance distribution

$$F(\beta_0 + \beta_1 x) = \frac{\exp\{\beta_0 + \beta_1 x\}}{1 + \exp\{\beta_0 + \beta_1 x\}}. \tag{6.2.3}$$

Suppose that it is known that $x^* < x_\gamma < x^{**}$. Thus, all dosages x should be in the interval (x^*, x^{**}). If we also know that $Q(x^*) = p_1$, where p_1 is obviously smaller than γ, we can rewrite the model as a one-parameter model

$$Q(x) = \frac{\exp\{\log([p_1/(1-p_1)]) + \beta(x - x^*)\}}{1 + \exp\{\log([p_1/(1-p_1)]) + \beta(x - x^*)\}}, \tag{6.2.4}$$

where $0 < \beta < \infty$. Let

$$G(\beta x) = \frac{p_1 \exp\{\beta(x - x^*)\}}{1 - p_1 + p_1 \exp\{\beta(x - x^*)\}}. \tag{6.2.5}$$

Notice that with this model, when x^* and p_1 are known, Eq. (6.2.2) of the MTD becomes

$$x_\gamma = x^* + \frac{\log(\gamma/(1-\gamma)) - \log(p_1/(1-p_1))}{\beta}. \tag{6.2.6}$$

Let $\mathcal{D}_k = \{(x_j, Y_j), j = 1, \ldots, k\}$ be the data of the first k trials. The likelihood function of β is then

$$L_k(\beta; \mathcal{D}_k) = \prod_{j=1}^{k} G(\beta x_j)^{Y_j}(1 - G(\beta x_j))^{1-Y_j}. \tag{6.2.7}$$

If p_1 is known, the kernel of this likelihood function is

(6.2.8)

$$L_k^*(\beta; \mathcal{D}_k) = \exp\left\{-\sum_{j=1}^{k}\left[\log\left(1 + \frac{p_1}{1-p_1}\exp\{\beta(x_j - x^*)\}\right) - \beta Y_j(x_j - x^*)\right]\right\}.$$

For a prior distribution $H(\beta)$ and the squared-error loss, the Bayesian estimator of x_γ after k trials is

(6.2.9)

$$\hat{x}_\gamma^{(k)} = x^* + \left(\log\left(\frac{\gamma}{1-\gamma}\right) - \log\left(\frac{p_1}{1-p_1}\right)\right) \cdot \frac{\int_0^\infty (1/\beta)L_k^*(\beta; \mathcal{D}_k)\, dH(\beta)}{\int_0^\infty L_k^*(\beta; \mathcal{D}_k)\, dH(\beta)}.$$

Typically CRM procedures assign the $(k+1)$st patient the dose close to the Bayesian estimator $\hat{x}_\gamma^{(k)}$.

We now illustrate the procedure numerically. For this purpose we simulate the response according to the $Q(x)$ function given in (6.1.2). For $\gamma = 1/3$ the MTD is $x_\gamma = 5.24$. We start at $x^* = 2.5$ with $p_1 = 0.1$. All dosages are in the interval $(2.5, 7.25)$. After each dose we compute the Bayesian estimator (6.2.9). For this purpose we consider the gamma prior distribution, $G(1, 1/2)$, for β. We evaluate the integrals in (6.2.9) by simulations with $M = 100$ (see Section 3.3). In Table 6.4 we present 51 estimates of the MTD computed according to this procedure.

Table 6.4: Simulated Values of $\hat{\mathbf{x}}_\gamma^{(\mathbf{k})}$, $\gamma = 1/3$

k	1	2	3	4	5	6	7	8	9	10
$\hat{x}_\gamma^{(k)}$	2.50	7.20	7.20	7.20	7.20	7.20	7.20	7.20	4.75	4.56
k	11	12	13	14	15	16	17	18	19	20
$\hat{x}_\gamma^{(k)}$	5.63	4.44	4.95	4.75	7.20	5.53	4.82	5.38	4.82	4.92
k	21	22	23	24	25	26	27	28	29	30
$\hat{x}_\gamma^{(k)}$	4.70	4.92	4.91	4.78	4.87	4.88	5.24	4.78	4.86	5.11
k	31	32	33	34	35	36	37	38	39	40
$\hat{x}_\gamma^{(k)}$	5.05	5.28	5.69	5.22	5.28	5.59	5.29	5.38	5.41	5.33
k	41	42	43	44	45	46	47	48	49	50
$\hat{x}_\gamma^{(k)}$	5.19	5.47	5.68	5.52	5.53	5.39	5.53	5.68	5.44	5.45

Derived using program bayesim3.

The striking feature of the results in this table is that doses 2–8 are extreme. Excluding these dosages, the proportion of dosages which are within the interval (0.9 MTD, 1.1 MTD) is 0.89. The median dose is 5.33. If we exclude the seven extreme dosages, the average distance between the dosages and the MTD is 0.382. In the following section we present a procedure developed by Babb, Rogatko, and Zacks (1998) of EWOC.

6.3 EFFICIENT DOSE ESCALATION WITH OVERDOSE CONTROL

Eichhorn and Zacks (1973) introduced the notion of a $1-\alpha$ feasible sequence of dosages. This was later extended to Bayesian feasibility.

A sequence $\{x_n^{(\alpha)}, n \geq 1\}$ is called *Bayesian feasible* at level $1-\alpha$ if

$$(6.3.1) \qquad P_H\{x_n^{(\alpha)} \leq x_\gamma \mid \mathcal{D}_{n-1}\} \geq 1-\alpha \quad \text{for all} \quad n \geq 1,$$

where $P_H\{\cdot \mid \mathcal{D}_{n-1}\}$ denotes the posterior probability for a prior H. Zacks, Rogatko, and Babb (1998) proved that the α-quantile of the posterior distribution of x_γ given $\mathcal{D}_{n-1}$ is the optimal Bayesian-feasible dose for stage n.

Let $\beta_{1-\alpha,n}$ denote the $1-\alpha$ quantile of the posterior distribution of β given $\mathcal{D}_{n-1}$. Then the α-quantile of the posterior distribution of x_γ given $\mathcal{D}_{n-1}$ is

$$(6.3.2) \qquad x_n^{(\alpha)} = x^* + \frac{\log(\gamma/(1-\gamma)) - \log(p_1/(1-p_1))}{\beta_{1-\alpha,n}}.$$

We approximate $\beta_{1-\alpha,n}$ by $E\{\beta \mid \mathcal{D}_{n-1}\} + \lambda(V\{\beta \mid \mathcal{D}_{n-1}\})^{1/2}$.

In Table 6.5 we present the values of $x_n^{(\alpha)}$ with $\lambda = 1.5$, $M = 100$, $x^* = 2.5$, $p_1 = 0.1$, $\gamma = 1/3$.

Table 6.5: Simulated Values of $\mathbf{x_k^{(\alpha)}}$

k	1	2	3	4	5	6	7	8	9	10
$x_k^{(\alpha)}$	2.50	3.51	3.86	3.54	3.38	3.53	3.73	3.90	4.11	4.70
k	11	12	13	14	15	16	17	18	19	20
$x_k^{(\alpha)}$	4.76	5.43	5.97	4.80	4.20	4.52	4.46	4.69	4.29	4.26
k	21	22	23	24	25	26	27	28	29	30
$x_k^{(\alpha)}$	4.26	4.31	4.44	4.54	4.81	4.49	4.24	4.19	4.18	4.31
k	31	32	33	34	35	36	37	38	39	40
$x_k^{(\alpha)}$	4.05	4.05	4.01	4.12	4.06	4.11	4.03	3.94	4.06	4.00
k	41	42	43	44	45	46	47	48	49	50
$x_k^{(\alpha)}$	3.97	4.12	4.13	3.94	3.94	4.08	3.98	3.98	4.01	3.99

Derived using program bayesim4.

We see in this table that most of the dosages are below the MTD. There are only two dosages above the MTD (estimate of α is 0.04). In contrast to the results in Table 6.4, in the present table there are no extreme dosages.

In Table 6.6 we present the results of 20 such simulation runs with $\lambda = 1.35$ and $n = 24$ patients. POD is the proportion of cases with dose above the MTD, and AVS is the average shortage, that is, $(1/n)\sum_{k=1}^{n}(x_\gamma - \hat{x}_k^{(\alpha)})^+$.

Table 6.6: Simulations of $\mathbf{\hat{x}_k^{(\alpha)}}$, $\gamma = 1/3$, $\lambda = 1.35$, n = 24

Run	POD	AVS	Run	POD	AVS
1	0.000	1.3054	11	0.167	0.7738
2	0.000	1.1434	12	0.292	0.4613
3	0.500	0.5770	13	0.125	0.8569
4	0.000	1.2649	14	0.042	0.8575
5	0.375	0.4045	15	0.042	0.8481
6	0.375	0.4119	16	0.375	0.3673
7	0.042	1.0236	17	0.042	0.9071
8	0.125	0.6650	18	0.000	2.1060
9	0.167	1.0797	19	0.292	1.0703
10	0.000	1.5044	20	0.667	0.2927

Derived using program bayesim5.

The average POD in Table 6.6 is 0.181 with S.E. = 0.044. The average of AVS is 0.8960 with S.E. = 0.0995. We see that this EWOC procedure reduces the POD from over 0.5 to about 0.2.

6.4 PATIENT-SPECIFIC DOSING

Babb and Rogatko (2001) published an interesting paper in which they show that the value of the MTD might be a function of the value c of an individual covariate. This has been observed earlier. In the study of Babb and Rogatko (2001) the dose levels of the drug PNU-214565 were adjusted according to each patient's plasma concentration of antibodies (PCA).

The tolerance distribution used, when the patient's covariate level is c, is

$$(6.4.1) \quad P\{\text{DLT} \mid \text{dose} = x,\ \text{PCA} = c\} = \frac{\exp\{\alpha + \beta \log(x) + \delta \log(c)\}}{1 + \exp\{\alpha + \beta \log(x) + \delta \log(c)\}}$$

with $\beta > 0$ and $\delta < 0$. The patient's specific MTD is given then for a probability threshold γ by

$$(6.4.2) \qquad x_\gamma(c) = \left(\frac{\gamma}{1-\gamma}\right)^{1/\beta} e^{-\alpha/\beta} c^{-\delta/\beta}.$$

The permissible dose range is also a function of c, namely $(x^*(c), x^{**}(c))$. Formulas are given for $x^*(c)$ and $x^{**}(c)$ which are specific to the PNU drug. Notice that since $0 < \beta < \infty$ and $-\infty < \delta < 0$, $-\delta/\beta > 0$ and $x_\gamma(c)$ is an increasing function of c. The parameters (β, α, δ) are, however, unknown and have to be adaptively estimated during the trials. The likelihood function of (α, β, δ) given the data $\mathcal{D}_k = \{(Y_j, x_j, c_j), j = 1, \ldots, k\}$ is
(6.4.3)

$$L(\alpha, \beta, \delta; \mathcal{D}_k) = \exp\left\{ \sum_{j=1}^{k} [Y_j(\alpha + \beta \log(x_j) + \delta \log(c_j)) - \log(1 + \exp\{\alpha + \beta \log(x_j) + \delta \log(c_j)\})] \right\}.$$

If $H(\alpha, \beta, \delta)$ denotes the prior distribution of (α, β, δ), then the posterior distribution of (α, β, δ) given $\mathcal{D}_k$ is

$$(6.4.4) \qquad dH(\alpha, \beta, \delta \mid \mathcal{D}_k) = \frac{L(\alpha, \beta, \delta; \mathcal{D}_k)\, dH(\alpha, \beta, \delta)}{\iiint L(\alpha, \beta, \delta; \mathcal{D}_k)\, dH(\alpha, \beta, \delta)}.$$

The log-dose for the $(k+1)$st patient is

$$(6.4.5) \qquad \log(x_\gamma(c_{k+1})) = \frac{\log(\gamma/(1-\gamma)) - \alpha - \delta \log(c_{k+1})}{\beta}.$$

If α and δ are known, the $(k+1)$st patient will be assigned a log-dose, according to EWOC,

$$\log(\hat{x}_{\gamma,\epsilon}(c_{k+1})) = \frac{\log(\gamma/(1-\gamma)) - \alpha - \delta\log(c_{k+1})}{\hat{\beta}_{1-\epsilon,k}}, \tag{6.4.6}$$

where $\hat{\beta}_{1-\epsilon,k}$ is the $1-\epsilon$, $0<\epsilon<1$, quantile of the posterior distribution of β given $\mathcal{D}_k$. If α and δ are unknown, the EWOC assignment would be

$$\log(\hat{x}_{\gamma,\epsilon}(c_{k+1})) = \frac{\log(\gamma/(1-\gamma)) - \hat{\alpha}_{1-\epsilon/3,k} - \hat{\delta}_{1-\epsilon/3,k}\log(c_{k+1})}{\hat{\beta}_{1-\epsilon/3,k}}, \tag{6.4.7}$$

where $\hat{\alpha}_{1-\epsilon/3,k}$, $\hat{\delta}_{1-\epsilon/3,k}$, and $\hat{\beta}_{1-\epsilon/3,k}$ are the $1-\epsilon/3$ quantiles of the posterior distribution of α, β, and δ given $\mathcal{D}_k$.

Interesting results of an actual CPICT conducted at Chase Fox Cancer Center with PNU are given in the paper of Babb and Rogatko (2001).

Individualized treatment rules are important in long treatments, in which different patients react differently to the same treatment. An interesting paper concerned with treatment of patients infected with HIV is that of Petersen, Deeks, and van der Loan (2007).

6.5 TOXICITY VERSUS EFFICACY

Generally, but not always, the efficacy of a drug as a cancer fighting agent can be assumed at a certain dose range to be a monotonically increasing function of the dose. The higher the dose, the more cancer cells die and the cancer size shrinks. In this case the drug is effectively fighting the cancer. The problem is that toxicity is also increasing monotonically with the dose. The drug often attacks various organs and high dosages may create untolerable toxicity. There are several studies connecting dose finding as a function of efficacy, E, and toxicity, T. In particular see Braun (2002), Ivanova (2003), Thall and Cook (2004), and Thall, Cook, and Estey (2006). The random variables (E,T) are binary, and the question is how to present the conditional joint probability $P(E=i, T=j \mid x, \mathbf{Z})$, where $i,j=0,1$; x is the dose level and $\mathbf{Z}$ is a vector of covariates.

If the marginal tolerance distributions are normal $\Phi(\gamma_E x + \boldsymbol{\beta}'_E\mathbf{Z})$ and $\Phi(\gamma_T x + \boldsymbol{\beta}_T\mathbf{Z})$, then a bivariate copula $\Phi_2(\Phi^{-1}(u), \Phi^{-1}(v); \rho)$ will yield a bivariate normal tolerance distribution $\Phi_2(\gamma_T x + \boldsymbol{\beta}'\mathbf{Z}, \gamma_E x + \boldsymbol{\beta}_E\mathbf{Z}; \rho)$, where $\Phi_2(z_1, z_2; \rho)$ is the standard bivariate normal c.d.f., with correlation $-1 < \rho < 1$. For logistic tolerance distributions, Thall and Cook (2004) propose the bivariate logistic distribution; that is, if $\text{logit}(\pi_E(x,\mathbf{Z})) = \gamma_E x + \boldsymbol{\beta}'_E\mathbf{Z}$ and

$\text{logit}(\pi_T(x, \mathbf{Z})) = \gamma_T x + \boldsymbol{\beta}_T' \mathbf{Z}$, then the joint probability function is

(6.5.1)

$$
\begin{aligned}
\pi_{E,T}(i, j; x, \mathbf{Z}) = {} & \pi_E(x, \mathbf{Z})^i \pi_T(x, \mathbf{Z})^j \cdot (1 - \pi_E(x, \mathbf{Z}))^{1-i} (1 - \pi_T(x, \mathbf{Z}))^{1-j} \\
& + (-1)^{i+j} \pi_E(x, \mathbf{Z})(1 - \pi_E(x, \mathbf{Z})) \pi_T(x, \mathbf{Z})(1 - \pi_T(x, \mathbf{Z})) \\
& \cdot \ (e^{\psi} - 1)/(e^{\psi} + 1),
\end{aligned}
$$

where ψ is an association parameter (correlation). Given a data set of n patients, a likelihood of $(\gamma_E, \boldsymbol{\beta}_E, \gamma_T, \boldsymbol{\beta}_T)$ can be constructed on the basis of (6.5.1), and one can apply a Bayesian approach to determine the desirable dose level x for a given patient having a vector of covariates $\mathbf{Z}$. For given thresholds $\underline{\pi}_E$ and $\overline{\pi}_T$ one would like to choose x so that both

$$
\pi_E(x, \mathbf{Z}) > \underline{\pi}_E \quad \text{and} \quad \pi_T(x, \mathbf{Z}) < \overline{\pi}_T.
$$

Additional design criteria should be imposed in order to select an "optimal" dose level. Notice that such a dose level depends on the individual covariate vector $\mathbf{Z}$, and this approach is a generalization of the one in the previous section.

CHAPTER 7

ADAPTIVE AND SEQUENTIAL PROCEDURES IN CLINICAL TRIALS, PHASES II AND III

7.1 RANDOMIZATION IN CLINICAL TRIALS

Randomization in Phase III of clinical trials is a very important feature of allocating the patients to the various treatments under comparison. Randomization means that patients entering the study are randomly assigned to the treatments. This is done in order to avoid biasing the results by some uncontrollable factors. There is a principle that should be followed in designing an experiment: Block over factors under control and randomize what cannot be controlled. If controllable patient characteristics like age, gender, and stage of the disease are relevant to the study, the patients should be grouped first into strata defined by such factors. Within each stratum the patients should be assigned to the different treatments at random, trying to avoid the creeping of unforeseen bias into the results. Various methods of randomly assigning patients to treatments have developed during the last 50 years. The reader is referred especially to the books of Rosenberger and Lachin (2002) and Hu and Rosenberger (2006). In the present chapter we present just the essentials.

Suppose there are only two treatments on test, a standard one and a new one. If there is a pool of N patients, and it is decided that M patients will be treated with the standard and $N-M$ with the new, one could choose a random sample of M patients out of N without replacement. In this case there are exactly M patients in one group (the control group) and $N-M$ in the second one (the test group). This should be executed also under double masking so that both the patients and the doctors will not know which treatment is given to whom. This is often impractical. Many Phase III clinical studies extend over several years. Patients arrive as candidates for treatments at random times, and the total number of patients entering the study is a random variable. Thus, in most studies an entering patient is assigned to a given treatment with certain probability vector $\boldsymbol{\psi}$. This probability vector might be the same for all patients or might change from one patient to another. For example, suppose that there are only two treatments, A and B. Let ψ be the probability of assigning a new patient to treatment A. In a "completely randomized" study $\psi = 1/2$ for all patients. But then, the number of patients assigned to treatment A, among the first n patients, is a random variable $J_n^{(A)}$ having a binomial distribution $\mathcal{B}(n, 1/2)$. With probability close to 1,

$$\frac{n}{2} - \frac{3}{2}\sqrt{n} < J_n^A < \frac{n}{2} + \frac{3}{2}\sqrt{n}.$$

Thus, if $n = 100$, $35 < J_{100}^A < 65$. This may result in a strongly imbalanced trial. We will list below several methods which have been devised in order to alleviate this problem. These methods change the probabilities ψ_n as a function of the observed values of $J_{n-1}^{(A)}$, that is, $\psi_n = \psi(J_{n-1}^{(A)})$, $n \geq 2$, where $\psi_1 = 1/2$. Another source of imbalance is *covariates imbalance*. We may find at the stage of analysis that more women were assigned at random to treatment A than men or some other type of imbalance (more older patients than young, etc.).

As mentioned earlier, Phase III clinical trials often last over a long period. Results of the treatments can be observed on the early entering patients. We will see later in this chapter reasons to terminate a trial early, when it becomes evident that the new treatment is worse than the standard one. On the other hand, if the number of "good" results of the new treatment is significantly larger than under the control, it might be ethically imperative to increase the probability of assigning new patients to the new treatment. Thus, the values of ψ_n, $n \geq 2$, might be changing adaptively to correct imbalances or to follow the better treatment.

7.2 ADAPTIVE RANDOMIZATION PROCEDURES

In the present section we discuss designs listed in Rosenberger and Lachin (2002, Chapter 2). We start with adaptive randomization designs, which attempt to keep the balance.

7.2.1 Random Allocation Rule

The following procedure was suggested by Lachin (1988). This procedure can be applied only if the total number of trials, N, is fixed and known from the beginning. In this case, the randomization probabilities are given by

$$\psi_n(J_{n-1}^{(A)}) = \frac{N/2 - J_{n-1}^{(A)}}{N-(n-1)}, \quad n \geq 1, \tag{7.2.1}$$

where $J_0^{(A)} \equiv 0$. Recall that $J_n^{(A)}$ denotes the random number of patients assigned to treatment A among the first n assignments. The problem with this rule is that if $J_m^{(A)} = N/2$ then $\psi_n = 0$ for all $n > m$. This creates a source of possible selection bias. We examine below whether this bias is serious. Notice that this random allocation rule (7.2.1) is equivalent to the sampling at random without replacement which was mentioned in the previous section. Accordingly, the distribution of $J_n^{(A)}$ following (7.2.1) is hypergeometric with p.d.f.

$$P\{J_n^{(A)} = j\} = \frac{\binom{N/2}{j}\binom{N/2}{n-j}}{\binom{N}{n}}, \quad n \geq 1, \quad j = 0, 1, \ldots, n. \tag{7.2.2}$$

It follows immediately that

$$E\{J_n^{(A)}\} = \frac{n}{2} \quad \text{for all } n \geq 1 \tag{7.2.3}$$

and

$$V\{J_n^{(A)}\} = \frac{n}{4}\left(1 - \frac{n-1}{N-1}\right), \quad n \geq 1. \tag{7.2.4}$$

Thus, $P\left\{J_N^{(A)} = \frac{N}{2}\right\} = 1$. This procedure is similar to the complete randomization for small values of n, but for large values of n it yields values of $J_n^{(A)}$ closer to $n/2$. It is interesting to investigate the probability distribution of the value of n at which either treatment A or treatment B gets the allotment of $N/2$ patients. For this we define the stopping variable

$$T_N = \min\left\{n \geq \frac{N}{2} : \max\left(J_n^A, n - J_n^A\right) = \frac{N}{2}\right\}. \tag{7.2.5}$$

Notice that $N/2 \le T_N \le N-1$.

Theorem 7.2.1 *The probability distribution of T_N is*

$$P\left\{T_N = \frac{N}{2} + j\right\} = \frac{2\binom{N/2+j-1}{j}}{\binom{N}{N/2}}, \quad j \ge 1, \tag{7.2.6}$$

and

$$P\left\{T_N = \frac{N}{2}\right\} = \frac{2}{\binom{N}{N/2}}. \tag{7.2.7}$$

Proof: To obtain (7.2.6) consider $J_n^{(A)}$. If $J_{N/2+j}^A = N/2$ for the first time,

$$P\left\{J_{\frac{N}{2}+j-1}^{(A)} = \frac{N}{2} - 1\right\}\psi_{\frac{N}{2}+j}\left(\frac{N}{2} - 1\right) = \frac{\binom{N/2}{N/2-1}\binom{N/2}{j}}{\binom{N}{N/2+j-1}(N/2-j+1)}$$

$$= \frac{N}{2} \cdot \frac{(N/2)!(N/2+j-1)!(N/2-j+1)!}{j!N!(N/2-j)!(N/2-j+1)}$$

$$= \frac{\binom{N/2+j-1}{j}}{\binom{N}{N/2}}.$$

Finally, due to symmetry, we obtain (7.2.6). ■

Due to symmetry, the probability that $\max\{J_{T_N}^{(A)}, T_N - J_{T_N}^{(A)}) = J_{T_N}^{(A)}$, that is, that $J_N^{(A)}$ gets to the level of $N/2$ before $J_n^{(B)}$ does, is $1/2$. Thus, if

$$T_N^{(A)} = \min\left\{n \ge \frac{1}{2}N : J_n^{(A)} = \frac{1}{2}N\right\},$$

then

$$P\left\{T_N^{(A)} = \frac{1}{2}N + j\right\} = \frac{1}{2}P\left\{T_N = \frac{1}{2}N + j\right\}, \quad j = 0, \ldots, \frac{1}{2}N - 1$$

and

$$P\{T_N^{(A)} = N\} = 1/2.$$

In Table 7.1 we present the distribution of T_N for $N = 20$. In this case $E\{T_N\} = 18.18$.

Table 7.1: Distribution of T_N, N = 20

n	10	11	12	13	14	15
$P\{T_N = n\}$	0.00001	0.00011	0.00059	0.00238	0.00774	0.02167
n	16	17	18	19	—	—
$P\{T_N = n\}$	0.05418	0.12384	0.26316	0.52632	—	—

Derived using program distm.

It is interesting that for $N = 100$ we have $P\{T_{100} = 97\} = 0.125$, $P\{T_{100} = 98\} = 0.253$, and $P\{T_{100} = 99\} = 0.505$. Thus, in the case of $N = 100$, $P\{T_{100} < 97\} = 0.117$. Similarly, if $N = 200$, $P\{T_{200} < 197\} = 0.121$. Thus, since T_N concentrates at $\{N-3, N-2, N-1\}$, the danger of bias is minimal. Notice that $E\{T_{200}\} = 198.02$.

The distribution of T_N is a special case of *fulfillment time distributions* studied by Rukhin (2004, 2006, 2007).

7.2.2 Truncated Binomial Design

This procedure was suggested by Blackwell and Hodges (1957):

$$\psi_n(J_{n-1}^{(A)}) = \begin{cases} \frac{1}{2} & \text{if } \max\{J_{n-1}^{(A)}, n-1-J_{n-1}^{(A)}\} < \frac{1}{2}N, \\ 0 & \text{if } J_{n-1}^{(A)} = \frac{1}{2}N, \\ 1 & \text{if } n-1-J_{n-1}^{(A)} = \frac{1}{2}N, \end{cases} \tag{7.2.8}$$

with $\psi_1 = 1/2$. Since the smallest value of n for which $\max\{J_n^{(A)}, n - J_n^{(A)}\} = \frac{1}{2}N$ is $\frac{1}{2}N$, according to (7.2.8), $\psi_n(J_{n-1}^{(A)}) = \frac{1}{2}$ for all $n = 1, 2, \ldots, T_N^*$, where

$$T_N^* = \min\left\{n \geq \frac{1}{2}N : \max\{J_n^{(A)}, n - J_n^{(A)}\} = \frac{1}{2}N\right\}. \tag{7.2.9}$$

Theorem 7.2.2 *The distribution of T_N^* is*

$$P\left\{T_N^* = \frac{1}{2}N + j\right\} = \binom{\frac{1}{2}N + j - 1}{j}\left(\frac{1}{2}\right)^{N/2+j-1}, \tag{7.2.10}$$

for $j = 0, 1, \ldots, \frac{1}{2}N - 1$. ∎

In Table 7.2 we provide the probability distribution of T_N^* for $N = 20$.

Table 7.2: Distribution of T^*_N, N = 20

n	$P\{T^*_N = n\}$	n	$P\{T^*_N = n\}$
10	0.00195	15	0.12219
11	0.00977	16	0.15274
12	0.02686	17	0.17456
13	0.05371	18	0.18547
14	0.08728	19	0.18547

Derived using program distm2.

The expected value of T^*_N is

(7.2.11)
$$E\{T^*_N\} = \frac{N}{2}\left(1 + \sum_{j=0}^{N/2-2} \binom{N/2+j}{j} \left(\frac{1}{2}\right)^{N/2+j}\right).$$

For example, for $N = 200$, $E\{T^*_{200}\} = 188.73$. Thus, under randomization rule (7.2.8), the danger of bias due to the fact that the last few assignments are all to one treatment is not negligible.

7.2.3 Efron's Biased Coin Design

Efron (1971) suggested a randomization procedure which is based on the difference $D_n = J_n^{(N)} - (n - J_n^{(A)}) = 2J_n^{(A)} - n$. This procedure is called the *biased coin design* and is given by

(7.2.12)
$$\psi_n(D_{n-1}) = \begin{cases} \frac{1}{2} & \text{if } D_{n-1} = 0, \\ p & \text{if } D_{n-1} < 0, \\ 1-p & \text{if } D_{n-1} > 0, \end{cases}$$

where $1/2 < p < 1$, and $D_0 \equiv 0$.

The process $\{D_n, n \geq 1\}$ is a birth-and-death process symmetric about $D_n = 0$ in the sense that, for n odd, $P\{D_n > 0\} = P\{D_n < 0\} = 1/2$. One can show then that $E\{\psi_n(D_{n-1})\} = 1/2$ for all $n \geq 1$.

In this procedure (7.2.12) $J_n^{(A)}$ (or $J_n^{(B)}$) could be anywhere between 0 and n. Thus, for values of n greater than $N/2$, $J_n^{(A)}$ could be substantially greater than $N/2$, resulting in a severe imbalance. Let $Y_n = |D_n|$, $n \geq 1$. The sequence $\{Y_n, n \geq 1\}$ is a periodic Markov chain with period 2 and transition matrix

(7.2.13)
$$P = \begin{bmatrix} 0 & 1 & 0 & 0 & 0 & 0 & \cdots \\ p & 0 & 1-p & 0 & 0 & 0 & \cdots \\ 0 & p & 0 & 1-p & 0 & 0 & \cdots \\ 0 & 0 & p & 0 & 1-p & 0 & \cdots \\ \vdots & & \ddots & & \ddots & & \end{bmatrix}.$$

Notice that, since $J_n^{(A)} = \frac{1}{2}(D_n + n)$, $J_n = \frac{1}{2}n$ only if $D_n = 0$. Moreover, since $p > 1 - p$, there is a drift of $\{Y_n, n \geq 1\}$ towards zero. The p.d.f. of Y_n on the set $\{0, 1, \ldots, n\}$ is given as the first row of the matrix P_{n+1}, where P_{n+1} is a submatrix of (7.2.13), consisting of the first $n+1$ rows and columns of P.

As given in Rosenberger and Lachin (2002, p. 44), the stationary distribution of P is $\{\pi_j, j \geq 0\}$, where

$$\pi_0 = \frac{r-1}{2r} \tag{7.2.14}$$

and

$$\pi_j = \frac{(r+1)(r-1)}{2r^{j+1}}, \quad j \geq 1, \tag{7.2.15}$$

where $r = p/(1-p)$. Here D_n is spanned over $\{-n, -n+1, \ldots, 0, \ldots, n-1, n\}$. Due to symmetry, the stationary distribution of D_n is $\{\pi_j^*, j = -n, \ldots, n\}$, where

$$\begin{aligned} \pi_0^* &= \pi_0, \\ \pi_j^* &= \frac{(r+1)(r-1)}{4r^{j+1}}, \quad |j| \geq 1. \end{aligned} \tag{7.2.16}$$

Thus, for large values of n,

$$P\{J_n^{(A)} = j\} \cong \pi_{2j-n}^*, \quad j = 0, \ldots, n. \tag{7.2.17}$$

In particular, for $p = 3/4$, $r = 3$ and

$$\begin{aligned} P\left\{J_n^{(A)} = \frac{n}{2}\right\} &\cong \frac{r-1}{2r} = \frac{1}{3}, \\ P\left\{J_n^{(A)} = \frac{n}{2} \pm 1\right\} &\cong \frac{2}{27}, \\ P\left\{J_n^{(A)} = \frac{n}{2} \pm 2\right\} &\cong \frac{2}{243}, \end{aligned} \tag{7.2.18}$$

and so on. Furthermore, the asymptotic variance of $J_n^{(A)}$ is

$$\begin{aligned} AV\{J_n^{(A)}\} &\cong \left(\frac{n}{2}\right)^2 \pi_0 + \frac{1}{2}\sum_{j=1}^{\infty} \pi_j \left[\left(\frac{n}{2} + j\right)^2 + \left(\frac{n}{2} - j\right)^2\right] - \left(\frac{n}{2}\right)^2 \\ &= \frac{(r+1)(r-1)}{2r} \sum_{j=1}^{\infty} j^2 \left(\frac{1}{r}\right)^j \\ &= \frac{r}{2}\left(\frac{r+1}{r-1}\right)^2. \end{aligned} \tag{7.2.19}$$

Thus, for $p = 3/4$, the asymptotic variance of $J_n^{(A)}$ is $AV = 6$. Thus, we expect $J_N^{(A)}$ for large values of N to be in the interval $(N/2 - 8, N/2 + 8)$.

This is a very good balancing. The advantage of this procedure over the random allocation rule is that randomized allocation continues until the last patient.

7.2.4 Wei's Urn Design

Wei (1977, 1978) developed a procedure with probabilities ψ_n which change from one patient to another. Starting with a pair of nonnegative integers (α, β) the conditional probability $\psi_n(J_{n-1}^{(A)})$ is

$$\psi_n(J_{n-1}^{(A)}) = \frac{\alpha + \beta(n-1-J_{n-1}^{(A)})}{2\alpha + \beta(n-1)}, \quad n \geq 1, \tag{7.2.20}$$

where $J_0^{(A)} \equiv 0$. Thus, if $J_n^{(A)} > J_{n-1}^{(A)}$, then $\psi_{n+1}(J_n^{(A)}) < \psi_n(J_{n-1}^{(A)})$, but if $J_n^{(A)} = J_{n-1}^{(A)}$, then $\psi_{n+1}(J_n^{(A)}) \geq \psi_n(J_{n-1}^{(A)})$. Such a design is designated as UD(α, β). If $\alpha = 0$ we define $\psi_1 = 1/2$. The UD$(\alpha, 0)$ is equivalent to complete randomization. Since $E\{J_1^{(A)}\} = 1/2$, we immediately obtain that $E\{\psi_2(J_1^{(A)})\} = 1/2$. Thus, we can prove by induction on n that $E\{\psi_n(J_{n-1}^{(A)})\} = 1/2$ for all $n \geq 1$; or $E\{J_n^{(A)}\} = n/2$ for all $n \geq 1$. One can show that this procedure is asymptotically (as $n \to \infty$) equivalent to complete randomization.

7.2.5 Response Adaptive Designs

Generally, Phase III trials are conducted in order to compare the probabilities of success (positive response) of different treatments. In particular, if a new treatment is compared to a standard one, it is ethically called to assign more patients to the treatment having a higher probability of success.

Let p_A denote the probability of success of the new treatment and p_B that of the standard. Given that $J_n^{(A)}$ patients have been assigned to the new treatment, let $X(J_n^{(A)})$ denote the number of successes among them and $X(n-J_n^{(A)})$ the number of successes among the patients assigned to treatment B. We assume that the conditional distribution of $X(J_n^{(A)})$ given $J_n^{(A)}$ is binomial $B(J_n^{(A)}, p_A)$. Similarly with the distribution of the number of successes in treatment B.

Let $\hat{p}_n^{(A)} = X(J_n^{(A)})/J_n^{(A)}$ and $\hat{p}_n^{(B)} = X(n-J_n^{(A)})/(n-J_n^{(A)})$. Moreover,

$$E\{\hat{p}_n^{(A)} - \hat{p}_n^{(B)} \mid J_n^{(A)}\} = p_A - p_B. \tag{7.2.21}$$

Thus $\hat{p}_n^{(A)} - \hat{p}_n^{(B)}$ is an unbiased estimator of $p_A - p_B$. The conditional variance of $\hat{p}_n^{(A)} - \hat{p}_n^{(B)}$ is

(7.2.22)

$$V\{\hat{p}_n^{(A)} - \hat{p}_n^{(B)} \mid J_n^{(A)}\} = \frac{p_A(1-p_A)}{J_n^{(A)}} + \frac{p_B(1-p_B)}{n-J_n^{(A)}} \quad \text{if } 0 < J_n^{(A)} < n-1.$$

Notice that if $J_n^{(A)} = 0$, $\hat{p}_n^{(A)} = 0$ with probability 1 and $V\{\hat{p}_n^{(A)} \mid J_n^{(A)} = 0\} = 0$. Similarly, $P\{\hat{p}_n^{(B)} = 0 \mid J_n^{(A)} = n\} = 1$ and $V\{\hat{p}_n^{(B)} \mid J_n^{(A)} = n\} = 0$. In testing the significance of $\hat{p}_n^{(A)} - \hat{p}_n^{(B)}$ we could use the statistic

$$(7.2.23) \qquad Z_n = \frac{\hat{p}_n^{(A)} - \hat{p}_n^{(B)}}{\sqrt{\hat{p}_n^{(A)}(1-\hat{p}_n^{(A)})/J_n^{(A)} + \hat{p}_n^{(B)}(1-\hat{p}_n^{(B)})/(n-J_n^{(A)})}}$$

when $0 < J_n^{(A)} < n$.

For the randomization methods we discussed before, J_n is either equal to $n/2$ or its distribution is concentrated near $n/2$. Thus, the asymptotic distribution of Z_n is the standard normal. To minimize the conditional variance $V\{\hat{p}_n^{(A)} - \hat{p}_n^{(B)} \mid J_n^{(A)}\}$, $J_n^{(A)}$ should be equal to

$$(7.2.24) \qquad n_A^0 = n\frac{\sqrt{p_A(1-p_A)}}{\sqrt{p_A(1-p_A)} + \sqrt{\hat{p}_B(1-\hat{p}_B)}}.$$

Thus, as long as we cannot reject the null hypothesis $H_0 : p_A = p_B$, the optimal allocation is $n_A = n/2$ and we should randomize the assignment to treatments with $\psi_n(J_{n-1}^{(A)})$ such that $E\{\psi_n(J_{n-1}^{(A)})\} = 1/2$. As soon as H_0 is rejected, one could switch to a randomization with

$$(7.2.25) \qquad \psi_{n+1}(J_n^{(A)}, X_n^{(A)}, X_n^{(B)}) = \frac{\sqrt{\hat{p}_n^{(A)}(1-\hat{p}_n^{(A)})}}{\sqrt{p_n^{(A)}(1-\hat{p}_n^{(A)})} + \sqrt{\hat{p}_n^{(B)}(1-\hat{p}_n^{(B)})}}.$$

Notice that $\hat{p}_n^{(A)}(1-p_n^{(A)})$ is greater than $\hat{p}_n^{(B)}(1-p_n^{(B)})$. Then $\psi_{n+1}(J_n^{(A)}, X_n^A, X_n^B) > 1/2$. This is satisfied only if $|\hat{p}_n^{(A)} - 1/2| < |\hat{p}_n^{(B)} - 1/2|$. Thus (7.2.25) does not answer the ethical request to allocate more patients to the treatment with the larger success probability. The randomization

$$(7.2.26) \qquad \psi_{n+1}(J_n^{(A)}, X_n^{(A)}, X_n^{(B)}) = \frac{\sqrt{\hat{p}_n^{(A)}}}{\sqrt{\hat{p}_n^{(A)}} + \sqrt{\hat{p}_n^{(B)}}}$$

satisfies the ethical demand but does not minimize the variance. Notice also that these kinds of randomization rules are only asymptotically stable.

7.3 FIXED-WIDTH SEQUENTIAL ESTIMATION OF THE SUCCESS PROBABILITY IN BERNOULLI TRIALS

In the present section we develop a sequential procedure for estimating the probabilities of success p_A and p_B with a prescribed precision. We start with a fixed-width confidence interval for p. Suppose that the prescribed width of the confidence interval is 2δ and the desired coverage probability is $1-\alpha$. For small values of δ we deal with large samples. We will therefore use the normal approximation. Thus, for large n,

$$P\{|\hat{p}_n - p| < \delta\} \cong 2\Phi\left(\frac{\sqrt{n}\,\delta}{\sqrt{p(1-p)}}\right) - 1 = (1-\alpha). \tag{7.3.1}$$

It follows that if

$$n \geq \frac{\chi^2_{1-\alpha}[1]}{\delta^2} p(1-p), \tag{7.3.2}$$

then the coverage probability of $\hat{p}_n - \delta, \hat{p}_n + \delta$ is approximately $1-\alpha$. Furthermore, since $p(1-p) \leq 1/4$, if $n \geq n^*$, where

$$n^* = \frac{\chi^2_{1-\alpha}[1]}{4\delta^2}, \tag{7.3.3}$$

then the coverage probability is guaranteed. We develop here a stopping variable which will always stop before n^*. We also derive the distribution of this stopping variable. Let X_n denote the number of successes among the first n trials and $\hat{p}_n = X_n/n$. The stopping variable is

$$N_k(\delta) = \min\left\{n \geq k : n \geq \frac{\chi^2_{1-\alpha}}{\delta^2}\hat{p}_n(1-\hat{p}_n)\right\}. \tag{7.3.4}$$

Notice that the event $n \geq 4n^*\hat{p}_n(1-\hat{p}_n)$ is equivalent to

$$n \geq 4n^* \frac{X_n}{n} \cdot \frac{n - X_n}{n}.$$

Let ξ_1 and ξ_2 be the roots of the quadratic equation

$$X_n^2 - nX_n + \frac{n^3}{4n^*} = 0, \tag{7.3.5}$$

which are

$$\xi_{1,2} = \frac{n}{2}\left(1 \pm \sqrt{1 - \frac{n}{n^*}}\right). \tag{7.3.6}$$

Define the boundaries

$$B_L(n) = \frac{n}{2}\left(1 - \sqrt{1 - \frac{n}{n^*}}\right), \quad n \leq n^*,$$

and

$$B_U(n) = \frac{n}{2}\left(1 + \sqrt{1 - \frac{n}{n^*}}\right), \quad n \leq n^*.$$

Thus $N_k(\delta)$ is equivalent to the stopping variable

$$N_k(\delta) = \min\{n \geq k : X_n \notin (B_L(n), B_U(n))\}. \tag{7.3.7}$$

Moreover, if $n = n^*$, then $B_L(n^*) = B_U(n^*) = n^*/2$. Thus,

$$P\{N_k(\delta) \leq n^*\} = 1. \tag{7.3.8}$$

Since n^* does not depend on unknown parameters, one can determine an initial sample size k so that $P\{N_k(\delta) = k\}$ is not too large. Notice that $X_k \sim B(k, p)$. Thus,

$$\begin{aligned} P\{N_k(\delta) = k\} &= B\left(\frac{k}{2}\left(1 - \sqrt{1 - \frac{k}{n^*}}\right); k, p\right) \\ &\quad + 1 - B\left(\frac{k}{2}\left(1 + \sqrt{1 - \frac{k}{n^*}}\right); k, p\right). \end{aligned} \tag{7.3.9}$$

For example, suppose $\alpha = 0.05$ and $\delta = 0.1$, $n^* = 96.04$. If $k = 20$ and $p = 0.3$, then $P\{N_k(\delta) = k\} = 0.007$; if $p = 0.2$, then $P\{N_K(\delta) = k\} = 0.069$. If we believe that $p = 0.1$ or smaller, we should use a smaller value of δ. Thus, if $k = 20$, $\alpha = 0.05$, and $\delta = 0.05$, $n^* = 384.16$ and $P\{N_\delta(k) = k\} = 0.122$. For further numerical examples we will use the values $\alpha = 0.05$ and $\delta = 0.01$. For these parameters, $n^* = 960.4$, and if $k = 30$, $p = 0.1$, $P\{N_\delta(k) = k\} = 0.042$.

We now develop the probability distribution of $N_k(\delta)$. Define the defective p.d.f.

$$g(j; n, p) = P_p\{X_n = j, N_k(\delta) \geq n\}. \tag{7.3.10}$$

In addition, for $n \geq k$, define the integers,

$$j_n^* = \min(j : B_L(n) < j < B_U(n)) \tag{7.3.11}$$

and

$$j_n^{**} = \max(j : B_L(n) < j < B_U(n)). \tag{7.3.12}$$

Hence, for each $k \leq n \leq n^*$,

$$P_p\{N_k(\delta) > n\} = \sum_{j=j_n^*}^{j_n^{**}} g(j; n, p). \tag{7.3.13}$$

The function $g(j; n, p)$ is computed recursively. Starting with $g(j; k, p) = b(j; k, p)$, we have, for each $j_n^* \leq j \leq j_n^{**}$,

(7.3.14)

$$g(j; n, p) = pI\{j_{n-1}^* \leq j - 1\}g(j - 1; n - 1, p) + (1 - p)I\{j \leq j_{n-1}^{**}\}g(j; n - 1, p).$$

Once these functions are computed for all $k \le n \le n^*$, we can determine

(7.3.15)
$$P_p\{N_k(\delta) = n\} = P_p\{N_k(\delta) > n-1\} - P_p\{N_k(\delta) > n\} \quad \text{for } n = k+1, \ldots, [n^*]-1,$$

and

$$P_p\{N_k(\delta) = [n^*]\} = P_p\{N_k(\delta) > [n^*] - 1\}. \tag{7.3.16}$$

Here $[x]$ designates the largest x smaller or equal to x.

Accordingly,

$$E_p\{N_k(\delta)\} = k + \sum_{n=k}^{[n^*]-1} P_p\{N(\delta) > n\}. \tag{7.3.17}$$

In Table 7.3 we compare $E_p\{N_k(\delta)\}$ to $n^0(p) = \chi^2_{1-\alpha}[1]p(1-p)/\delta^2$. Notice that $n^0(p)$ and $E_p\{N_k(\delta)\}$ are symmetric in p around $p = 1/2$.

Table 7.3: Values of $\mathbf{n^0(p)}$ and $\mathbf{E_p\{N_k(\delta)\}}$ for $\boldsymbol{\alpha} = \mathbf{0.05}$, $\boldsymbol{\delta} = \mathbf{0.1}$ and $\mathbf{k = 10}$

p	$n^0(p)$	$E_p\{N_R(\delta)\}$
0.1	34.573	26.745
0.2	61.463	53.406
0.3	80.671	77.195
0.4	92.195	90.885
0.5	96.037	95.204

Derived using program exbnk.

We see in Table 7.3 that $E_p\{N_k(\delta)\}$ is smaller than $n^0(p)$. The difference between the two diminishes as p gets closer to 0.5. It is important to determine the coverage probability of the interval $(\hat{p}_{N_k(\delta)} \pm \delta)$, where $\hat{p}_{N_k(\delta)} = x_{N_k(\delta)}/N_k(\delta)$. In Table 7.4 we present estimates of $E_p\{N_k(\delta)\}$ and of CP $= P_p\{|\hat{p}_{N_k(\delta)} - p| < \delta\}$. These estimates are based on $M = 1000$ simulation runs. Although we have computed the exact values of $E_p\{N_k(\delta)\}$, the comparison with the simulation estimates shows that the computations of the exact values are correct.

Table 7.4: Simulation Estimates of $\mathbf{E_p\{N_k(\delta)\}}$ and CP, $\mathbf{k = 10, \alpha = 0.05, \delta = 0.1, M = 1000}$

p	$E_p\{N_k(\delta)\}$	CP
0.1	27.325 ± 0.999	0.994 ± 0.005
0.2	53.099 ± 1.289	0.804 ± 0.025
0.3	77.559 ± 0.896	0.907 ± 0.018
0.4	91.324 ± 0.333	0.942 ± 0.015
0.5	95.216 ± 0.196	0.937 ± 0.015

Derived using program exbnks.

We see in Table 7.4 that the coverage probabilities when $0.2 < p < 0.3$ are smaller than the nominal. It is interesting that when $p = 0.1$ the coverage probability is close to 1.

7.4 SEQUENTIAL PROCEDURE FOR ESTIMATING THE PROBABILITY OF SUCCESS IN BERNOULLI TRIALS WITH PRESCRIBED PROPORTIONAL CLOSENESS

It is often not meaningful to estimate the probability of success, p, with a fixed-width confidence interval. For example, if $p = 0.1$ and $\delta = 0.1$, the width of the confidence interval is twice the value of p. For this reason we introduce the *prescribed proportional closeness* of level $1 - \alpha$. In other words, let $0 < \lambda < 1$. We wish to estimate p by $\hat{p}_n$ so that

$$P_p\{|\hat{p}_n - p| \leq \lambda p\} \geq 1 - \alpha \quad \text{for all } p. \tag{7.4.1}$$

This criterion requires considerably larger samples when $p < 1/2$. For large n, using the normal approximation to the binomial, with $\hat{p}_n = X_n/n$,

$$P_p\{(1-\lambda)p \leq \hat{p}_n \leq (1+\lambda)p\} \cong 2\Phi\left(\frac{\sqrt{n}\,\lambda\sqrt{p}}{\sqrt{1-p}}\right) - 1. \tag{7.4.2}$$

Or, for proportional closeness equal to $1 - \alpha$, n should be greater than

$$n^*(p) = \frac{\chi^2_{1-\alpha}[1]}{\lambda^2} \cdot \frac{1-p}{p}. \tag{7.4.3}$$

Thus, if $p = 1/2$ and $\lambda = 0.1$, with $\alpha = 0.05$, $n^*(1/2) = 384.15$, while for estimating $p = 1/2$ with fixed-width interval and $\delta = 0.1$ we need $n^*(1/2)/4$ observations. Moreover, if $p = 0.1$, $n^*(0.1) = 9n^*(1/2) = 3457.35$. On the other hand, if $p = 0.9$, $n^*(0.9) = n^*(1/2)/9 = 42.68$.

Consider a sequential procedure with a stopping variable

$$N_k(\lambda) = \min\left\{n \geq k : n \geq \frac{\chi^2_{1-\alpha}[1]}{\lambda^2}\frac{(1-\hat{p}_n)}{\hat{p}_n}\right\}. \tag{7.4.4}$$

Let $\gamma_\alpha^2 = \chi_{1-\alpha}^2[1]/\lambda^2$. Then (7.4.4) is equivalent to

$$N_k(\lambda) = \min\left\{n \geq k : X_n \geq \gamma_\alpha^2 \frac{n}{n+\gamma_\alpha^2}\right\}. \tag{7.4.5}$$

Let $B^*(n)$ be the boundary of the continuation region, that is,

$$B^*(n) = \gamma_\alpha^2 \frac{1}{1+\gamma_\alpha^2/n}. \tag{7.4.6}$$

This is a monotonically increasing, concave function of n, with

$$\lim_{n\to\infty} B^*(n) = \gamma_\alpha^2. \tag{7.4.7}$$

Indeed, if $B(x) = \gamma^2(1+\gamma^2/x)^{-1}$, $x \geq 1$, $B'(x) = (\gamma^2/2x^2)(1+\gamma^2/x)^{-2} > 0$ for all $x \geq 1$, and $B''(x) = -(\gamma^2/x^3)(1+\gamma^2/x)^{-2}(1-(1/x^2)(1+\gamma^2/x)^{-1})$. Since $(1/x^2)(1+\gamma^2/x)^{-1} < 1$ for all $x \geq 1$, $B''(x) < 0$ for all $x \geq 1$. Thus, the boundary $B^*(n)$ is concave for $n \geq 1$.

In Table 7.5 we present simulation estimates of $E_p\{N_k(\lambda)\}$ and of the coverage probability

$$\text{CP}(p;\lambda) = P\left\{(1-\lambda)p \leq \frac{X_{N_k}(\lambda)}{N_k(\lambda)} \leq (1+\lambda)p\right\}. \tag{7.4.8}$$

Table 7.5: Simulation Estimates of $\mathbf{E_p\{N_k(\lambda)\}}$ and CP, $\mathbf{k = 10}$, $\boldsymbol{\alpha = 0.05}$, $\boldsymbol{\lambda = 0.1}$

p	$n^*(p)$	$E_p\{N_k(\lambda)\}$	CP
0.4	576.23	574.07 ± 3.08	0.956 ± 0.01
0.5	384.15	383.00 ± 3.74	0.950 ± 0.02
0.6	256.10	254.75 ± 3.31	0.942 ± 0.02
0.7	164.60	158.67 ± 2.34	0.907 ± 0.02
0.8	96.04	84.34 ± 3.29	0.804 ± 0.04

Derived using program expros.

We see in Table 7.5 that for $p \leq 0.5$ the stopping variable $N_k(\lambda)$ yields the desired results. However, when $p > 0.6$, it tends to stop somewhat early. This results in loss of CP.

7.5 SEQUENTIAL COMPARISON OF SUCCESS PROBABILITIES

One of the main objectives of Phase III clinical trials is to compare the success probabilities of the test and the control groups, p_A and p_B, respectively. As discussed in Section 7.2, patients are assigned to the two groups at random.

Although one tries to balance the randomization, the actual size of the groups, n_A and n_B, might not be equal. The commonly used test statistic for testing the significance of the difference of the estimates, $\hat{p}_A - \hat{p}_B$, is

$$(7.5.1) \qquad Z = \frac{\hat{p}_A - \hat{p}_B}{\sqrt{\hat{p}_A(1-\hat{p}_A)/n_A + \hat{p}_B(1-\hat{p}_B)/n_B}}.$$

For large values of n_A and n_B, the statistic Z is asymptotically normally distributed. Thus, one rejects the null hypothesis $H_0 : p_A = p_B$ when the alternative is $H_1 : p_A > p_B$ if $Z \geq Z_{1-\alpha}$, where $Z_{1-\alpha} = \Phi^{-1}(1-\alpha)$ and α is a level of significance. For small values of n_A and n_B (in Phase II trials) one can use the Fisher exact test, which is a most powerful unbiased test of level α (see Lehmann and Romano, 2006).

A large sample confidence interval for $D = p_A - p_B$ of level $1 - \alpha$ is given by the confidence limits

$$(7.5.2) \qquad \hat{p}_A - \hat{p}_B \pm Z_{1-\alpha/2}\sqrt{\frac{\hat{p}_A(1-\hat{p}_B)}{n_A} + \frac{\hat{p}_B(1-\hat{p}_B)}{n_B}}.$$

If n_A and n_B are greater than

$$(7.5.3) \qquad n^* = \left\lfloor \frac{\chi^2_{1-\alpha}[1]}{2\delta^2} \right\rfloor + 1,$$

then the width of the confidence interval is smaller than 2δ. If this confidence interval does not cover the value $D = 0$, we reject the two-sided null hypothesis $H_0 : D = 0$ versus the alternative hypothesis $H_1 : D \neq 0$. If we wish that $\min(n_A, n_B) = n^*$, the best randomization procedure is the random allocation rule, where the total number of patients is $N = 2n^*$ and where n^* patients are chosen from N at random *without replacement*. This can be performed even if the patients arrive to the trial sequentially.

The total number of patients, N, can be reduced if we allocate to each group $M = N/2$ patients, where

$$(7.5.4) \qquad M = \min\left(n \geq k : n \geq \frac{\chi^2_{1-\alpha}[1]}{\delta^2}(\hat{p}_n^A(1-\hat{p}_n^{(A)}) + \hat{p}_n^{(B)}(1-\hat{p}_n^{(B)}))\right),$$

where $\hat{p}_n^{(A)}$ and $\hat{p}_n^{(B)}$ are the proportion of successes in the groups after n trials at each one. This kind of balanced allocation of patients can be achieved if we randomize the patients in pairs when one of each pair is randomly assigned to group A and the other is sent to group B. Notice that, for $\alpha = 0.05$ and $\delta = 0.1$, $n^* = 193$. In Table 7.6 we present simulation runs for estimating $E\{M\}$ and the coverage probability $\text{CP} = P\{|\hat{p}_M^{(A)} - \hat{p}_M^{(B)} - (p_A - p_B)| < \delta\}$.

Table 7.6: Simulation Estimates of E{M} and CP with $\alpha = 0.05$, $\delta = 0.1$, and k = 10

p_A	p_B	$n^*(p_A, p_B)$	$E\{M\}$	CP
0.4	0.1	126.77	126.12 ± 1.80	0.97 ± 0.03
0.3	0.1	115.24	113.44 ± 2.13	0.93 ± 0.05
0.2	0.1	96.04	93.02 ± 3.77	0.95 ± 0.04
0.5	0.2	157.50	157.39 ± 1.56	0.93 ± 0.05
0.4	0.2	153.66	153.38 ± 1.63	0.95 ± 0.04
0.3	0.2	142.14	142.50 ± 2.06	0.94 ± 0.05
0.8	0.6	153.66	152.31 ± 1.55	0.94 ± 0.05
0.8	0.5	157.50	155.32 ± 3.32	0.92 ± 0.05
0.7	0.5	176.71	176.68 ± 1.14	0.97 ± 0.03
0.6	0.5	188.23	187.06 ± 0.72	0.92 ± 0.05

Derived using program dexbnks.

If p_A and p_B were known, the required number of trials in each group would have been $\lfloor n^*(p_A, p_B) \rfloor + 1$, where

$$(7.5.5) \qquad n^*(p_A, p_B) = \frac{\chi^2_{1-\alpha}[1]}{\delta^2}(p_A(1-p_A) + p_B(1-p_B)).$$

We see in Table 7.6 that all the estimates of $E\{M\}$ are not significantly different from $n^*(p_A, p_B)$. We see also that all estimates of CP are not significantly different than $1 - \alpha = 0.95$. Furthermore $E\{M\}$ is generally considerably smaller than n^* given by (7.5.3).

7.6 GROUP SEQUENTIAL METHODS

The so-called group sequential method is actually a multistage testing procedure. Instead of evaluating the results after each observation, we wait until a whole group of m patients are tested on the two treatments. Afterwards, the hypothesis $H_0 : p_A = p_B$ is tested. If H_0 is rejected, then the trial is stopped; otherwise, another group of m patients is treated on each one of the treatments, and so on. In other words, the total number of N patients is tested in K stages. In each stage m patients are assigned at random to treatment A and m patients to treatment B. If in *all* K stages the hypothesis H_0 is not rejected, the trial terminates after K stages, with a total of $N = 2mK$ patients treated. On the other hand, if H_0 is rejected after the kth stage, $1 \leq k < K$, the trial is terminated with $N_k = 2mk$ patients treated. The problem is to devise the repetitive tests so that the level of significance will not exceed a prescribed value α. There are many papers on the subject. The reader is referred to the book of Jennison and Turnbull (2000) for details and tables.

Let $X_{m,i}^{(A)}$ and $X_{m,i}^{(B)}$, $i = 1, \ldots, K$, denote the number of successes among the patients who have received treatment A or B at the ith stage. The test statistic at the kth stage is based on the partial sums $\sum_{i=1}^{k} X_{m,i}^{(A)}$ and $\sum_{i=1}^{k} X_{m,i}^{(B)}$ and the statistic

$$Z_k = \frac{\sqrt{mk}(\hat{p}_k^{(A)} - \hat{p}_k^{(B)})}{\sqrt{\hat{p}_k^{(A)}(1 - \hat{p}_k^{(A)}) + \hat{p}_k^{(B)}(1 - \hat{p}_k^{(B)})}}, \tag{7.6.1}$$

where $\hat{p}_k^{(A)} = \sum_{i=1}^{k} X_{m,i}/mk$ and $\hat{p}_k^{(B)}$ is similarly defined. For a group size m which is large, Z_k is approximately distributed like $N(0, 1)$. Another way to construct approximately standard normal statistics is to use the angular transformation (see Johnson and Kotz, 1969, p. 69). This is the well-known variance stabilizing transformation

$$Y_i^{(A)} = 2 \arcsin \sqrt{X_{m,i}^{(A)}/m}, \quad i = 1, \ldots, k. \tag{7.6.2}$$

If $\eta^{(A)} = 2 \arcsin \sqrt{p^{(A)}}$, then for large values of m, $Y_i^{(A)} - \eta^{(A)} \sim N(0, 1/m)$. Let $\bar{Y}_k^{(A)} = (1/k) \sum_{i=1}^{k} Y_i^{(A)}$. Since $Y_1^{(A)}, \ldots, Y_k^{(A)}$ are independent, $\bar{Y}_k^{(A)} - \eta^{(A)} \sim N(0, 1/(km))$, $k = 1, \ldots, K$, for large m. Thus, one could use the statistics

$$\tilde{Z}_k = \sqrt{\frac{mk}{2}}(\bar{Y}_k^{(A)} - \bar{Y}_k^{(B)}), \quad k = 1, \ldots, K. \tag{7.6.3}$$

If $\delta = \eta^{(A)} - \eta^{(B)}$, then $(\tilde{Z}_k - \sqrt{mk/2}\ \delta)$ is distributed approximately like $N(0, 1)$.

Notice that, for $1 \leq k < l \leq K$,

$$\begin{aligned}
\operatorname{Cov}(\tilde{Z}_k, \tilde{Z}_l) &= \frac{m}{2}\sqrt{kl}\ \operatorname{Cov}(\bar{Y}_k^{(A)} - \bar{Y}_k^{(B)}, \bar{Y}_l^{(A)} - \bar{Y}_l^{(B)}) \\
&= \frac{m}{2}\frac{\sqrt{kl}}{k \cdot l}\operatorname{Cov}\left(\sum_{i=1}^{k}(Y_i^{(A)} - Y_i^{(B)}), \sum_{j=1}^{l}(Y_j^{(A)} - Y_j^{(B)})\right) \\
&= \frac{m}{2}\frac{1}{\sqrt{kl}} V\left\{\sum_{i=1}^{k}(Y_i^{(A)} - Y_i^{(B)})\right\} \\
&= \frac{m}{2}\frac{2k}{\sqrt{kl}\ m} = \sqrt{\frac{k}{l}}.
\end{aligned} \tag{7.6.4}$$

Thus, $\tilde{\mathbf{Z}} = (\tilde{Z}_1, \ldots, \tilde{Z}_k)'$ is distributed for large values of m approximately like a K-variate normal with expected value $E\{\tilde{\mathbf{Z}}\} = \delta\sqrt{m/2}\ \boldsymbol{\mu}_K$ and covariance matrix

$$R_K = (\rho_{kl}; k, l = 1, \ldots, K), \tag{7.6.5}$$

where $\boldsymbol{\mu}_K = (1, \sqrt{2}, \sqrt{3}, \ldots, \sqrt{K})'$ and $\rho_{kl} = (k/l)^{1/2}$ if $k \leq l$ and $\rho_l = (l/k)^{1/2}$ if $l < k$.

We are testing the hypothesis $H_0 : \delta = 0$ versus $H_1 : \delta \neq 0$. Notice that, under H_0, $\tilde{\mathbf{Z}}_K \sim N(\mathbf{0}, R_K)$. The vector $\mathbf{Z}_K = (Z_1, \ldots, Z_K)'$ has the same asymptotic distribution for large values of m as that of $\tilde{\mathbf{Z}}_K$. Let $\mathbf{U}_K = (U_1, \ldots, U_K)'$ be distributed like $N(\mathbf{0}, R_K)$. To test H_0 versus H_1 in K stages, one needs to find critical values $(C_1, \ldots, C_K)$ such that H_0 is rejected at the kth stage if $|U_k| \geq C_k$ and if $k < K$; one continues to stage $k+1$ if $|U_k| < C_k$. Thus, H_0 is not rejected only if K stages were performed, and $|U_K| < C_K$. Define the stopping variable

$$K_s = \min\{k, 1 \leq k \leq K : |U_k| > C_k\}. \tag{7.6.6}$$

We have to determine $(C_1, \ldots, C_K)$ so that

$$P\{|U_K| < C_K, K_s = K\} \geq 1 - \alpha. \tag{7.6.7}$$

One way to do it is to apply the Bonferroni inequality with $C_k = Z_{1-\alpha/2K}$ for all $k = 1, \ldots, K$. Indeed, under these critical values the probability of accepting H_0 is

$$\begin{aligned} P\left\{\bigcap_{k=1}^{K}\{|U_k| \leq Z_{1-\alpha/2K}\}\right\} &= 1 - P\left\{\bigcup_{k=1}^{K}\{|U_k| > Z_{1-\alpha/2K}\}\right\} \\ &\geq 1 - \sum_{k=1}^{K} P\{|U_k| > Z_{1-\alpha/2K}\} \\ &= 1 - \alpha. \end{aligned} \tag{7.6.8}$$

However, these critical values might be too conservative, leading to loss of power. Another approach is based on the following. As in the O'Brein and Fleming (1979) test, let $C_k = \gamma_{\alpha,K}\sqrt{K/k}$, $k = 1, \ldots, K$. This reduces the number of parameters to one. We further define the defective densities

$$g_k(x; \gamma_{\alpha,K}) = \frac{d}{dx} P\{U_k \leq x, K_s \geq k\}, \quad k = 1, \ldots, K. \tag{7.6.9}$$

Since $Z_k \mid Z_{k-1} \sim N(\rho_{k-1,k} Z_{k-1}, (1 - \rho^2_{k-1,k}))$ for all $k \geq 2$, we can determine $g_k(x; \gamma_{\alpha,K})$ recursively. Starting with

$$g_1(x; \gamma_{\alpha,K}) = \frac{1}{\sqrt{2\pi}} e^{-\frac{1}{2}x^2}, \quad -\infty < x < \infty, \tag{7.6.10}$$

we have, for $k \geq 2$,

$$\begin{aligned} g_k(x; \gamma_{\alpha,K}) = &\int_{-\gamma_{\alpha,K}\sqrt{K/(k-1)}}^{\gamma_{\alpha,K}\sqrt{K/(k-1)}} g_{k-1}(y; \gamma_{\alpha,K}) \\ &\cdot \frac{1}{\sqrt{1 - \rho^2_{k-1,k}}} \phi\left(\frac{x - \rho_{k-1,k} y}{\sqrt{1 - \rho^2_{k-1,k}}}\right) dy, \end{aligned} \tag{7.6.11}$$

where $\phi(z)$ is the p.d.f. of $N(0,1)$. Notice that, for $1 \leq k \leq K-1$,

$$P\{K_s > k; \gamma_{\alpha,K}\} = \int_{-\gamma_{\alpha,K}\sqrt{K/k}}^{\gamma_{\alpha,K}\sqrt{K/k}} g_k(x;\gamma_\alpha)\,dx. \tag{7.6.12}$$

Furthermore, $\gamma_{\alpha,K}$ should be determined so that

$$\int_{-\gamma_{\alpha,K}}^{\gamma_{\alpha,K}} g_K(x;\gamma_{\alpha,K})\,dx = 1-\alpha. \tag{7.6.13}$$

The value of $\gamma_{\alpha,K}$ depends on α and on K. Its determination requires delicate numerical analysis. Values of $\gamma_{\alpha,K}$ for $K = 1(1)20$ and $\alpha = 0.01, 0.05, 0.10$ can be found in Jennison and Turnbull (2000, p. 29). We have tested the effectiveness of these boundaries on the statistics Z_k and $\tilde{Z}_k$ defined in (7.6.1) and (7.6.3) by simulations. The results are presented in Table 7.7. We restrict the computations to the case of $K = 4$ and $\alpha = 0.05$ with group size of $m = 50$. According to O'Brein and Fleming, $\gamma_{0.05,4} = 2.024$. We denote by K_s the number of stages till stopping based on Z_k and by $\tilde{K}_s$ that based on $\tilde{Z}_k$. The corresponding levels of significance or powers are denoted by α and $\tilde{\alpha}$, respectively.

Table 7.7: Simulation Estimates of $\mathbf{E\{K_s\}}$ and $\mathbf{E\{\tilde{K}_s\}}$ and Associated Significance Levels, $\alpha = 0.05$, K = 4, m = 50, $\gamma_{0.05,4} = 2.024$

p_A	p_B	$E\{K_s\}$	$E\{\tilde{K}_s\}$	α	$\tilde{\alpha}$
0.3	0.3	3.99 ± 0.02	3.98 ± 0.04	0.02 ± 0.03	0.05 ± 0.04
0.4	0.4	4.00 ± 0.00	3.98 ± 0.03	0.04 ± 0.04	0.05 ± 0.04
0.6	0.6	3.97 ± 0.03	3.98 ± 0.03	0.06 ± 0.05	0.10 ± 0.06
0.7	0.7	4.00 ± 0.00	3.96 ± 0.04	0.04 ± 0.04	0.07 ± 0.05
				Power	Power
0.8	0.5	1.82 ± 0.09	1.82 ± 0.09	1.00 ± 0.00	1.00 ± 0.00
0.7	0.5	2.45 ± 0.13	2.43 ± 0.15	0.97 ± 0.03	0.98 ± 0.03
0.6	0.5	3.72 ± 0.11	3.63 ± 0.13	0.45 ± 0.10	0.52 ± 0.10

Derived using program exgs.

In the upper part of Table 7.7 we see estimates of the expected number of stages and the level of significance when $p_A = p_B$. The lower part of the table provides estimates of these characteristics when $p_A > p_B$. Notice that in these cases α and $\tilde{\alpha}$ designate the power of the tests. We see that the procedures based on Z_k or $\tilde{Z}_k$ yield very close results.

The recursive equations (7.6.10) and (7.6.11) are not suitable for an exact computation of the power of the test, since these equations are based on the assumption that $E\{U_k\} = 0$, all k. In the general case, let

$$E\{U_k\} = \theta\sqrt{\frac{1}{2}mk}, \quad k = 1, \ldots, K. \tag{7.6.14}$$

In this case,

$$\begin{aligned} E\{U_k \mid U_{k-1}\} &= \theta\left(\sqrt{\frac{1}{2}mk} - \rho_{k-1,k}\sqrt{\frac{1}{2}m(k-1)}\right) + \rho_{k-1,k}U_{k-1} \\ &= \theta\sqrt{\frac{1}{2}mk}(1 - \rho_{k-1,k}^2) + \rho_{k-1}U_{k-1}. \end{aligned} \tag{7.6.15}$$

The g-functions become

$$g_1(x; \gamma_{\alpha,K}, \theta) = \phi\left(x - \theta\sqrt{\frac{1}{2}m}\right), \tag{7.6.16}$$

and, for $k \geq 2$,

$$\begin{aligned} g_k(x; \gamma_{\alpha,K}, \theta) &= \frac{1}{\sqrt{1 - \rho_{k-1,k}^2}} \cdot \int_{-\gamma_{\alpha,K}\sqrt{K/(k-1)}}^{\gamma_\alpha\sqrt{K/(k-1)}} g_{k-1}(y; \gamma_{\alpha,K}, \theta) \\ &\quad \cdot \phi\left(\frac{x - \rho_{k-1}y}{\sqrt{1 - \rho_{k-1,k}^2}} - \theta\sqrt{\frac{1}{2}mk}(1 - \rho_{k-1,k}^2)\right) dy. \end{aligned} \tag{7.6.17}$$

Let K_s be the stopping variable (7.6.6) with $C_k = \gamma_{\alpha,K}\sqrt{K/k}$. The power function is

$$\psi_K(\theta) = \sum_{k=1}^{K-1} P_\theta\{K_s = k\} + \left(\int_{-\infty}^{-\gamma_{\alpha,K}} + \int_{\gamma_{\alpha,K}}^{\infty}\right) g_K(x; \gamma_{\alpha,K}, \theta)\, dx. \tag{7.6.18}$$

Moreover,

$$\begin{aligned} P_\theta\{K_s = 1\} &= \Phi\left(-\gamma_{\alpha,K}\sqrt{K} - \theta\sqrt{\frac{1}{2}m}\right) \\ &\quad + 1 - \Phi\left(\gamma_{\alpha,K}\sqrt{K} - \theta\sqrt{\frac{1}{2}m}\right) \\ &= 2 - \Phi\left(\gamma_{\alpha,K}\sqrt{K} + \theta\sqrt{\frac{1}{2}m}\right) \\ &\quad - \Phi\left(\gamma_{\alpha,K}\sqrt{K} - \theta\sqrt{\frac{1}{2}m}\right). \end{aligned} \tag{7.6.19}$$

Furthermore, for $k = 2, \dots, K-1$,

(7.6.20)
$$P_\theta\{K_s = k\} = P_\theta\{K_s > k-1\} - P_\theta\{K_s > k\}.$$

Substituting in (7.6.18) we get
(7.6.21)
$$\begin{aligned}\psi_K(\theta) &= 1 - P_\theta\{K_s > K-1\} + \left(\int_{-\infty}^{-\gamma_{\alpha,K}} + \int_{\gamma_{\alpha,K}}^{\infty}\right) g_K(x; \gamma_{\alpha,K}, \theta)\, dx \\ &= 1 - \int_{-\gamma_{\alpha,K}}^{\gamma_{\alpha,K}} g_K(x; \gamma_{\alpha,K}, \theta)\, dx.\end{aligned}$$

Notice that, according to (7.6.13), $\psi_K(0) = \alpha$.

7.7 DYNAMIC DETERMINATION OF STAGE-WISE SAMPLE SIZE

In the group sequential designs discussed in the previous section, all groups have a fixed sample size m. The question is whether one could increase the power of the tests when the groups size can be dynamically changed as a function of the observed results. This is especially important in Phase II clinical trials, in which the trials focus just on a new drug with relatively small samples. The objective in Phase II is to determine the antidisease activity of the drug. In this stage the probability of successful response is generally unknown. Clinicians often give a possible range (p_0, p_1) for the success probability and a minimum, m, and maximum, M, for the sample size. It is important to conduct the trial in stages to increase its efficiency. There are several papers which address the question of adaptively determining the sample size of the various stages. If there is evidence after any stage that the probability of success is smaller than p_0, the trial may terminate early. The reader is referred to the papers of Bartoff and Lai (2008), Bauer (1989), Bauer and Einfalt (2006), Birkett and Day (1994), Cui, Hung, and Wang (1999), Denne and Jennison (2000), Fisher (1998), Jennison and Turnbull (2003), Lai and Shih (2004), Simon (1989), Thall, Simon, Ellenberg, and Shrager (1988), and Wittes and Brittain (1990).

We present here a three-stage procedure which is based only on a prescribed value of p_0 and the minimum and maximum sample sizes m, M. We then compare it to the three-stage procedure of Bartoff and Lai.

7.7.1 Truncated Three-Stage Procedure for Power (TTSP)

Let X_n be a random variable having a binomial distribution $\mathcal{B}(n, p)$. Suppose we wish to test the hypothesis $H_0 : p \le p_0$ against $H_1 : p \ge p_1$, where $0 < p_0 < p_1 < 1$. What should be the sample size so that the uniformly most powerful test of size α will have power $1 - \beta$ when $p = p_1$? A normal approximation for large samples yields the formula

$$(7.7.1)\quad n_{\text{opt}}(p_0, p_1, \alpha, \beta) = \left\lfloor \frac{(Z_{1-\alpha}\sqrt{p_0(1-p_0)} + Z_{1-\beta}\sqrt{p_1(1-p_1)}\,)^2}{(p_1 - p_0)^2} \right\rfloor + 1.$$

For example, if $p_0 = 0.3$, $\alpha = 0.05$, $\beta = 0.20$, we obtain the following values of n_{opt} as p_1 varies:

p_1	0.35	0.40	0.45	0.50
n_{opt}	534	136	62	35

The following is a three-stage adaptive procedure, TTSP, when the value of p_1 is unknown.
Stage 1: Take a random sample of size $N_1 = m$. Let $\hat{p}_m = X_m/m$ denote the MLE of p. For a specified value of the size α, compute the critical value

$$q_1 = B^{-1}(1 - \alpha; m, p_0),$$

where $B^{-1}(\gamma; m, p_0)$ is the γ-quantile of the binomial $\mathcal{B}(m, p_0)$. If $X_m < q_1$, accept H_0 and stop sampling; else, compute for a specified value of β,

$$(7.7.2)\qquad N_2 = \min(n_{\text{opt}}(p_0, \hat{p}_m, \alpha, \beta), M),$$

according to (7.7.1). If $N_2 \leq N_1$, stop sampling and reject H_0. If $N_2 > N_1$, go to Stage 2.
Stage 2: Take additional $N_2 - N_1$ observations, independent of the first-stage sample. Compute the MLE p_{N_2} based on all the N_2 observations. Compute

$$q_2 = B^{-1}(1 - \alpha; N_2, p_0).$$

If $N_2\hat{p}_{N_2} < q_2$, stop sampling and accept H_0; else, compute

$$(7.7.3)\qquad N_3 = \min(n_{\text{opt}}(p_0, \hat{p}_{N_2}, \alpha, \beta), M).$$

If $N_3 \leq N_2$, reject H_0 and stop sampling. If $N_3 > N_2$, go to Stage 3.
Stage 3: Take additional $N_3 - N_2$ independent observations. Compute the MLE $\hat{p}_{N_3}$ and

$$q_3 = B^{-1}(1 - \alpha; N_3, p_0).$$

If $N_3\hat{p}_{N_3} < q_3$, accept H_0 and stop sampling; else reject H_0 and stop sampling. ■

For example, suppose $p_0 = 0.3$, $\alpha = 0.05$, $\beta = 0.20$, $M = 100$, and $p = 0.4$. Let $N_1 = m = 20$. By simulation from $B(20, 0.4)$ we obtain $X_{N_1} = 7$ and $\hat{p}_{N_1} = 7/20 = 0.35$. Now, $q_1 = 11$. Since $X_1 < q_1$ we stop sampling and accept H_0. Notice that under $N_1 = 20$ the power of this test is $1 - B(10; 20, 0.4) = 0.1275$. Thus, if $N_1 = 20$, most of the samples will stop after

Stage 1 and accept H_0. On the other hand, if $N_1 = 40$, then $q_1 = 18$ and $1 - B(17, 40, 0.4) = 0.3115$. The smallest value of $\hat{p}_{n_0}$ is $18/40 = 0.45$. For this value, $n_{\text{opt}}(0.3, 0.45, 0.05, 0.2) = 62$. This will be the maximal size of N_2. On the other hand, if $X_{40} \geq 20$, $\hat{p}_{40} \geq 0.5$. Moreover, $n_{\text{opt}}(0.3, 0.5, 0.05, 0.2) = 35$ and we stop after the first stage and reject H_0. The size of N_2 depends on X_{40}. If $X_{40} = 18$, then $\hat{p}_{40} = 0.45$ and $N_2 = 62$. If $X_{40} = 19$, then $\hat{p}_{40} = 0.475$ and $N_2 = 46$. Furthermore, if $N_2 = 62$, $q_2 = 26$. Thus, if $X_{62} \leq 25$, we accept H_0 and stop. If $X_{62} = 26$, then $N_3 = 95$, and if $X_{62} = 27$, then $N_3 = 75$. If $X_{62} \geq 28$, then $N_3 < N_2$ and we stop and reject H_0; and so on. Thus, the probability of stopping after Stage 1 is $1 - b(18, 40, 0.4) - b(19, 40, 0.4) = 0.818$. We stop after Stage 2 with probability

$$b(18, 40, 0.4)[1 - b(26, 62, 0.4) - b(27, 62, 0.4)] + b(19, 40, 0.4)[1 - b(21, 46, 0.4) - b(22, 46, 0.4)] = 0.1507.$$

The probability of reaching Stage 3 in this design is 0.0313. The expected number of stages is 1.446. ■

We develop now the formula for the probability of accepting H_0 under p. Let $q_1 = B^{-1}(1 - \alpha, N_1, p_0)$, and for $q_1 \leq j \leq N_1$,

$$N_2(j) = \min\left\{M, n_{\text{opt}}\left(p_0, \frac{j}{N_1}, \alpha, \beta\right)\right\}. \tag{7.7.4}$$

Define the set $A_1 = \{j : N_2(j) > N_1\}$, and let

$$q_2(j) = B^{-1}(1 - \alpha, N_2(j), p_0). \tag{7.7.5}$$

For $q_2(j) \leq k_j \leq N_2(j)$, let

$$N_3(k_j; j) = \min\left\{M, n_{\text{opt}}\left(p_0, \frac{k_j}{N_2(j)}, \alpha, \beta\right)\right\}, \tag{7.7.6}$$

and $A_2(j) = \{k_j : N_3(k_j; j) > N_2(j)\}$,

$$q_3(k_j; j) = B^{-1}(1 - a; N_3(k_j; j), p_0). \tag{7.7.7}$$

The probability of accepting H_0 is then

(7.7.8)

$$\begin{aligned}
\pi(p) &= B(q_1 - 1; N_1, p) \\
&\quad + \sum_{j=0}^{N_1} I\{N_2(j) > N_1\} b(j; N_1, p) B(q_2(j) - 1 - j; N_2(j) - N_1, p) \\
&\quad + \sum_{j=0}^{N_1} \sum_{k=0}^{N_2(j)} I\{N_2(j) > N_1\} I\{N_3(k; j) > N_2(j)\} \\
&\quad \cdot b(j; N_1, p) b(k - j; N_2(j) - N_1, p) \\
&\quad \cdot B(q_3(k; j) - 1 - j - k; N_3(k; j) - N_2(j), p).
\end{aligned}$$

The power of the test is $\psi(p) = 1 - \pi(p)$. The expected sample size is (7.7.9)

$$E_p\{N\} = N_1 \cdot B(q_1 - 1; N_1, p) + \sum_{j=0}^{N_1} [I\{N_2(j) \leq N_1\} N_1 b(j; N_1, p) + I\{N_2(j) > N_1\} N_2(j) b(j; N_1, p) \cdot B(q_2(j) - 1 - j; N_2(j) - N_1, ; p)]$$

$$+ \sum_{j=0}^{N_1} \sum_{k=0}^{N_2(j)} I\{N_2(j) > N_1\} [I\{N_3(k; j) \leq N_2(j)\} \cdot N_2(j) b(j; N_1, p) b(k - j; N_2(j) - N_1, p) + I\{N_3(k; j) > N_2(j)\} N_3(k; j) \cdot b(j; N_1, p) \cdot b(k - j; N_2(j) - N_1 p)].$$

The expected number of stages $E_P\{K\}$ is obtained by replacing in (7.7.9) N_1 by 1, $N_2(j)$ by 2 and $N_3(k; j)$ by 3 whenever they appear as sample size factors (free terms). In Table 7.8 we present some numerical results.

Table 7.8: Power, Expected Sample Size, and Expected Number of Stages for $p_0 = 0.3$, $m = 30$, $M = 82$, $\alpha = \beta = 0.1$ of TTSP

p	Power, $\psi(p)$	$E_P\{N\}$	$E_P(K)$
0.30	0.0701	37.47	1.176
0.35	0.2519	44.88	1.382
0.44	0.7138	51.87	1.668
0.50	0.8476	46.51	1.570
0.60	0.9916	34.23	1.184

Derived using program Octs.

7.7.2 Bartoff–Lai GLR Procedure

The generalized likelihood ratio (GLR) procedure of Bartoff and Lai (2008) is based on the properties of GLR testing of the hypothesis $H_0 : p = p_0$ against the composite hypothesis $H_1 : p > p_0$. The likelihood function of the binomial parameter p, given $X_n = \sum_{i=1}^{n} J_i$, where $J_1, \ldots, J_n$ are i.i.d. $\mathcal{B}(1, p)$, is

$$L_n(p; X_n) \alpha \left(\frac{p}{1-p}\right)^{X_n} (1-p)^n. \tag{7.7.10}$$

Accordingly, the GLR for testing H_0 against H_1 is

$$\Lambda_n(\hat{p}_n; p_0) = n \left[(1 - \hat{p}_n) \log\left(\frac{1 - \hat{p}_n}{1 - p_0}\right) + \hat{p}_n \log\left(\frac{\hat{p}_n}{p_0}\right)\right], \tag{7.7.11}$$

where $\hat{p}_n = X_n/n$ is the MLE of p. Notice that $\Lambda_n(\hat{p}_n; p_0)$ is a monotone increasing function of $\hat{p}_n$ on the interval (p_0, ∞). Thus, H_0 is rejected if

$\hat{p}_n$ is sufficiently large. A size α test of H_0 against H_1 is: Reject H_0 if $n \cdot \hat{p}_n > B^{-1}(1-\alpha; n, p_0)$. The level of significance of this test is $\tilde{\alpha} \leq \alpha$.

Since the sample size is restricted to the interval (m, M), we define p^* to be the smallest p such that $P_p\{M\hat{p}_M > B^{-1}(1-\alpha; m, p_0)\} \geq 1-\beta$, that is,

$$p^* = \inf\{0 < p < 1 : B(B^{-1}(1-\alpha; m, p_0); M, p) \leq \beta\}. \tag{7.7.12}$$

The value of p^* has a special role in the GLR procedure. The sample size determination of the GLR procedure is based on some optimal properties of the sequential probability ratio test (SPRT) which are discussed in Chapter 10.

As proven by Siegmund (1985, p. 21), for any stopping rule T of any test $H_0 : f = f_0$ against $H_1 : f = f_1$ with error probabilities α and β, respectively, if $E_i\{T\} < \infty$, then

$$E_1\{T\} \geq \frac{(1-\beta)\log((1-\beta)/\alpha) + \beta\log(\beta/(1-\alpha))}{I(f_1, f_0)}, \tag{7.7.13}$$

and

$$E_0\{T\} \geq \frac{(1-\alpha)\log((1-\alpha)/\beta) + \alpha\log(\alpha/(1-\beta))}{I(f_0, f_1)}, \tag{7.7.14}$$

where $I(f_1, f_0)$ is the Kullback–Liebler information to discriminate f_1 from f_0 and $I(f_0, f_1)$ is that to discriminate f_0 from f_1. Thus, asymptotically, as $\alpha \to 0$ and $\beta \to 0$, the optimal procedure satisfies

$$E_0\{T\} \approx \frac{|\log(\beta)|}{I(f_0, f_1)} \tag{7.7.15}$$

and

$$E_1\{T\} \approx \frac{|\log \alpha|}{I(f_1, f_0)}. \tag{7.7.16}$$

The Kullback–Liebler information function for the binomial case is

$$I(p, \theta) = (1-p)\log\left(\frac{1-p}{1-\theta}\right) + p\log\left(\frac{p}{\theta}\right). \tag{7.7.17}$$

For a sample of size m, define

$$N(\hat{p}_m) = \min\left\{\frac{|\log \alpha|}{I(\hat{p}_m, p_0)}, \frac{|\log \beta|}{I(\hat{p}_m, p^*)}\right\}, \tag{7.7.18}$$

where $\hat{p}_m$ is the MLE of p. The GLR three-stage sampling procedure follows the decision rules:

Stage 1: Sample m independent observations. If $X_m > B^{-1}(1-\alpha\epsilon_1; m, p_0)$, stop and reject H_0; if $X_m < B^{-1}(\alpha\epsilon_1; m, p^*)$, stop and accept H_0. Compute

$$N_2 = \min\{M, N(\hat{p}_m)\}. \tag{7.7.19}$$

If $B^{-1}(\alpha\epsilon_1, m, p^*) \leq X_m \leq B^{-1}(1-\alpha\epsilon_1; m, p_0)$ *and* $N_2 > m$, go to Stage 2. Else, stop sampling. If $X_m \geq B^{-1}(1-\alpha; m, p_0)$, reject H_0; otherwise accept H_0.

Stage 2: Sample additional $N_2 - m$ independent observations. Let X_{N_2} be the total number of "successes" in the first two stages. If $X_{N_2} > B^{-1}(1-\alpha\epsilon_2; N_2, p_0)$, stop and reject H_0; if $X_{N_2} < B^{-1}(\alpha\epsilon_2; N_2, p^*)$, stop and accept H_0. Else, if $N_2 < M$, go to Stage 3; otherwise stop.

Stage 3: Take additional $M - N_2$ independent observations, and let X_M be the total number of "successes." If $X_M > B^{-1}(1-\alpha\epsilon_3; M, p_0)$, reject H_0; otherwise, accept H_0.

The characteristics of this procedure (Table 7.9) are given in their paper.

Table 7.9: Power, Expected Sample Size, and Expected Number of Stages for $\mathbf{p_0 = 0.3}$, $\mathbf{m = 30}$, $\mathbf{M = 82}$, $\boldsymbol{\alpha = \beta = 0.1}$ of GLR

p	Power, $\psi(p)$	$E_P\{N\}$	$E_P\{K\}$
0.30	0.100	51.8	1.5
0.35	0.350	60.4	1.7
0.44	0.887	52.9	1.5
0.50	0.984	42.4	1.3
0.60	0.999	31.9	1.0

The value of p^* is 0.44 for three parameters. Comparing Tables 7.8 and 7.9 we see the following apparent differences between the two procedures: The GLR is more powerful than the TTSP. On the other hand, the expected size is considerably smaller in TTSP than in the GLR for $p < p^*$ and almost the same for larger values of p.

CHAPTER 8

SEQUENTIAL ALLOCATION OF RESOURCES: ONE- AND MULTIARMED BANDITS APPLIED TO CLINICAL TRIALS

8.1 BERNOULLI BANDITS

We start with the one-armed bandit (OAB) problem. In this problem we have two experiments: $\mathcal{E}_1$ (arm A_1) consists of Bernoulli trials with an unknown probability of success, θ, $0 < \theta < 1$, and $\mathcal{E}_2$ (arm A_2) consists of Bernoulli trials with a *known* probability of success, λ. Berry and Friestedt (1985, p. 100) proved:

Theorem 8.1.1 *If the discounting sequence α is regular and $\alpha_1 > 0$, then for any prior distribution H for θ on $[0,1]$ there exists an index $\Lambda(\boldsymbol{\alpha}, H)$ such that, if $\Lambda(\boldsymbol{\alpha}, H) > \lambda$, arm A_1 is initially optimal.*

It is also shown that

$$\Lambda(\boldsymbol{\alpha}, H) = \sup_{\{\tau(\phi)=1\}} \frac{E_\tau\left\{\sum_{i=1}^{M_\tau} \alpha_i X_{1i} \mid H\right\}}{E_\tau\left\{\sum_{i=1}^{M_\tau} \alpha_i \mid H\right\}}, \tag{8.1.1}$$

where $\{\boldsymbol{\tau}(\phi) = 1\}$ *is the set of all strategies with* $\tau_1 = 1$ *and* M_τ *is a stopping variable for* A_1 *associated with* $\boldsymbol{\tau}$. ■

The problem is reduced to that of finding the optimal stopping variable. We remark also that after each trial on A_1 the prior distribution H has to be converted to the posterior distribution given the total number of successes on A_1 during the previous trials.

A commonly applied prior distribution for θ is the beta distribution or its special case of a uniform prior on $(0, 1)$. If after n trials on A_1 we have observed X_n successes, the posterior distribution for the uniform prior is the beta$(X_n + 1, n + 1 - X_n)$. For the Bernoulli OAB, Gittins (1989, p. 138) determined $\Lambda(\boldsymbol{\alpha}, H)$ by dynamic programming with a finite horizon N. In this case, the discounting values are $\alpha_n = 1$ for $n \leq N$ and $\alpha_n = 0$ for $n > N$. To illustrate this finite-horizon dynamic programming, we first mention that for a uniform prior the predictive distribution of the result of the $(n + 1)$st trial, J_{n+1}, given X_n is

$$P_H(J_{n+1} = 0 \mid X_n) = \frac{n - X_n + 1}{n + 2}, \tag{8.1.2}$$

and

$$P_H(J_{n+1} = 1 \mid X_n) = \frac{X_n + 1}{n + 2}. \tag{8.1.3}$$

Accordingly,

$$E_H\{J_{n+1} \mid X_n\} = \frac{X_n + 1}{n + 2}. \tag{8.1.4}$$

Suppose that we have already performed $N - 1$ trials on A_1 and we have to decide on which arm to conduct the last trial.

The conditional expected reward of the last trial is

$$R_N(X_{N-1}) = \begin{cases} \lambda & \text{if } A_2 \text{ is chosen,} \\ \dfrac{X_{N-1} + 1}{N + 1} & \text{if } A_1 \text{ is chosen.} \end{cases} \tag{8.1.5}$$

Define

(8.1.6)

$$\begin{aligned} \rho^{(0)}(X_{N-1}) &= \max\left\{\lambda, \frac{X_{N-1} + 1}{N + 1}\right\} \\ &= \lambda I\{X_{N-1} < \lambda(N + 1) - 1\} + \frac{X_{N-1} + 1}{N + 1} I\{X_{N-1} \geq \lambda(N + 1) - 1\}. \end{aligned}$$

Thus, we choose A_1 if $X_{N-1} \geq \lambda N - (1 - \lambda)$ and A_2 otherwise.

Recall that if after $N - 2$ trials on A_1 it is optimal to choose A_2, then the last trial should also be on A_2. Accordingly, after $N - 2$ trials on A_1,

(8.1.7)

$$R_{N-1}(X_{N-2}) = \begin{cases} 2\lambda & \text{if } A_2 \text{ is chosen,} \\ \dfrac{X_{N-2} + 1}{N} + E_H\{\rho^{(0)}(X_{N-2} + J_{N-1}) \mid X_{N-2}\} & \text{if } A_1 \text{ is chosen.} \end{cases}$$

The maximal expected conditional reward is

$$\rho^{(1)}(X_{N-2}) = \max\left(2\lambda, \frac{X_{N-2}+1}{N}\rho^{(0)}(X_{N-2}+1) + \frac{N-1-X_{N-1}}{N}\rho^{0}(X_{N-2}) + \frac{X_{N-2}+1}{N}\right). \tag{8.1.8}$$

By backward induction, we define, for all $1 \le n \le N-2$,

$$\begin{aligned}\rho^{(n)}(X_{N-n-1}) = \max\Bigg((n+1)\lambda, &\frac{X_{N-n-1}+1}{N-n+1}\cdot\rho^{(n-1)}(X_{N-n-1}+1)\\ &+ \frac{N-n-X_{N-n-1}}{N-n+1}\rho^{(n-1)}(X_{N-n-1})\\ &+ \frac{X_{N-n-1}+1}{N-n+1}\Bigg).\end{aligned} \tag{8.1.9}$$

Finally, since the first trial is on A_1,

$$\rho^{(N-1)}(X_1) = \max\left(N\lambda, \frac{X_1+1}{3}\rho^{(N-2)}(X_1+1) + \frac{2-X_1}{3}\rho^{(N-2)}(X_1) + \frac{X_1+1}{3}\right). \tag{8.1.10}$$

Since $P_H(X_1 = 0) = P_H(X_1 = 1) = \frac{1}{2}$, the maximal expected reward is $\rho^{(N)} = \frac{1}{2}\rho^{(N-1)}(0) + \frac{1}{2}\rho^{(N-1)}(1)$. The optimal stopping variable is

$$\begin{aligned}M^0 = \min\Bigg(m \ge 1 : &\frac{X_m+1}{m+2}\rho^{(N-m-1)}(X_m+1)\\ &+ \frac{m-X_m+1}{m+2}\rho^{(N-m-1)}(X_m) + \frac{X_m+1}{m+2} \le (N-m+1)\lambda\Bigg).\end{aligned} \tag{8.1.11}$$

The dynamic allocation index in the Bernoulli OAB case with a uniform prior for θ and N-truncated uniform discount is

$$\begin{aligned}\Lambda_n(N, X_n) = \frac{1}{N-n+1}\Bigg[&\frac{X_n+1}{n+2} + \frac{X_n+1}{n+2}\rho^{(N-n-1)}(X_n+1)\\ &+ \frac{n+1-X_n}{n+2}\rho^{(N-n-1)}(X_n)\Bigg], \quad n = 1, \ldots, N-1.\end{aligned} \tag{8.1.12}$$

In Table 8.1 we present some values of $\rho^{(n)}(\cdot)$ for $N = 10$, $\lambda = 0.5$.

Table 8.1: Values of $\rho^{(N-n)}(X_{N-n-1})$, $N = 10$, $\lambda = 0.5$

n	X_n = 0	1	2	3	4	5	6	7	8	9	10
10	0.500	0.500	0.500	0.500	0.500	0.545	0.636	0.727	0.818	0.909	1.000
9	1.000	1.000	1.000	1.000	1.023	1.200	1.400	1.600	1.800	2.000	
8	1.500	1.500	1.500	1.500	1.677	2.000	2.333	2.667	3.000		
7	2.000	2.000	2.000	2.088	2.504	3.000	3.500	4.000			
6	2.500	2.500	2.500	2.897	3.573	4.286	5.000				
5	3.000	3.000	3.199	4.014	5.000	6.000					
4	3.500	3.500	4.288	5.603	7.000						
3	4.000	4.394	6.024	8.000							
2	4.500	6.147	9.000								
1	5.382	10.000									

Derived using program ropt.

Thus, in such $N = 10$ trials the total expected maximal gain is $\rho^{(10)} = 7.691 = (10+5.382)/2$. Notice that if we apply A_2 to all the 10 trials the expected gain is 5. Moreover, $\Lambda_n(N, X_n) = \rho^{(N-n)}(X_n)/(N-n+1)$. Thus, for example, if $X_6 = 4$, $\Lambda_6(10, 4) = 3.573/5 = 0.7146$, and it is optimal to continue on A_1. On the other hand, if $X_6 = 2$, $\Lambda_6(10, 2) = 2.5/5 = 0.5$, and it is optimal to switch from A_1 to A_2. Berry and Friestedt (1985, pp. 115–119) derive lower and upper bounds for $\Lambda(\boldsymbol{\alpha}, H)$. In Section 8.2 we develop the lower bound for $\Lambda(\boldsymbol{\alpha}, H)$. Although this lower bound is for the case of geometric $\boldsymbol{\alpha}$ and infinite horizon, it is interesting to note that for $X_6 = 4$ and uniform prior with $\alpha = 0.99$ the lower bound is 0.7020, which is quite close to $\Lambda_6(10, 4) = 0.7146$. The exact computations, as illustrated before, can be performed quickly even for large values of N.

Another Bayesian stopping rule for the OAB problem in the Bernoulli case which is not optimal but is easy to apply is to stop when the posterior probability of $\{\theta \leq \lambda\}$ is greater than some value γ. Notice that $P_H(\theta \leq \lambda \mid X_n, n) = I_\lambda(X_n + 1, n + 1 - X_n)$, where $I_x(\nu_1, \nu_2)$ is the incomplete beta function ratio, or the c.d.f. of beta(ν_1, ν_2). The proposed stopping variable is

$$M_\gamma = \min\{n \geq k : I_\lambda(X_n + 1, n + 1 - X_n) \geq \gamma\}. \tag{8.1.13}$$

Furthermore, $I_\lambda(X_n+1, n+1-X_n) \geq \gamma$ if and only if $H^{-1}(\gamma; X_n+1, n+1-X_n) \leq \lambda$, where $H^{-1}(\gamma; \nu_1, \nu_2)$ is the γ-quantile of beta(ν_1, ν_2). This stopping variable is not optimal; however, it is easily applicable. We will study its efficiency below. As shown in Table 8.1, the optimal value of $\Lambda_5(10, 3) = 0.669$. Here, for $\gamma = 0.90$, $H^{-1}(0.90; 4, 3) = 0.7991$. Both indices lead to continuation on A_1. In Table 8.2 we present estimates of the 0.25-, 0.5-, and 0.75-quantiles (Q_1, Me, Q_3) of M_γ for several cases of p_1 and λ. All estimates are based on $N_s = 1000$ simulation runs. Here M_γ is truncated at N, that is, we estimate the quantiles of $M_\gamma^* = \min(M_\gamma, N)$.

Table 8.2: Simulation Estimates of $\mathbf{Q_1}$, Me, $\mathbf{Q_3}$, Mean, STD, and Eff. of $\mathbf{M_\gamma^*}$, N = 100, $\gamma = 0.9$, $\mathbf{N_s} = 1000$

p_1	λ	Q_1	Me	Q_3	Mean	STD	Eff.
0.6	0.5	100	100	100	94.361	20.942	0.991
0.5	0.5	34	100	100	75.422	36.657	1.000
0.45	0.5	13	50	100	55.049	38.224	0.946
0.40	0.5	11	20	52	35.136	29.737	0.927

Derived with program simsr1, sr1.

If we knew which arm has the maximal probability, we would have used it during all N trials. The expected payoff in this case is $N \max(p_1, \lambda)$. If, on the other hand, we use arm 1 only during M_γ^* trials, the expected payoff is $E_{p_1}\{p_1 M_\gamma^* + \lambda(N - M_\gamma^*)\}$. Accordingly, the efficiency index of the procedure which applies M_γ^* is given by

$$\text{Eff.}(p_1, \lambda) = E_{p_1}\left\{\frac{p_1 M_\gamma^* + \lambda(N - M_\gamma^*)}{N \max(p_1, \lambda)}\right\}. \tag{8.1.14}$$

We see in Table 8.2 that the stopping variable M_γ^* is quite efficient.

If both θ_1 and θ_2 are unknown, we are in the case of the *two-armed bandit* (TAB), which is more complicated than the OAB. After n trials, let $N_1(n)$ be the number of times A_1 was chosen and $N_2(n)$ that of A_2. Assume $N_1(n) + N_2(n) = n$. Moreover, let $X_{N_1(n)}$ be the number of success on A_1 and $Y_{N_2(n)}$ those on A_2. The sequentially sufficient statistic is $S_n = (N_1(n), X_{N_1(n)}, N_2(n), Y_{N_2(n)})$. We could consider the prior distribution of (θ_1, θ_2) to be the product of two beta priors, which implies that θ_1 and θ_2 are priorly independent. In principle one could obtain the optimal strategy for a finite horizon, N, by dynamic programming. It is, however, considerably more complicated than the dynamic programming in the OAB case. Gittins and Jones (1974) proved that if $\boldsymbol{\alpha} = (1, \alpha, \alpha^2, \ldots)$ is a geometric discounting sequence, we can compute an index $\Lambda(\boldsymbol{\alpha}, H_i)$, $i = 1, 2$, for each arm separately and apply in the next trial the arm having a maximal index. We discuss this in the following section.

8.2 GITTINS DYNAMIC ALLOCATION INDICES

Consider a bandit problem with K arms. The reward from using arm A_k is $R(X_k)$, where $X_{k1}, X_{k2}, \ldots$ are i.i.d. random variables associated with A_k, $k = 1, 2, \ldots, K$. Also the K arms are independent. Gittins (1979) and Gittins and Jones (1974, 1979) developed a solution to the problem of maximizing

$$(8.2.1) \quad W_\tau(H_1, \ldots, H_K; \alpha) = \sum_{n=1}^{\infty} \alpha^{n-1} E\left\{\sum_{k=1}^{K} E\{I\{\tau_n = k\} R(X_k) \mid H_k\}\right\}$$

when the discounting sequence is geometric $\boldsymbol{\alpha} = (1, \alpha, \alpha^2, \ldots)$, $0 < \alpha < 1$, where H_k is the posterior distribution after $m_k(n)$ trials on A_k. They proved that after n trials one should compute, for each arm separately, an index $\Lambda_n(H_k, \alpha)$ and choose for the $(n+1)$st trial the arm whose index is maximal. That is, if $\Lambda_n(H_{k^*}, \alpha) = \max_{1 \le k \le K}\{\Lambda_n(H_k, \alpha)\}$, then the $(n+1)$st trial should be on A_{k^*}. Other proofs of this result were given throughout the years by Varaiya, Warland, and Bruyukkoc (1985), Weiss (1988), Whittle (1980), Glazebrook (1990), Tsitsiklis (1994), Weber (1992), Bertsimas and Nino-Mora (1993), and more. The so-called *Gittins dynamic allocation* is given by the general formula

$$(8.2.2) \qquad \Lambda(H_k, \alpha) = \sup_{\tau \ge 0} \frac{E\left\{\sum_{n=0}^{\tau-1} \alpha^n R(X_n) \mid H_k\right\}}{E\left\{\sum_{n=0}^{\tau-1} \alpha^n \mid H_k\right\}},$$

where τ is a stopping variable. Generally, it is difficult to determine this index. Explicit formulas for the index are given in Berry and Friestedt (1985, Chapter 5) for special cases of Bernoulli bandits. Kaspi and Mandelbaum (1995) developed explicit expressions for multiarmed bandits driven by Levy processes. For example, if the Levy process $X(t) = -ct + Y(t)$, where $Y(t)$ is a compound Poisson process with exponentially distributed jumps with parameters μ, then the Gittins index, when $X(t) = x$ and $R(x)$ is the reward, is

$$(8.2.3) \qquad \Lambda(x) = pR(x) + q \int_0^\infty e^{-y} R\left(x + \frac{y}{p\alpha}\right) dy,$$

where

$$(8.2.4) \qquad q = \frac{\mu c - \lambda - \beta + \sqrt{(\lambda + \beta - c\mu)^2 + 4\mu c\beta}}{2\mu c},$$

$p = 1 - q$, λ is the intensity of the Poisson process, and β is a positive parameter. There are a few algorithms to compute the Gittins index (Varaiya et al.

(1985); Katehakis and Veinott, 1987, Bertsimas and Nino-Mora, 1993). Sonin (1999a,b) developed algorithms when the bandits are governed by Markov chains.

Berry and Friestedt (1985, p. 111) proposed to approximate the Gittins index in the Bernoulli bandits in the following manner. Consider the stopping rule τ_r for an integer $r \geq 1$ of the following nature. If *all* the first r trials are successful, then continue the trials on the same arm irrespective of the outcomes. If, on the other hand, the first failure occurs before the rth trial, stop the trials and switch to an arm having a larger index. Notice that, since the trials are Bernoulli with probability of success θ, the number of trials, M, until the first failure has the geometric distribution

$$P_\theta(M = m) = (1-\theta)\theta^{m-1}, \quad m = 1, 2, \ldots. \tag{8.2.5}$$

Let H be a prior distribution for θ. The index $\Lambda_r(H, \alpha)$ for this stopping rule is

(8.2.6)

$$\Lambda_r(H,\alpha) = \frac{E\left\{\sum_{m=1}^{r} \alpha^{m-1}(1-\theta)\theta^{m-1}E_\theta(J_m) + \frac{\alpha^r}{1-\alpha}P_\theta\{M > r\}E_\theta(J) \mid H\right\}}{E\left\{\sum_{m=1}^{r} \alpha^{m-1}(1-\theta)\theta^{m-1} + \frac{\alpha^r}{1-\alpha}P_\theta\{M > r\} \mid H\right\}}.$$

Notice that $P_\theta\{M > r\} = 1 - \sum_{m=1}^{r}(1-\theta)\theta^{m-1} = 1 - (1-\theta^r) = \theta^r$. Accordingly, if H has the beta(a, b) distribution, where $X_n = \sum_{i=1}^{n} J_i$, $a = X_n + 1$, and $b = n + 1 - X_n$, then

(8.2.7)

$$\Lambda_r((a,b),\alpha) = \frac{\sum_{m=0}^{r-1} \alpha^m B(a+m+1, b+1) + \frac{\alpha^r}{1-\alpha}B(a+r+1, b+1)}{\sum_{m=0}^{r-1} \alpha^m B(a+m, b+1) + \frac{\alpha^r}{1-\alpha}B(a+r, b+1)}.$$

Berry and Friestedt (1985, p. 111) proved that, for any H, $\Lambda_r(H, \alpha)$ is unimodal as $r = 1, 2, \ldots$. Thus, if $\Lambda_{r^*}(H,\alpha) = \max_{r \geq 1} \Lambda_r(H, \alpha)$, then $\Lambda_{r^*}(H, \alpha)$ is also a lower bound for the Gittins index, which is close to the true value. For example, below we give seven values of $\Lambda_r((2,2), 0.99)$ for the beta$(2, 2)$ prior:

r	1	2	3	4	5	6	7
Λ_r	0.4975	0.5619	0.6025	0.6251	0.6341	0.6335	0.6267

Derived with program gindx.

Thus, $r^* = 5$ and $\Lambda_5((2,2), 0.99) = 0.6341$. The SPLUS program gindx$(r, a1, a, b)$ computes $\Lambda_r((a,b),\alpha)$ according to (8.2.7) and program gittlb$(a1, a, b)$ computes $\Lambda_{r^*}((a,b),\alpha)$. In Table 8.3 we present a few values of $\Lambda_{r^*}((a,b), 0.99)$.

Table 8.3: Values of $\Lambda_{r^*}((a,b), 0.99)$ for $n = 1, \ldots, 10$ and X_n Simulated from $B(n, 0.6)$

n	X_n	a	b	$\Lambda_{r^*}((a,b), 0.99)$
1	1	2	1	0.7601
2	1	2	2	0.6341
3	1	2	3	0.5364
4	2	3	3	0.6110
5	2	3	4	0.5371
6	3	4	4	0.5941
7	3	4	5	0.5354
8	3	4	6	0.4878
9	4	5	6	0.5332
10	5	6	6	0.5719

Derived with program gittlb.

Notice that for the uniform prior $a = 1$, $b = 1$, before starting the trials $\Lambda_{r^*}((1,1), 0.99) = 0.6636$. Thus, if Table 8.3 illustrates what happened on A_1, we would have switched to A_2 after the second trial. As long as we continue on A_2, A_1 does not change. If after a few trials on A_2, its index Λ_{r^*} falls below 0.6341, we switch back to A_1, and so on. Notice also that $\Lambda_{r^*}((a,b),\alpha)$ is an increasing function of α. For example, $\Lambda_{r^*}((1,1), 0.98) = 0.6125 < \Lambda_{r^*}((1,1), 0.99) = 0.6636$. This monotonicity can be easily proven from Eq. (8.2.2), and in particular Eq. (8.2.7) implies that $\Lambda_r((a,b),\alpha) \nearrow \alpha$ for all $r \geq 1$ and all (a,b).

8.3 SEQUENTIAL ALLOCATIONS IN CLINICAL TRIALS

Sequential allocation of patients to two or more treatments is a very important feature in clinical trials, as has already been discussed in Chapter 7. We emphasized in that chapter allocation problems associated with randomization procedure to maintain balance and valid inference. From ethical considerations it is desired to maximize the expected number of patients receiving the better treatment. The question is whether optimal procedures for bandit problems can be applied to clinical trials. As we have seen before, in bandit problems the result of each trial should be available before the next trial can be allocated. This is often not the case in clinical trials, where the success or failure of treatments takes a long time to be established. Also, when one arm (treatment) is being applied, other arms are generally not frozen, as it is in the multiarmed bandit procedures. One could develop, however, stopping rules according to which trials on a certain arm terminate as soon as it is realized that the treatments on that arm yield inferior results relative to the other arms. The OAB could sometimes be applied when a new treatment with an unknown probability of success is tested against a standard treatment with a *known* probability of success. In this case one could start with allocating patients one by one to the new treatment. The stopping rule of Section 7.2.1 could be applied. If trials on the new treatment (arm A_1) are stopped, all future patients are sent to the standard treatment (A_2). Many papers (see Wang, 1991; Bather, 1981; Hardwick, 1995; Jones, Lewis, and Hartley, 1995; and others) formulate additional criteria for clinical trials, like probability of correct selection, expected number of patients receiving an inferior treatment, and more. Jones, Lewis, and Hartley (1995) considered the following stopping rule: After n_1 trials on A_1 and n_2 trials on A_2, they compute the predictive probabilities $\hat{p}_i = (X_i + 1)/(n_i + 2)$ $(i = 1, 2)$. As soon as $|\hat{p}_1 - \hat{p}_2| > \Delta$, they switch all the remaining observations to the arm having the larger value of $\hat{p}_i$. Suppose that N is the total number of trials allowed. If (a_1, b_1, a_2, b_2) is the state of the system, the posterior probability that $\theta_1 < \theta_2$ for the independent beta priors is

$$\begin{aligned}\psi(a_1, b_1, a_2, b_2) &= P_H\{\theta_1 < \theta_2 \mid (a_1, b_1, a_2, b_2)\} \\ &= \sum_{j=a_1}^{a_1+b_1-1} \binom{a_1 + b_1 - 1}{j} \frac{B(a_2 + j, a_1 + b_1 + b_2 - j - 1)}{B(a_2, b_2)},\end{aligned} \tag{8.3.1}$$

where $a_i = X_i + 1$ and $b_i = n_i - X_i + 1$ $(i = 1, 2)$. Indeed,

$$\begin{aligned}P\{\theta_1 &< \theta_2 \mid a_1, b_1, a_2, b_2\} \\ &= \frac{1}{B(a_2, b_2)} \int_0^1 v^{a_2-1}(1 - v)^{b_2-1} I_v(a_1, b_1)\, dv.\end{aligned} \tag{8.3.2}$$

Furthermore,

$$I_v(a_1, b_1) = \sum_{j=a_1}^{n_1+1} \binom{n_1 + 1}{j} v^j (1 - v)^{n_1+1-j}. \tag{8.3.3}$$

Substituting (8.3.3) in (8.3.2), we obtain (8.3.1). Define the stopping variables

$$M_1 = \min\{n \geq k : \psi(a_1, b_1, a_2, b_2) \geq 1 - \alpha_1\} \tag{8.3.4}$$

and

$$M_2 = \min\{n \geq k : \psi(a_1, b_1, a_2, b_2) \leq \alpha_2\}. \tag{8.3.5}$$

Notice that $n = n_1 + n_2$. Here α_1 and α_2 are small values, for example, $\alpha_1 = \alpha_2 = 0.01$. We stop at $M = \min(M_1, M_2)$. Suppose also that, for $n \leq M$, $n_1 = n_2 = n/2$.

If $M = M_1$, then all the additional $N - M$ trials are allocated to A_2. On the other hand, if $M = M_2$, all the additional $N - M$ trials are on A_1. Let N_1 denote the number of trials on A_1. This is given by

$$N_1 = I\{M = M_1\}\frac{M_1}{2} + I\{M = M_2\}\left(N - \frac{M_2}{2}\right). \tag{8.3.6}$$

For example, in a simulation of $N = 100$ trials, with $k = 40$, when $\theta_1 = 0.5$ and $\theta_2 = 0.8$, we obtained $M = M_1 = 50$. In this case $N_1 = 25$. In Table 8.4 we present simulation estimates of $E\{N_1\}$ under different values of p_1 and p_2 with $k = 20$, 40. Each estimate is based on 100 runs.

Table 8.4: Simulation Estimates of $\mathbf{E\{N_1\}}$, $\mathbf{N = 100}$, $\boldsymbol{\alpha_1 = \alpha_2 = 0.05}$, $\mathbf{k = 20, 40}$

p_1	p_2	$k = 20$ $E\{N_1\}$	$k = 40$ $E\{N_1\}$
0.5	0.6	39.1	40.8
0.5	0.7	25.8	33.6
0.5	0.8	17.7	24.4

Derived with programs simpgr, pgr, awr.

In the above simulations we estimated also the *probability of correct selection* of the superior arm. Let $\widehat{\text{PCS}}(p_1, p_2)$ denote the estimator of this probability. Thus, for the case of $\alpha_1 = \alpha_2 = 0.05$, $N = 100$, and $k = 40$, we obtained $\widehat{\text{PCS}}(0.5, 0.6) = 0.55$, $\widehat{\text{PCS}}(0.5, 0.7) = 0.92$, and $\widehat{\text{PCS}}(0.5, 0.8) = 1.00$. In order to minimize $E\{N_1\}$ and maximize PCS one should use an optimal allocation determined by dynamic programming with uniform discounting truncated at N. This, however, is impractical. Bather and Simons (1985) showed that if we start with $M_1 = M_2 \cong 0.3\sqrt{N}$ and then use for the rest of the trials the arm with the maximal value of $\hat{p}_i$, then the risk is minimax. Notice that if $N = 100$, $0.3\sqrt{N} = 3$. In Table 8.5 we present simulation estimates of $E\{N_1\}$ and of $\text{PCS}(p_1, p_2)$ following the Bather and Simons procedure. These are also based on 1000 simulation runs.

Table 8.5: Simulation Estimates of $\mathbf{E\{N_1\}}$ and PCS, $\mathbf{N = 100}$, $\mathbf{p \leq 0.5}$

p_2	$E\{N_1\}$	PCS
0.6	27.6	0.74
0.65	22.6	0.79
0.70	18.3	0.84
0.75	16.3	0.86
0.80	11.8	0.91

Comparing Tables 8.4 and 8.5, the indication is that the Bather–Simons procedure is better than that of Jones et al. (1995) with respect to minimizing the expected number of trials on the inferior arm, while the Jones et al. procedure yields higher PCS if $p \geq 0.7$.

8.4 BERNOULLI BANDITS WITH CHANGE POINT

8.4.1 Introduction

The material of this section is based on the paper of Lamprecht and Zacks (1998). It deals with a Bernoulli OAB with a change point in arm A_2. Arm A_1 has a fixed *known* probability of success $p_1 = \lambda$. Arm A_2 has a *known* probability of success, θ, before the change and probability of success ϕ after the change. Both θ and ϕ are *known* and $0 < \theta < \lambda < \phi < 1$. However, the point of change, τ, is unknown. We further assume that, conditionally on $(\theta, \lambda, \phi, \tau)$, the observed values of the binary random variables are independent. The question is how to allocate the trials between the two arms when τ is unknown when the objective is to maximize the total expected payoff. If τ were known, the optimal strategy is obviously to allocate the first $\tau_N = \min(\tau, N)$ trials to A_1 and the remaining $N - \tau_N$ trials to A_2. In this case, the maximal expected total yield, assuming $\alpha_n = 1$ for $n \leq N$ and $\alpha_n = 0$ for $n > N$, is

$$W^0(\tau_N) = \tau_N \lambda + (N - \tau_N)\phi. \tag{8.4.1}$$

In a Bayesian framework we assume the modified geometric prior for τ, namely,

$$\pi(\tau) = \begin{cases} \pi & \text{if } \tau = 0, \\ (1-\pi)p(1-p)^{\tau-1} & \text{if } \tau > 0. \end{cases} \tag{8.4.2}$$

The event $\{\tau = 0\}$ signifies that the change point has occurred before the beginning of the trials. The event $\{\tau > N\}$ signifies that the change has not occurred before the N trials terminated. The event $\{\tau = i\}$, $i = 1, \ldots, N$, signifies that $i - 1 < \tau \leq i$. The maximal expected total yield according to this prior of τ is

$$\begin{aligned} E_{(\pi,p)}\{W^0(\tau_N)\} = N\phi - \frac{\phi - \lambda}{p}(1-\pi)(1-(1-p)^N) \\ - \lambda(1-\pi)(1-p)^{N-1}(N - p(1-p)). \end{aligned} \tag{8.4.3}$$

The expected payoff of any strategy is compared to (7.4.3).

Generally speaking, our strategy consists of a sequence of *surveillance cycles* followed by a *final cycle.* A surveillance cycle starts for a while on A_1 and then switches to A_2. In A_2, if the number of successes is too low, the cycle terminates by switching back to A_1. If the change point τ occurred prior to switching to A_2, there is a considerable chance that the trials will conclude with one cycle only. The surveillance cycle becomes a final cycle. Let $n^{(1)}$ denote the number of initial trials on A_1. Since trials on A_1 do not yield information on τ, $n^{(1)}$ is determined optimally before the trials on A_1 start, according to the prior distribution $\pi(\tau)$. Let $X_i^{(2)} = 1$ if the ith trial on A_2 is successful and $X_i^{(2)} = 0$ otherwise. Let $S_n = \sum_{i=1}^{n} X_i^{(2)}$. We consider a stopping rule based on

$$N_2^* = \min\{1 \le n \le N - n^{(1)} : S_n \le -a + bn\}, \tag{8.4.4}$$

where a and b determine the lower boundary in the Wald SPRT of $H_0 : p = \theta$ versus $H_1 : p = \phi$ in the Bernoulli case. More explicit formulas for a and b will be given later. The random time $\min(N, n^{(1)} + N_2^*)$ is the end of the surveillance cycle. If $n^{(1)} + N_2^* < N$, the prior distribution $\pi(\tau)$ is converted to a posterior distribution $\pi_{\text{sc}}(\tau)$ and a new surveillance cycle starts. In the following paragraphs we develop these ideas.

8.4.2 Optimizing the Final Cycle

In the final cycle, one can perform n out of N trials on arm 1 ($0 \le n \le N$) and then switch to arm 2, on which all the remaining $(N-n)$ trials are performed. The loss due to choosing n different than τ is

$$L_f(n, \tau; N) = (n - \tau_N)^+(\phi - \lambda) + (\tau_N - n)^+(\lambda - \theta), \tag{8.4.5}$$

where $a^+ = \max(0, a)$. Notice that the loss function is the shortage from the maximal payoff $W_0(\tau_N)$ due to not knowing τ_N. The prior (posterior) risk of choosing n for the final stage under the modified geometric prior (posterior) is

(8.4.6)

$$\begin{aligned} R_f(n; \pi, N) = (\phi - \lambda)&\left[n\pi + I\{n \ge 1\}(1-\pi)p\sum_{t=1}^{n}(n-t)(1-p)^{t-1}\right] \\ &+ (\lambda - \theta)\left[I\{n \le N-1\}(1-\pi)p\sum_{t=n}^{N-1}(t-n)(1-p)^{t-1}\right. \\ &\left. + (1-\pi)(1-p)^{N-1}(N-n)\right]. \end{aligned}$$

Thus, if $1 \le n \le N-1$, then

$$\begin{aligned} R_f(n; \pi, N) = &\frac{\phi - \lambda}{p}[n\pi p + (1-\pi)((1-p)^n + np - 1)] \\ &+ (1-\pi)\frac{\lambda - \theta}{p}(1-p)^n(1-(1-p)^{N-n}). \end{aligned} \tag{8.4.7}$$

For $n = 0$ and $n = N$, the risk function is, respectively,

$$R_f(0;\pi,N) = (1-\pi)\frac{\lambda-\theta}{p}[1-(1-p)^N], \tag{8.4.8}$$

and

$$R_f(N;\pi,N) = \frac{\phi-\lambda}{p}[Np-(1-\pi)(1-(1-p)^N)]. \tag{8.4.9}$$

Let $\tilde{R}_f(x;\pi,N)$ be an extension of $R_f(n;\pi,N)$ such that

(i) $\tilde{R}_f(x;\pi,N)$ is continuous in x on $[0,N]$ and

(ii) $\tilde{R}_f(n;\pi,N) = R_f(n;\pi,N)$ for $n = 0,\ldots,N$.

The function $\tilde{R}_f(x;\pi,N)$ is convex in x. Indeed,

$$\frac{\partial^2}{\partial x^2}\tilde{R}_f(x;\pi,N) = (1-\pi)\left(\frac{\phi-\theta}{p}\right)(1-p)^n(\log(1-p))^2. \tag{8.4.10}$$

Hence $\tilde{R}_f(x;\pi,N)$ has a unique minimum at

$$x_f^0(\pi,N) = \frac{\log\left(p\dfrac{\phi-\lambda}{\phi-\theta}\right) - \log((1-p)(-\log(1-p)))}{\log(1-p)}. \tag{8.4.11}$$

This value is approximately equal to
(8.4.12)

$$n_f^0(\pi,N) = \text{least } n \geq 1 \text{ such that } R_f(n+1;\pi,N) - R_f(n;\pi,N) \geq 0.$$

In Table 8.6 we present a few values of $n^0(\pi,N) = \min(n_f^0(\pi,N),N)$ as well as the associated minimal risk $R_f^*(\pi,N) = R_f(n^0(\pi,N);\pi,N)$.

Table 8.6: Minimal Prior Risk of a Final Cycle and $\mathbf{n^0(\pi,N)}$, for $\theta = 0.35$, $\lambda = 0.50$, $\phi = 0.65$, $\pi = 0.1$

		p		
N		0.05	0.025	0.01
50	n^0	12	24	50*)
	R_f^*	1.810	2.559	2.168
70	n^0	12	24	59
	R_f^*	1.943	3.164	3.592
90	n^0	12	24	59
	R_f^*	1.991	3.529	4.809

The dependence of $n^0(\pi,N)$ on the parameter p is very pronounced. It is obviously a decreasing function of p.

8.4.3 Surveillance Cycle

A surveillance cycle starts with $n^{(1)}$ trials on arm 1. After switching to arm 2, a stopping rule is required for deciding when, if at all, to terminate the cycle and return back to arm 1. In the next two sections, we study the performance of simpler stopping rules. We construct a linear lower boundary $b_L(n) = -a_L + b_L n$ and switch back to arm 1 (terminate) the cycle as soon as $S_n \le -a_L + b_L n$, where $S_n = \sum_{i=1}^n X_i^{(2)}$, $n \ge 1$, is the number of successes on arm 2. Such a stopping rule is not optimal but might yield results close to optimal. The problem is that of choosing a good lower boundary. Obviously, if S_{n-1} is above the boundary and $X_n = 1$, one should not stop. Therefore, b_L should be smaller than 1. We propose here the slope of the lower boundary of Wald's SPRT for testing $H_0 : p = \theta$ versus $H_1 : p = \phi$ in Bernoulli trials. This slope is given by the formula (see Siegmund, 1985)

$$b_L = \frac{\log \dfrac{1-\theta}{1-\phi}}{\log\left(\dfrac{\phi(1-\theta)}{\theta(1-\phi)}\right)}. \tag{8.4.13}$$

The intercept $-a_L$ should be negative, and its magnitude can be adjusted to avoid stopping too fast or too late. In our computations we have chosen the intercept of the lower boundary of Wald's SPRT, namely,

$$a_L = -\frac{\log\left(\dfrac{\beta}{1-\beta}\right)}{\log\left(\dfrac{\phi(1-\theta)}{\theta(1-\phi)}\right)} \quad \text{with} \quad \beta = 0.03. \tag{8.4.14}$$

8.4.3.1 Distribution of the Stopping Time $\mathbf{N^{(2)}}$ Consider a sequence of independent Bernoulli trials $X_1, X_2, X_3, \ldots$. Let $p_i^{(\tau)} = P_\tau[X_i = 1]$ be the success probability when the change point is at τ, that is,

$$p_i^{(\tau)} = \begin{cases} \theta & \text{if } i \le \tau, \\ \phi & \text{if } i > \tau. \end{cases}$$

Let $S_n = \sum_{i=1}^n X_i$. Let $b(j; n, p)$ denote the p.d.f. of the binomial distribution with parameters (n, p), that is, $b(j; n, p) = \binom{n}{j} p^j (1-p)^{n-j}$, $j = 0, 1, \ldots, n$. The p.d.f. of S_n under a change point at τ is

(8.4.15)

$$P_\tau\{S_n = j; n, \theta, \phi\} = \begin{cases} b(j; n, \phi) & \text{if } \tau = 0, \\ \displaystyle\sum_{l=0}^{j} b(l; \tau, \theta) b(j-l; n-\tau, \phi) & \text{if } 1 \le \tau \le n-1, \\ b(j; n, \theta) & \text{if } \tau \ge n \end{cases}$$

(for) $j = 0, 1, \ldots, n$. Denote the p.d.f. (8.4.15) by $f_{\theta,\phi}^{(\tau)}(j; n)$.

A sample path of S_n, $n = 1, 2, \ldots$, may cross the given lower boundary on or just before the time points $\{n(j); j = 0, 1, 2, \ldots\}$ given by

$$n(j) = \text{smallest integer } \geq \left(\frac{a_L + j}{b_L}\right). \tag{8.4.16}$$

As defined in (8.4.4),

$$N_2^* = \text{ least } n, \; n \geq 1 \text{ such that } S_n \leq -a_L + b_L n. \tag{8.4.17}$$

Here N_2^* is the number of trials on arm 2 until the *first* crossing of $b_L(n)$. Notice that, for each $j = 0, 1, 2, \ldots$,

$$\{N_2 = n(j)\} = \{S_{N_2} = j\}.$$

We consider the random variable

$$N_2^* = \min\{N_2, N_1\}, \tag{8.4.18}$$

where $N_1 = N - n^{(1)}$. We denote by n^* the maximal value of $n(j)$ smaller than or equal to N_1. Let

$$\begin{aligned} \psi_{\theta,\phi}^{(\tau)}(j) &= P_\tau\{N_2^* = n(j)\} \\ &= P_\tau\{S_{N_2^*} = j\}. \end{aligned} \tag{8.4.19}$$

These probabilities can be computed recursively by the formula

$$\psi_{\theta,\phi}^{(\tau)}(j) = f_{\theta,\phi}^{(\tau)}(j; n(j)) - \sum_{i=0}^{j-1} \psi_{\theta,\phi}^{(\tau)}(i) f_{\theta,\phi}^{(\tau - n(i))}(j - i; n(j) - n(i)) \tag{8.4.20}$$

for $j = 1, 2, \ldots$ with

$$\psi_{\theta,\phi}^{(\tau)}(0) = f_{\theta,\phi}^{(\tau)}(0; n(0)). \tag{8.4.21}$$

Furthermore, we set

$$P_\tau\{N_2^* = N_1\} = 1 - \sum_{j=0}^{j^*} \psi_{\theta,\phi}^{(\tau)}(j), \tag{8.4.22}$$

where j^* is the j-value corresponding to n^*. According to Eq. (8.4.15), $f_{\theta;\phi}^{(\tau)}(j; n) = b(j; \theta, n)$ if $\tau \geq n$. Hence, if $\tau \geq n(j)$, then, according to Eq. (8.4.20), $\psi_{\theta,\phi}^{(\tau)}(j)$ depends only on θ and j and is given, for all $\tau \geq n(j)$, by

$$\psi_\theta^*(j) = b(j; n(j), \theta) - \sum_{i=0}^{j-1} \psi_\theta^*(i) b(j - i; n(j) - n(i)). \tag{8.4.23}$$

8.4.3.2 Predictive Distribution of N_2^* and the Posterior Distribution of $(\tau - N_{sc})^+$ Let $\psi_{\theta,\phi}^{(p)}(j;\pi_1)$, $j = 0, 1, \ldots$, denote the predictive first crossing probabilities, that is,

$$
\begin{aligned}
\psi_{\theta,\phi}^{(p)}(j;\pi_1) &= E_{\pi_1}\{\psi_{\theta,\phi}^{(\tau)}(j)\} \\
&= \pi_1 \psi_{\theta,\phi}^{(0)}(j) + (1-\pi_1)p \sum_{t=1}^{n(j)-1} (1-p)^{t-1}\psi_{\theta,\phi}^{(t)}(j) \\
&\quad + (1-\pi_1)(1-p)^{n(j)-1}\psi_\theta^*(j),
\end{aligned} \tag{8.4.24}
$$

where $\psi_\theta^*(j)$ is as in (8.4.23) and π_1 is given by

$$\pi_1 = \pi + (1-\pi)(1-(1-p)^{n^{(1)}}). \tag{8.4.25}$$

Notice that π_1 is the prior probability that the change occurred before the switch to arm 2. Also, we have

$$(1-\pi_1) = (1-\pi)(1-p)^{n^{(1)}}. \tag{8.4.26}$$

Moreover,

$$P_{\theta,\phi}^{(p)}\{N_2^* = N_1\} = 1 - \sum_{j=0}^{j^*} \psi_{\theta,\phi}^{(p)}(j;\pi). \tag{8.4.27}$$

We now develop the formulas for the posterior distribution of $\tau_2 = (\tau - N_{sc})^+$ given $(n^{(1)}, N_2^*)$, where $N_{sc} = n^{(1)} + N_2^*$. If one returns to arm 1 at the end of a surveillance cycle, the posterior probability distribution of τ_2, given the statistics of the surveillance cycle $(n^{(1)}, N_2^*)$, is

$$P\{\tau_2 = j \mid n^{(1)}, N_2^*\} = \begin{cases} \pi_{sc}, & \text{if } j = 0, \\ (1-\pi_{sc})p(1-p)^{j-1} & \text{if } j \geq 1, \end{cases} \tag{8.4.28}$$

where π_{sc} is the posterior probability that the change happened during or before the surveillance cycle. According to Bayes's theorem,

$$\pi_{sc} = 1 - \frac{(1-\pi_1)(1-p)^{N_2^*-1}\psi_\theta^*(J_2^*)}{\psi_{\theta,\phi}^{(p)}(J_2^*;\pi_1)}, \tag{8.4.29}$$

where $J_2^* = j(N_2^*)$. In Table 8.7 we present the values of π_{sc} as a function of N_2^*.

Table 8.7: Posterior Probabilities π_{sc}, $n^{(1)} = 10$, $N_1 = 50$, $\theta = 0.35$, $\phi = 0.65$.

		$\pi = 0.1$	$\pi = 0.5$	$\pi = 0.1$	$\pi = 0.5$
J^*	N_2^*	$p = 0.01$	$p = 0.01$	$p = 0.05$	$p = 0.05$
0	6	0.021509	0.064754	0.102699	0.170726
1	8	0.025256	0.059111	0.125948	0.181436
2	10	0.031067	0.062003	0.157394	0.209145
3	12	0.037174	0.066880	0.189657	0.240105
4	14	0.043197	0.072339	0.221232	0.271364
5	16	0.049021	0.077924	0.251734	0.302038
6	18	0.054611	0.083456	0.281109	0.331852
7	20	0.059963	0.088861	0.309416	0.360746
8	22	0.065085	0.094109	0.336746	0.388744
9	24	0.069990	0.099193	0.363195	0.415894
10	26	0.074694	0.104115	0.388856	0.442252
11	28	0.079212	0.108881	0.413807	0.467870
12	30	0.083559	0.113501	0.438114	0.492790
13	32	0.087749	0.117984	0.461832	0.517045
14	34	0.091795	0.122342	0.485003	0.540659
15	36	0.095709	0.126583	0.507658	0.563648
16	38	0.099502	0.130718	0.529819	0.586019
17	40	0.103184	0.134754	0.551498	0.607773
18	42	0.106764	0.138701	0.572701	0.628908
19	44	0.110250	0.142565	0.593429	0.649416
20	46	0.113651	0.146354	0.613674	0.669286
21	48	0.116973	0.150074	0.633427	0.688506
22	50	0.120222	0.153732	0.652675	0.707063

8.4.3.3 Predictive Risk of the Surveillance Cycle The loss associated with the surveillance cycle due to $n^{(1)}$ and N_2^*, when τ is unknown, is

$$
\begin{aligned}
L_{\text{sc}}(n^{(1)}, N_2^*, \tau) = {} & I\{\tau \le n^{(1)}\}(\phi - \lambda)(n^{(1)} - \tau) \\
& + I\{0 < \tau_1 < N_2^*\}\tau_1(\lambda - \theta) \\
& + I\{\tau_1 \ge N_2^*\}(\lambda - \theta)N_2^*,
\end{aligned} \tag{8.4.30}
$$

where $\tau_1 = (\tau - n^{(1)})^+$.

The predictive risk of the surveillance cycle is

$$
\begin{aligned}
R_{\text{sc}}(n^{(1)}, N_1, \pi) &= E_\pi\{L_{\text{sc}}(n^{(1)}, N_2^*, \tau)\} \\
&= (\phi - \lambda)E_\pi\{(n^{(1)} - \tau)I\{\tau \le n^{(1)}\}\} \\
&\quad + (\lambda - \theta)E_{\pi_1}\{\tau_1 P_{\theta,\phi}\{N_2^* > \tau_1 \mid \tau_1\}\} \\
&\quad + (\lambda - \theta)E_{\pi_1}\{E_\pi\{N_2^* I\{N_2^* \le \tau_1\} \mid \tau_1\}\}.
\end{aligned} \tag{8.4.31}
$$

The first term on the r.h.s. of Eq. (8.4.31) is as in Eq. (8.4.7). For $n^{(1)} \geq 1$,

(8.4.32)
$$(\phi-\lambda)E_{\pi}\{(n^{(1)}-\tau)I\{\tau \leq n^{(1)}\}\} = \frac{\phi-\lambda}{p}[n^{(1)}p-(1-\pi)(1-(1-p)^{n^{(1)}})].$$

Let $j(n)$ denote the value of j, $j=0,1,\ldots$, corresponding to $n \in \{n(0), n(1),\ldots\}$, that is,

$$j(n) = [(-a_L+b_Ln)^+], \quad n > 0,1,\ldots. \tag{8.4.33}$$

From the definition of N_2^*, we have

$$P_{\theta,\phi}\{N_2^* > \tau_1 \mid \tau_1\} = \begin{cases} 1, & \tau_1 < n(0), \\ \displaystyle\sum_{j=j(\tau_1)+1}^{j*} \psi_{\theta,\phi}^{(\tau_1)}(j), & n(0) \leq \tau_1 \leq N_1-1, \\ 0 & \text{if } \tau_1 \geq N_1. \end{cases} \tag{8.4.34}$$

Hence,

(8.4.35)
$$\begin{aligned} E_{\pi_1}\{\tau_1 P_{\theta,\phi}\{N_2^* > \tau_1 \mid \tau_1\}\} &= \frac{1-\pi_1}{p}[1-(1-p)^{n(0)-1}(1+p(n(0)-1))] \\ &\quad + (1-\pi_1)p\sum_{t=n(0)}^{N_1-1} t(1-p)^{t-1}\sum_{j=j(t)+1}^{j*}\psi_{\theta,\phi}^{(t)}(j). \end{aligned}$$

Also,

$$E\{N_2^*I\{N_2^* \leq \tau_1\} \mid \tau_1\} = \begin{cases} 0 & \text{if } \tau_1 < n(0), \\ \displaystyle\sum_{j=0}^{j(\tau_n)} n(j)\psi_\theta^*(j) & \text{if } n(0) \leq \tau_1 \leq N_1-1, \\ \displaystyle\sum_{j=0}^{j*} n(j)\psi_\theta^*(j) & \text{if } N_1 \leq \tau_1. \end{cases} \tag{8.4.36}$$

Hence,

(8.4.37)
$$\begin{aligned} E_{\pi_1}\{E\{N_2^*I\{N_2^* \leq \tau_1\} \mid \tau_1\}\} &= (1-\pi_1)p\sum_{t=n(0)}^{N_1-1}(1-p)^{t-1}\sum_{j=0}^{j(t)} n(j)\psi_\theta^*(j) \\ &\quad + (1-\pi_1)(1-p)^{N_1-1}\sum_{j=0}^{j*} n(j)\psi_\theta^*(j). \end{aligned}$$

Finally, from (8.4.31), (8.4.32), (8.4.35), and (8.4.37), the predictive risk of the surveillance cycle is
(8.4.38)

$$
\begin{aligned}
R_{\text{sc}}(n^{(1)}, N_1, \pi) = {} & \frac{\theta-\lambda}{p}[n^{(1)}p - (1-\pi)(1-(1-p)^{n^{(1)}})] \\
& + \frac{\lambda-\theta}{p}(1-\pi_1)\Bigg[1-(1-p)^{n(0)-1}(1+p(n(0)-1)) \\
& + p^2 \sum_{t=n(0)}^{N_1-1}(1-p)^{t-1}\left(t\sum_{j=j(t)+1}^{j*}\psi_{\theta,\phi}^{(t)}(j) + \sum_{j=0}^{j(t)} n(j)\psi_\theta^*(j)\right) \\
& + p(1-p)^{N_1-1}\sum_{j=0}^{j*} n(j)\psi_\theta^*(j)\Bigg].
\end{aligned}
$$

8.4.3.4 Combining the Surveillance and the Final Cycles After a surveillance cycle, $N_f = (N - N_{\text{sc}})^+$ trials are left. If $N_f > 0$, we design the final cycle according to the values of π_{sc} and N_f. The optimal number of trials on arm 1 is $n_f^0(\pi_{\text{sc}}, N_f)$, obtained by rounding the result of (8.4.12) with $\pi = \pi_{\text{sc}}$ and $N = N_f$. The ensuing minimal posterior risk of the final cycle is computed by Eq. (8.4.7), substituting $n = n_f^0(\pi_{\text{sc}}, N_f)$ and $\pi = \pi_{\text{sc}}$, $N = N_f$. Let $R_f^*(\pi_{\text{sc}}, N_f) = I\{N_f > 0\}R_f(n_f^0(\pi_{\text{sc}}), \pi_{\text{sc}}, N_f)$ denote the minimal posterior risk of the final cycle. Notice that if $N_f = 0$, then $R_f^*(\pi_{\text{sc}}, 0) \equiv 0$. The predictive risk of the surveillance cycle combined with an optimal final cycle is

$$
(8.4.39) \qquad \rho_{\text{cb}}(n^{(1)}; \pi, N) = R_{\text{sc}}(n^{(1)}; N_1, \pi) + E_{\pi_1}^{(p)}\{R_f^*(\pi_{\text{sc}}, N_f)\},
$$

where

$$
(8.4.40) \qquad E_{\pi_1}^{(p)}\{R_f^*(\pi_{\text{sc}}, N_f)\} = E_{\pi_1}^{(p)}\{R_f^*(\pi_{\text{sc}}, (N - n^{(1)} - N_2^*)^+)\}.
$$

Thus, the predictive risk of the final cycle is
(8.4.41)

$$
E_{\pi_1}^{(p)}\{R_f^*(\pi_{\text{sc}}, N_f)\} = \sum_{j=0}^{j*}\psi_{\theta,\phi}^{(p)}(j;\pi_1)R_f^*(\pi_{\text{sc}}(\pi_1, n(j)), (N - n^{(1)} - n(j))^+),
$$

where $\psi_{\theta,\phi}^{(p)}(j;\pi_1)$ are the predictive probabilities of $\{N_2^* = n(j)\}$, as given by Eq. (8.4.24).

Let $n_{\text{opt}}^{(1)}$ be the value of $n^{(1)}$ minimizing the combined predictive risk $\rho_{\text{cb}}(n^{(1)}; \pi, N)$. In Table 8.8, we present the values of $n_{\text{opt}}^{(1)}$ and $\rho_{\text{cb}}^*(\pi, N) = \rho_{\text{cb}}(n_{\text{opt}}^{(1)}; \pi, N)$.

Table 8.8: Minimal Prior Combined Risk, $\rho^*_{\text{sc}}(\pi, \mathbf{N})$ and the Associated Values of $\mathbf{n}^{(1)}_{\text{opt}}$, for $\theta = 0.35$, $\lambda = 0.50$, $\phi = 0.65$, $\alpha = \beta = 0.03$ and $\pi = 0.10$

		p		
N		0.05	0.025	0.01
50	$n^{(1)}_{\text{opt}}$	9	19	35
	ρ^*_{cb}	1.676	2.040	2.314
70	$n^{(1)}_{\text{opt}}$	10	20	27
	ρ^*_{cb}	1.726	2.641	2.772
90	$n^{(1)}_{\text{opt}}$	10	20	30
	ρ^*_{cb}	1.731	2.935	3.439

Comparing Table 8.8 to Table 8.6, we see the intuitively expected results that $\rho^*_{\text{cb}}(\pi, N) < R^*_f(\pi, N)$. The only case in which this does not hold is that of $N = 50$ and $p = 0.01$. Here, p is so small that often $n^{(0)}_{\text{opt}}(\pi, N) > N$, and the constrained result is taken, namely $n^{(0)} = N$. This causes the constrained minimal ρ_{cb} to be greater than R^*_f. Moreover, similar to the case of the final cycle, $n^{(1)}_{\text{opt}}$ varies little with N but depends strongly on p.

8.4.4 Multiple Surveillance Cycles

Suppose that at most k surveillance cycles are allowed, $k \geq 1$. If k such cycles are completed and there are remaining trials to perform, then a final cycle is planned and executed.

Let $n^{(l)}_1$, $l = 1, \ldots, k$, denote the number of trials on arm 1 in the lth cycle. Let $\pi^{(l)}_{\text{sc}}$, $l = 1, \ldots, k$, denote the posterior probability that the change point is before the end of the lth cycle. Let $N^{(l)}_2$ denote the number of trials on arm 2 in the lth cycle. The length of the lth surveillance cycle is $N^{(l)}_{\text{sc}} = n^{(l)}_1 + N^{(l)}_2$. The number of remaining trials after l cycles is $N^{(l)}_r = N - \sum_{j=1}^{l} N^{(j)}_{\text{sc}}$. Notice that $N^{(l)}_r$ is a random variable, and if $N^{(j)}_r = 0$ for $j = 1, 2, \ldots, k$, then $N^{(l)}_r = 0$ for all $l \geq j$, and the trials terminate. Let

$$\pi^{(l)}_1 = \pi^{(l-1)}_{\text{sc}} + (1 - \pi^{(l-1)}_{\text{sc}})(1 - (1-p)^{n^{(l)}_1}). \tag{8.4.42}$$

We set $N^{(0)}_r = N$. Let $\rho^{(l)}(\pi, N)$ denote the minimal prior risk when l surveillance cycles are allowed, $l = 1, 2, \ldots, k$. The following recursive relationship

holds:
(8.4.43)

$$\rho^{(l)}(\pi, N) = \min_{0 \le n \le N} E^{(p)}_{\pi_1(n)}\{L_{sc}(n, N_2^{(1)}, \tau) + \rho^{(l-1)}(\pi_{sc}^{(1)}(n, N_2^{(1)}), N - n - N_2^{(1)})\},$$

$$l = 1, \ldots, k.$$

Notice that $\rho^{(1)}(\pi, N) = \min_{0 \le n \le N}\{\rho_{cb}(n; \pi, N)\}$ and $\rho^{(0)}(\pi, N) = R_f^*(\pi, N)$. The value of n minimizing $\rho^{(l)}(\pi, N)$ is the optimal $n_1^{(1)}$.

The determination of the minimal risk functions $\rho^{(l)}(\pi, N)$ according to (8.4.43) requires lengthy computations when $l \ge 2$. We therefore simplify the procedure and consider the myopic procedure in which, after the lth surveillance cycle, if there is a return to arm 1 ($N_r^{(l)} > 0$), one determines the next $n_{l+1}^{(1)}$ by minimizing $\rho_{cb}(n; \pi_{sc}^{(l)}(n_1^{(l)}, N_2^{(l)}), N_r^{(l)})$. To evaluate this procedure, we use the previously defined functions with simulation according to the following computing algorithm:

Step 0. Set π, p, N, θ, λ, ϕ, α, β, trisk $\leftarrow 0$, $nc \leftarrow 0$, nrep, $k \leftarrow 1$.

Step 1. Generate a uniformly $(0,1)$ distributed random deviate U.

Step 2. Determine the predictive crossing probabilities $\psi^{(p)}_{\theta,\phi}(j; \pi_1)$, $j = 0, 1, \ldots, j^*$, and

$$T^{(p)}_{\theta,\phi}(j; \pi_1) = \sum_{l=0}^{j} \psi^{(p)}_{\theta,\phi}(l; \pi_1).$$

Step 3. Determine $n_1^{(1)}$ by minimizing $\rho_{cb}(n; \pi, N)$.

Step 4. Determine the random deviate J = smallest nonnegative integer j such that

$$T^{(p)}_{\theta,\phi}(j; \pi_1) \ge U$$

and $N_2^* = n(J)$.

Step 5. IF $J = j^*$ THEN
set: nc $\leftarrow$ nc + 1; trisk $\leftarrow$ trisk $+\tilde{R}_{sc}(n^{(1)}, N_2^*, \pi)$
GO TO Step 6
ELSE
Compute:
$\tilde{R}^*_{sc}(n^{(1)}, N_2^*, \pi)$
π_{sc} as a function of $n^{(1)}, N_2^{(1)}, \pi$ (Eq. (3.17))
set:
$\pi \leftarrow \pi_{sc}$; $N \leftarrow N_r^{(1)}$; nc $\leftarrow$ nc + 1;
trisk $\leftarrow$ trisk + $\tilde{R}_{sc}(n^{(1)}, N_2^*)$; $N_r^{(1)} = N - n_1^{(1)} - N_2^*$;
IF $k <$ nrep THEN

GO TO Step 1
ELSE STOP

Step 6. If $k <$ nrep THEN
set:
$k \leftarrow k+1$; $\pi \leftarrow \pi$; $N \leftarrow N$;
GO TO Step 1
ELSE STOP.

The term nrep in the algorithm is the number of independent simulation runs (repetitions). At the end of these runs, the empirical frequency distribution of the number of cycles (nc) is computed, and the average of conditional total risks is denoted as trisk. This function is the sum over the random number of cycles of the conditional (posterior) risks,

$$\tilde{R}_{\text{sc}}(n^{(1)}, N_2^*, \pi) = E_\pi\{L_{\text{sc}}(n^{(1)}, N_2^*, \tau) \mid n^{(1)}, N_2^*\}. \tag{8.4.44}$$

This posterior risk is given by

$$\begin{aligned}\tilde{R}_{\text{sc}}(n^{(1)}, N_2^*, \pi) = & \frac{\phi-\lambda}{p}[n^{(1)}p - (1-\pi)(1-(1-p)^{n^{(1)}})] \\ & + \frac{\lambda-\phi}{p}(1-\pi_1)(1-(1-p)^{N_2^*}).\end{aligned} \tag{8.4.45}$$

In Table 8.9, we present the statistics of 50 independent simulation runs of this multicycle procedure.

Table 8.9: Statistics of 50 Independent Simulation Runs of the Multicycle Procedure, $\theta = 0.35$, $\lambda = 0.50$, $\phi = 0.65$, $\alpha = \beta = 0.03$, $\pi = 0.1$

		Frequency Distribution of ncycles						
N	p	1	2	3	4	5	Average Risk [a]	Risk Index
50	0.050	31	14	4	1	0	0.7474 (0.1070)	0.028
	0.025	27	18	5	1	0	0.9593 (0.0821)	0.048
	0.010	18	17	12	3	0	0.8079 (0.0456)	0.067
70	0.050	34	10	4	2	0	0.7060 (0.1190)	0.018
	0.025	24	14	10	2	0	1.4857 (0.1420)	0.045
	0.010	19	17	13	1	0	1.3208 (0.0723)	0.063
90	0.050	30	13	4	3	0	1.0166 (0.1620)	0.019
	0.025	29	10	6	2	3	1.6540 (0.2010)	0.036
	0.010	20	11	12	5	2	1.9146 (0.1080)	0.062

[a] The standard error of the average risk is given in parentheses.

Comparing Tables 8.8 and 8.9, we see that the multicycle procedure suggested in the present section is expected to reduce the risk considerably over that of the optimal one-combined-cycle procedure. Even when $p = 0.05$, the probability of terminating after one combined cycle is estimated to be approximately 0.6. In the case of $p = 0.01$, the median number of surveillance cycles is estimated to be 2. How good is the procedure? An answer can be given by comparing the estimates of the prior risk in Table 8.8 to the maximal expected payoff $E_{(\pi,p)}\{W^0(\tau)\}$ given by Eq. (8.4.3). The ratio of the average risk to $E_{(\pi,p)}\{W^0(\tau)\}$ is called the risk index in Table 8.9. We see that the risk index ranges from 3 to 7 percent as p varies from 0.05 to 0.01. These results will obviously vary with π, ϕ, and λ.

8.5 SEQUENTIAL DESIGNS FOR ESTIMATING THE COMMON MEAN OF TWO NORMAL DISTRIBUTIONS: ONE VARIANCE KNOWN

In the present section we present an example of a sequential estimation problem in which two alternative experiments are available and the objective is to minimize the expected total number of trials. This problem can be considered an OAB problem. We follow the exposition and results of Zacks (1973).

Two experiments are available: $\mathcal{E}_1$ yields a sequence of i.i.d. $N(\mu, \sigma)$ random variables, while $\mathcal{E}_2$ yields a sequence of $N(\mu, 1)$ random variables, where $-\infty < \mu < \infty$ and $0 < \sigma < \infty$ are unknown parameters. The objective is to construct a fixed-width confidence interval for the common mean μ, with the minimal expected total sample size. If one knows that $\sigma > 1$, then the solution is to perform

$$n_1(\delta) = \text{ least integer } n \geq \frac{\chi^2_{1-\alpha}[1]}{\delta^2} \tag{8.5.1}$$

observations on $\mathcal{E}_2$ and construct the interval $(\bar{Y}^{(2)}_{n_1(\delta)} - \delta, \bar{Y}^{(2)}_{n_1(\delta)} + \delta)$, where

$$\bar{Y}^{(2)}_{n_1(\delta)} = \frac{1}{n_1(\delta)} \sum_{j=1}^{n_1(\delta)} Y_{2i}.$$

This interval has coverage probability at least $1 - \alpha$, $0 < \alpha < 1$, and $n_1(\delta)$ is the smallest integer for which the required coverage is attained. If $\sigma < 1$ and known, one can attain the objective by performing $n' = n_1(\delta)\sigma$ trials on $\mathcal{E}_1$ and using the interval $\bar{Y}^{(1)}_{n'} - \delta, \bar{Y}^{(1)}_{n'} + \delta$. The following is a procedure for unknown σ.

We start the trials on $\mathcal{E}_1$. After n observations we compute $\bar{Y}^{(1)}_n$ and $Q_n = \sum_{i=1}^{n}(Y_{1i} - \bar{Y}^{(1)}_n)^2$. Let N be a stopping variable which depends on $\mathbf{Y}_1$ only through Q_n. Furthermore, if $\sigma < 1$, the number of observations required from $\mathcal{E}_1$ is not greater than $n_1(\delta)$. We therefore truncate N to be smaller or equal to $n_1(\delta)$. Moreover, when $\sigma^2 < 1$, N should not exceed much the value of $\sigma^2 n_1(\delta)$. Thus, we use for N a stopping variable of the form

$$N(\delta) = \min\{N_1(\delta), N_2(\delta), n_1(\delta)\}, \tag{8.5.2}$$

where $N_1(\delta)$ is a stopping variable for immediate estimation and $N_2(\delta)$ is a stopping variable for testing the hypothesis $H_0 : \sigma \le 1 - \delta$ against $H_1 : \sigma \ge 1+\delta$. If $N(\delta) = N_1(\delta)$, we stop and construct the interval $\bar{Y}^{(1)}_{N_1(\delta)} - \delta, \bar{Y}^{(1)}_{N_1(\delta)} + \delta$. If $N(\delta) = N_2(\delta)$, we stop the trials on $\mathcal{E}_1$ and add $M(\delta)$ observations on $\mathcal{E}_2$, where

$$M(\delta) = \text{ least integer } m \ge 0 \text{ such that } m \ge n_1(\delta) - N_2^2(\delta)/Q_{N_2(\delta)}. \tag{8.5.3}$$

The interval estimator is $\hat{\mu} - \delta, \hat{\mu} + \delta$, where

$$\hat{\mu} = \frac{M(\delta)(Q_{N_2(\delta)}/N_2(\delta))\bar{Y}^{(2)}_{M(\delta)} + N_2(\delta)\bar{Y}^{(1)}_{N_2(\delta)}}{(M(\delta)/N_2(\delta))Q_{N_2}(\delta) + N_2(\delta)}. \tag{8.5.4}$$

For $N_1(\delta)$ we use the Chow–Robbins stopping variable (see Chow and Robbins, 1965)

$$N_1(\delta) = \text{ least integer } n \ge 1 \text{ such that } Q_n \le \frac{\delta^2}{\chi^2_{1-\alpha}} n^2. \tag{8.5.5}$$

Zacks (1973) considered three types of stopping variables for $N_2(\delta)$, called parabolic (P), Wald (W), and Chernoff (C). For the rational leading to each one of these variables see Zacks (1973). The formulas of these stopping variables are

$$\begin{aligned} N_2^{(P)}(\delta) = &\text{ least } n,\ n \ge 2 \text{ such that} \\ &Q_n \ge n e^{1/n} \Phi\left(\sqrt{\frac{n}{2}} \ln\left(\frac{n_1(\delta) Q_n}{n^2}\right) - \sqrt{\frac{2}{n}}\right), \end{aligned} \tag{8.5.6}$$

$$\begin{aligned} N_2^{(W)}(\delta) = &\text{ least } n,\ n \ge 2 \text{ such that} \\ &Q_n \ge n \exp\left\{\frac{\log(n_1(\delta))}{n}\right\}, \end{aligned} \tag{8.5.7}$$

and

$$\begin{aligned} N_2^{(C)}(\delta) = &\text{ least } n,\ n \ge 2 \text{ such that} \\ &Q_n \ge \begin{cases} n \exp\left\{\sqrt{\dfrac{2}{n}}\left[\log\left(\dfrac{n_1^3(\delta)}{n^3 8\pi}\right)\right]^{1/2}\right\} & \text{if } n \le \dfrac{n_1(\delta)}{(8\pi)^{1/3}}, \\ n & \text{otherwise.} \end{cases} \end{aligned} \tag{8.5.8}$$

The performance of these procedures with respect to coverage probability and expected sample size was evaluated by simulations. The results are given in Table 8.10.

Table 8.10: Simulation Estimates of $\mathbf{EN_2^{(\cdot)}(\delta)}$, $\mathbf{E\{M(\delta)\}}$, and Coverage Probability, $\mathbf{n_1(\delta) = 50}$, $\boldsymbol{\gamma} = \mathbf{0.95}$

σ	$E\{N_2(\delta)\}$			$E\{M(\delta)\}$			$P\{\lvert\hat{\mu}-\mu\rvert<\delta\}$		
	P	W	C	P	W	C	P	W	C
0.25	3.72	2.32	2.32	0.00	0.00	0.00	0.9329	0.8976	0.8976
0.50	9.11	5.82	5.82	0.00	0.00	0.00	0.8223	0.7153	0.7153
0.75	17.75	15.07	14.48	2.30	0.00	0.93	0.8115	0.6995	0.6993
1.00	16.16	23.22	19.10	22.57	11.08	15.65	0.8424	0.7612	0.7629
1.25	8.41	12.90	12.67	36.47	29.19	29.39	0.8492	0.7826	0.7825
1.50	5.24	7.96	8.81	42.23	35.98	35.54	0.8725	0.7978	0.7972
1.75	4.24	6.11	7.50	44.15	39.68	39.26	0.8839	0.8235	0.8236
2.00	3.71	5.04	6.28	45.83	41.00	40.73	0.8989	0.8279	0.8281

It seems that $N_2^{(P)}(\delta)$ is the best for the coverage probability $P\{|\hat{\mu}-\mu| < \delta\}$. Also $E\{N_2^{(P)}(\delta)\}$ is the smallest when $\sigma \geq 1$. The Wald and Chernoff stopping rules yield similar results.

CHAPTER 9

SEQUENTIAL DETECTION OF CHANGE POINTS

9.1 BAYESIAN DETECTION WHEN THE DISTRIBUTIONS BEFORE AND AFTER THE CHANGE ARE KNOWN

9.1.1 Problem

Consider a sequence of independent observable random variables $X_1, X_2, \ldots, X_{\tau-1}, X_\tau, \ldots$. It is assumed that:

1. $X_1, \ldots, X_{\tau-1}$ have an identical distribution function $F_0(x)$.

2. $X_\tau, X_{\tau+1}, \ldots$ have an identical distribution function $F_1(x)$.

3. $F_0(x) \neq F_1(x)$.

The two specified distributions are completely known, and the index of shift (change point) τ is *unknown*. The sequence of variables is observed sequentially. We wish to apply a stopping rule which will stop soon after the shift occurs without too many "false alarms." It is generally assumed that observations resume immediately on the same process if the alarm is false; a correct alarm terminates the process.

Let N be a *stopping variable* associated with a detection procedure. We look for a procedure which attains the following objectives (optimality criteria):

(i) *Bayesian criterion:* If $\pi(\cdot)$ denotes the prior distribution of the shift index τ, then the prior risk

$$R(\pi, N) = P_\pi(N < \tau) + cP_\pi(N \geq \tau) \cdot E_\pi\{N - \tau \mid N \geq \tau\} \tag{9.1.1}$$

is minimized with respect to all proper stopping rules (Markov times).

(ii) *Variational criterion:* $E_\pi\{N - \tau \mid N \geq \tau\}$ is minimized under the constraint

$$P_\pi\{N < \tau\} \leq \alpha, \quad 0 < \alpha < 1. \tag{9.1.2}$$

9.1.2 Bayesian Framework

Shiryaev (1963a) developed the following theory (see also Shiryaev, 1973, Chapter 4; 1978): The shift index m is considered a realization of a random variable τ having a prior distribution $\pi(\tau)$ concentrated on the set of nonnegative integers $\{0, 1, 2, \ldots\}$. Specifically, it is assumed that the prior probability function of θ is

$$\pi(\theta) = \begin{cases} \pi & \text{if } \tau = 0, \\ (1-\pi)p(1-p)^{j-1} & \text{if } \tau = j \geq 1, \end{cases} \tag{9.1.3}$$

$0 < \pi < 1$, $0 < p < 1$.

The observable random variables $X_1, X_2, \ldots$ are defined on a probability space $(\Omega, \mathcal{F})$ on which a family of probability measures $\{P_\pi, 0 < \pi < 1\}$ induce, for $(X_1, \ldots, X_n)$ with $n \geq 1$, a joint predictive c.d.f.

$$\begin{aligned} F_\pi(x_1, \ldots, x_n) &= (\pi + (1-\pi)p) \prod_{i=1}^{n} F_1(x_i) \\ &\quad + (1-\pi)p \sum_{j=1}^{n-1} (1-p)^j \cdot \prod_{i=1}^{j} F_0(x_i) \prod_{i=j+1}^{n} F_1(x_i) \\ &\quad + (1-\pi)(1-p)^n \prod_{i=1}^{n} F_0(x_i). \end{aligned} \tag{9.1.4}$$

Let $X_0 \equiv 0$ and $\mathcal{F}_n = \sigma\{\pi, X_0, X_1, \ldots, X_n\}$, be the σ-field generated by the first n observations. Let $\mathcal{M}$ denote the class of all *Markov times*, $\tau(\omega, \pi)$, which are nonnegative r.v's such that $\{\tau(\omega, \pi) \leq n\} \in \mathcal{F}_n$ for all $n = 0, 1, 2, \ldots$. Let $f_0(x)$ and $f_1(x)$ denote the p.d.f.'s corresponding to F_0 and F_1, respectively.

After observing $x_1, \ldots, x_n$, the prior probability function $\pi(\tau)$ is converted into a *posterior* probability function on $\{n, n+1, \ldots\}$,

$$\pi_n(\tau) = \begin{cases} \pi_n, & \tau \le n, \\ (1-\pi_n)p(1-p)^{\tau-n-1}, & \tau \ge n+1, \end{cases} \tag{9.1.5}$$

where

(9.1.6)

$$\pi_n = P_\pi\{\tau \le n \mid \mathcal{F}_n\}$$

$$= \frac{(\pi + p(1-\pi))\prod_{i=1}^{n} f_1(x_i) + (1-\pi)p\sum_{j=1}^{n-1}(1-p)^{j-1}\prod_{i=1}^{j} f_0(x_i)\prod_{i=j+1}^{n} f_1(x_i)}{D_n}$$

in which

$$\begin{aligned} D_n = {} & (\pi + p(1-\pi))\prod_{i=1}^{n} f_1(x_i) + (1-\pi)p\sum_{j=1}^{n-1}(1-p)^{j-1}\prod_{i=1}^{j} f_0(x_i) \\ & \cdot \prod_{i=j+1}^{n} f_1(x_i) + (1-\pi)(1-p)^n \prod_{i=1}^{n} f_0(x_i). \end{aligned} \tag{9.1.7}$$

Let $R(x_i) = f_1(x_i)/f_0(x_i)$ be the likelihood ratio. Dividing the numerator and the denominator of π_n by $(1-\pi)\prod_{j=1}^{n} f_0(x_j)$ we obtain the formula

$$\pi_n = \frac{[\pi/(1-\pi)]\prod_{i=1}^{n} R(x_i) + p\sum_{j=0}^{n-1}(1-p)^{j-1}\prod_{i=j+1}^{n} R(x_i)}{[\pi/(1-\pi)]\prod_{i=1}^{n} R(x_i) + p\sum_{j=0}^{n-1}(1-p)^{j-1}\prod_{i=j+1}^{n} R(x_i) + (1-p)^n}. \tag{9.1.8}$$

Let $q_n = 1 - \pi_n$. For $n = 0, 1, \ldots$ one can write

$$q_{n+1} = \frac{(1-\pi)(1-p)^{n+1}}{R(x_{n+1})[D_n - (1-\pi)(1-p)^n] + B_{n+1}}, \tag{9.1.9}$$

where

$$B_{n+1} = R(x_{n+1})(1-\pi)(1-p)^n p + (1-\pi)(1-p)^{n+1}. \tag{9.1.10}$$

But $(1-\pi)(1-p)^n = q_n D_n$. Hence, we obtain the recursive formulas

$$q_{n+1} = \frac{q_n(1-p)}{R(x_{n+1})(1 - q_n(1-p)) + q_n(1-p)}, \tag{9.1.11}$$

or, for $n = 0, 1, \ldots,$

$$\pi_{n+1} = \frac{(\pi_n + (1-\pi_n)p)R(x_{n+1})}{(\pi_n + (1-\pi_n)p)R(x_{n+1}) + (1-\pi_n)(1-p)}, \tag{9.1.12}$$

where $\pi_0 = \pi$, $q_0 = 1 - \pi$.

If $\mathcal{F}_n^* = \sigma\{\pi_0, \pi_1, \ldots, \pi_n\}$ is the σ-field generated by the posterior probabilities, $\mathcal{F}_n^* \subseteq \mathcal{F}_n$, and

$$P_\pi\{\tau \le n \mid \mathcal{F}_n\} = P_\pi\{\tau \le n \mid \mathcal{F}_n^*\}. \tag{9.1.13}$$

The posterior probability function $\pi_n(\omega, \pi) = \pi_n$ is a *Markov random function*; that is:

1. $\pi_n(\omega, \pi) \in \mathcal{F}_n^*$.

2. For any Borel set $B \subseteq [0, 1]$

$$P_\pi\{\pi_n \in B \mid \mathcal{F}_{n-1}^*\} = P_\pi\{\pi_n \in B \mid \pi_{n-1}\}, \quad n \ge 1. \tag{9.1.14}$$

Shiryaev (1963a) proved that the optimal Bayesian stopping time is

$$\tau^* = \min(n : \pi_n \ge A^*), \tag{9.1.15}$$

where $0 < A^* < 1$ is a function of (c, π, p). The proof is based on the fact that $\{\pi_n, \mathcal{F}_n^*, n \ge 1\}$ is a *submartingale*. Indeed, the predictive p.d.f. of X_{n+1}, given $\mathcal{F}_n^*$, is

$$f_\pi(x_{n+1} \mid \mathcal{F}_n^*) = (\pi_n + (1 - \pi_n)p)f_1(x_{n+1}) + (1 - \pi_n)(1 - p)f_0(x_{n+1}). \tag{9.1.16}$$

Hence

$$E_\pi\{X_{n+1} \mid \mathcal{F}_n^*\} = \pi_n + p(1 - \pi_n) \quad \text{a.s.} \tag{9.1.17}$$

Using the martingale convergence theorem and Faton's lemma, we prove that

$$\lim_{n \to \infty} \pi_n = 1 \quad \text{a.s.}$$

Thus, $P_\pi\{\tau^* < \infty\} = 1$.

The minimal Bayesian risk function $\rho(\tau)$ satisfies the equation

$$\rho(\pi) = \min(1 - \pi, E_\pi\{\rho(\pi_1)\}). \tag{9.1.18}$$

Then, $\rho(\pi)$ is continuous and concave on $(0, 1)$. Moreover, at the time of stopping $\rho(\pi_{\tau^*}) = 1 - \pi_{\tau^*}$. This establishes (9.1.15)

Explicit expression of A^* in terms of (c, π, p) is not given by Shiryaev. A Wiener process approximation to A^* is presented in the next section. Bather (1967) proved that, for the variational problem, if the expected number of false alarms is bounded by B, then $A^* = 1/(B + 1)$. See also Pollak and Siegmund (1985).

9.1.3 Application in System Reliability

A system starts functioning with a constant (known) failure rate λ. At an unknown epoch the failure rate function of the system starts to increase in a polynomial fashion. We are interested in detecting the time of shift from constant failure rate to increasing failure rate (Zacks, 1984).

Initially, the life length T of such a system is exponentially distributed, that is, $T \sim \mathcal{E}(\lambda)$, where $\mathcal{E}(1/\mu)$ designates an exponential r.v. with mean μ. At an unknown time point τ, $0 < \tau < \infty$, the life length becomes a Weibull r.v. $T^\alpha \sim \mathcal{E}(\lambda)$, $1 < \alpha < \infty$; that is,

$$P_\lambda[T \geq t+s \mid T \geq t] = \begin{cases} e^{-\lambda s}, & t+s < \tau, \\ e^{-\lambda(t+s)^\alpha + \lambda t}, & t < \tau \leq t+s \\ e^{-\lambda(t+s)^\alpha + \lambda t^\alpha}, & \tau \leq t. \end{cases} \tag{9.1.19}$$

According to a preventive maintenance policy, the system is replaced by a new one either after a predetermined time interval Δ or at failure. The observations are therefore censored, that is,

$$X_i = \min(\Delta, T_i), \quad i = 1, 2, \ldots,$$

$X_1, X_2, \ldots$ are conditionally independent.

Let $t_0 = 0$, $t_1 = X_1$, $t_2 = X_1 + X_2, \ldots, t_n = \sum_{i=1}^n X_i$ be the recorded times of replacement and $\Delta_i = t_i - t_{i-1}$; $i = 1, \ldots, n$. Let

$$J_i = \begin{cases} 1 & \text{if } X_i = T_i, \\ 0 & \text{if } X_i < T_i, \end{cases} \quad i = 1, \ldots, n,$$

and let $K_i^{(n)} = \sum_{j=i}^n J_j$ be the number of failures in $(t_i, t_n]$. Let $I\{\cdot\}$ designate an indicator variable assuming the value 1 if the relation in braces is true and the value zero otherwise. The likelihood function of τ is then

$$\begin{aligned} L(\tau) &= I\{\tau > t_n\} \exp\{-\lambda t_n\} \lambda^{K_0^{(n)}} \\ &\quad + \lambda^{K_0^{(n)}} \sum_{i=0}^{n-1} I\{t_i < \tau \leq t_{i+1}\} \alpha^{K_i^{(n)}} \prod_{j=i+1}^{n} [1 - J_j + J_j \Delta_j]^{\alpha-1} (t_{i+1} - \tau)^{\alpha-1} \\ &\quad \cdot \exp\left\{ -\lambda(\tau - t_{i-1}) - \lambda(t_{i+1} - \tau)^\alpha - \lambda \sum_{j=i+1}^{n} \Delta_j^\alpha \right\}. \end{aligned} \tag{9.1.20}$$

Let $\xi(\tau)$ be the prior p.d.f. of τ. Let $q(t) = P_\xi\{\tau \geq t\}$,

$$q(t_n \mid \mathbf{x}_n^*) = \frac{\lambda^{K_0^{(n)}} \exp\{-\lambda t_n\} G(t_n)}{\lambda^{K_0^{(n)}} \exp\{-\lambda t_n\} G(t_n) + B_n}, \tag{9.1.21}$$

where
(9.1.22)

$$
\begin{aligned}
B_n &= \int_0^{t_n} \xi(\tau) L(\tau; \mathbf{x}_n^*)\, d\tau \\
&= \lambda^{K_0^{(n)}} \sum_{i=0}^{n-1} \alpha^{K_i^{(n)}} \exp\left\{ -\lambda \sum_{j=i+1}^{n} \Delta_j^{\alpha} \right\} \prod_{j=i+1}^{n} [1 - J_j + J_j \Delta_j]^{\alpha - 1} \\
&\quad \cdot \int_{t_i}^{t_{i+1}} \xi(\tau)(t_{i+1} - \tau)^{\alpha - 1} \exp\{-\lambda\tau - \lambda(t_{i+1} - \tau)^{\alpha}\}\, d\tau.
\end{aligned}
$$

We consider now a prior exponential p.d.f. for τ,

$$\xi(\theta) = \frac{1}{\mu} e^{-\tau/\mu}, \quad \tau \geq 0, \quad \mu > 0.$$

The integral in (9.1.22) can be expressed as

$$E_{i+1} = \frac{1}{\mu\lambda\alpha} \exp\{-(\lambda + \mu)t_{i+1}\} \sum_{v=0}^{\infty} \frac{(\mu\lambda + 1)^v}{v!\lambda^{v/\alpha}\mu^{\nu}} \Gamma(\lambda\Delta_{i+1}^{\alpha}; \frac{\nu}{\alpha} + 1), \tag{9.1.23}$$

where $\Gamma(x; \alpha) = \int_0^x y^{\alpha-1} e^{-y}\, dy$.

We illustrate now Shiryaev's stopping rule (9.1.15) with two simulated sequences. In these simulations we shift from the exponential to the Weibull interfailure times after $\tau = 1750$ hr. The interfailure times are simulated with the parameters:

$$\lambda^{-1} = 200 \text{ hr}, \quad \alpha = 2, \quad \Delta = 400 \text{ hr}.$$

The parameter of the prior distribution of τ is $\mu = 1/2000$ hr. The values of the replacement times t_n and the posterior probabilities q_n for the two simulation runs are given in Table 9.1. We see in this table that if the cost and prior parameters (c, π, p) are such that $A^* = 0.5$ then in run 1 we detect the shift 88.9 hr, and in run 2 38.2 hr after its occurrence.

Table 9.1: Two Simulation Runs of Replacement Times and the Associated q_n Values, $\tau = 1750$ hr, $\lambda^{-1} = 200$ hr, $\Delta = 400$ hr, $\mu^{-1} = 2000$ hr

Replacement No.	Run 1		Run 2	
	t_n	q_n	t_n	q_n
1	298.2	1.000	31.0	0.974
2	639.7	1.000	273.9	1.000
3	695.4	1.000	300.1	0.920
4	915.5	1.000	439.4	1.000
5	1214.8	1.000	477.4	0.997
6	1570.1	1.000	877.4	1.000
7	1659.2	1.000	1277.4	1.000
8	1765.2	1.000	1564.7	1.000
9	1769.1	0.975	1757.3	1.000
10	1801.7	0.974	1760.9	0.979
11	1826.4	0.840	1782.9	0.779
12	1838.9	0.274	1788.2	0.264
13	1851.9	0.030	1802.1	0.030

9.1.4 Optimal Stopping for Detecting a Change Point in the intensity of a Poisson Process

The results reported in the present section are based on the paper of Brown and Zacks (2006).

Let $\{N(t), t \geq 0\}$ be an ordinary Poisson process with arrival intensity

$$\lambda(t;\tau) = \begin{cases} \lambda_1 & \text{if } t \leq \tau, \\ \lambda_2 & \text{if } t > \tau, \end{cases} \tag{9.1.24}$$

where $0 < \lambda_1 < \lambda_2 < \infty$ and τ is a random change point having a prior distribution

$$H(\tau) = \pi + (1-\pi)(1-e^{-\mu\tau}), \quad \tau \geq 0. \tag{9.1.25}$$

Notice that $H(0) = \pi$ and $H(0-) = 0$. The event $\{\tau = 0\}$ designates that the change point has happened before time $t = 0$. The loss function consists of two components: (i) a penalty for early stopping (false alarm) and (ii) a cost per unit time of delayed stopping. Without loss of generality, the penalty for false alarm is one cost unit, and the cost for delayed stopping is c cost units per time unit. Thus, the risk associated with a stopping time θ is

$$R_{\pi,\mu}(\theta) = E_{\pi,\mu}\{I(\theta < \tau)\} + cE_{\pi,\mu}\{(\theta - \tau)^+\}. \tag{9.1.26}$$

The objective is to find a stopping time which minimizes (9.1.26). For $N(t) = n$, let $0 < s_1 < \cdots < s_n < t$ denote the jump points of $N(t)$, that is, $N(s_i) = i$,

$1 \le i \le n$. Also, let $s_0 \equiv 0$, $N(0) \equiv 0$. The conditional likelihood of τ given $\{N(s), 0 < s \le t\}$ is

(9.1.27)
$$L_t(\tau) = I(\tau \le 0)\lambda_2^n e^{-\lambda_2 t} + \sum_{i=0}^{n-1} I\{s_i < \tau \le s_{i+1}\}\lambda_1^i \lambda_2^{n-i} e^{-\lambda_1\tau - \lambda_2(t-\tau)} + I\{s_n < \tau \le t\}\lambda_1^n e^{-\lambda_1\tau-\lambda_2(t-\tau)} + I(\tau > t)\lambda_1^n e^{-\lambda_1 t}.$$

Let $\bar{\Psi}_n(t,\pi) = P_{\pi,p}(\tau > t \mid \{N(s), 0 < s \le t\})$. We denote this posterior probability by $\bar{\pi}_t$. We have

(9.1.28)
$$\bar{\pi}_t = \frac{(1-\pi)e^{-(\mu+\lambda_1-\lambda_2)t}(\lambda_1/\lambda_2)^n}{D_n(t,\pi)},$$

where

(9.1.29)
$$D_n(t,\pi) = \pi + I(n \ge 1)(1-\pi)\frac{\mu}{\zeta}\sum_{i=0}^{n-1}\rho^i(e^{\zeta s_{i+1}} - e^{\zeta s_i}) + (1-\pi)\frac{\mu}{\zeta}\rho^n(e^{\zeta t} - e^{\zeta s_n}) + (1-\pi)\rho^n e^{\zeta t}, \quad n \ge 0,$$

where $\zeta = \lambda_2 - \lambda_1 - \mu$ and $\rho = \lambda_1/\lambda_2$.

Define the embedded sequence

(9.1.30)
$$\psi_n = \begin{cases} \pi & \text{if } n = 0, \\ \Psi_n(s_n, \pi) & \text{if } n \ge 1, \end{cases}$$

where $\Psi_n(s_n,\pi) = 1 - \bar{\Psi}_n(s_n,\pi)$. We also have $\bar{\psi}_n = 1 - \psi_n$. Let $\mathcal{S}_t = \sigma\{N(s), 0 < s < t\}$ be the σ-field generated by the process. We proved that $\{\bar{\psi}_n, \mathcal{S}_{s_n}; n \ge 0\}$ is a supermartingale, and

(9.1.31)
$$E\{\bar{\psi}_n \mid \psi_{n-1}\} = \bar{\psi}_{n-1}\frac{\lambda_1}{\mu + \lambda_1} \quad \text{a.s.}$$

Moreover, the predictive density of $T_n = s_n - s_{n-1}$ given $\mathcal{S}_{s_n-1}$ is

(9.1.32)
$$f_n(t) = \psi_{n-1}\lambda_2 e^{-\lambda_2 t} + \bar{\psi}_{n-1}\lambda_2\frac{\mu}{\zeta}(e^{-(\mu+\lambda_1)t} - e^{-\lambda_2 t}) + \bar{\psi}_{n-1}\lambda_1 e^{-(\mu+\lambda_1)t}.$$

From Eq. (9.1.31) we get that

(9.1.33)
$$\lim_{n\to\infty} \bar{\psi}_n = 0 \quad \text{a.s.}$$

Peskir and Shiryaev (2002) proved that the optimal stopping is

(9.1.34)
$$\theta^* = \inf\{t > 0 : \pi_t > B^*\},$$

where

$$(9.1.35) \qquad B^* = \begin{cases} \dfrac{\mu}{\mu + c} & \text{if } c \geq \lambda_2 - \lambda_1 - \mu, \\ \dfrac{\mu(\lambda_2 - c)}{\mu\lambda_2 + c\lambda_1} & \text{if } \lambda^* \leq c \leq \lambda_2 - \lambda_1 - \mu, \end{cases}$$

with

$$(9.1.36) \qquad \lambda^* = \frac{\lambda_1\lambda_2(\lambda_2 - \lambda_1 - \mu)}{\lambda_1\lambda_2 + (\lambda_2 - \lambda_1)(\mu + \lambda_1)}.$$

We extended the investigation to the case of $c < \lambda^*$. For this Brown and Zacks (2006) applied dynamic programming with finite horizon. They proved that if $c < \lambda^*$ the optimal stopping boundary is random. Let $q^* = 1 - B^*$. If at the nth arrival s_n we decide to continue until the next arrival and then stop, the additional predictive risk is

$$(9.1.37) \qquad R_n^{(1)} = \frac{c}{\lambda_2}\psi_n + \left(\frac{c}{\lambda_2} \cdot \frac{\mu}{\mu + \lambda_1} + \frac{\lambda_1}{\mu + \lambda_1}\right)\bar{\psi}_n.$$

For proof see Brown and Zacks (2006). Define recursively

$$(9.1.38) \quad M_n^{(j)}(\psi_n) = E\{\min(0, R_{n+1}^{(1)} - \bar{\psi}_{n+1} + M_{n+1}^{(j-1)}(\psi_{n+1})) \mid \mathcal{S}_{s_n}\}, \quad j \geq 1,$$

where $M_n^{(0)}(\psi_n) \equiv 0$. The minimal predictive risk at s_n when j more observations are allowed is

$$(9.1.39) \qquad R_n^{(j)} = \bar{\psi}_n + \min(0, R_n^{(1)} - \bar{\psi}_n + M_n^{(j-1)}(\psi_n)), \quad j \geq 1.$$

The j-step-ahead stopping rule is

$$(9.1.40) \qquad N^{(j)} = \min\left\{n \geq 1 : \bar{\psi}_n \leq q^*\left(1 + \frac{\lambda_2}{c}M_n^{(j-1)}(\psi_n)\right)\right\}.$$

We proved that if $c < \lambda^*$ then $M_n^{(j)} < 0$ for all $j \geq 1$. Explicit expression for $M_n^{(1)}$ was found and the corresponding two-step-ahead boundary is

$$q_{2,n}^* = \max\left(0, q^*\left(1 + \frac{\lambda_2}{c}M^{(1)}(\psi_n)\right)\right).$$

9.2 BAYESIAN DETECTION WHEN THE DISTRIBUTIONS BEFORE AND AFTER THE CHANGE ARE UNKNOWN

In many practical cases the distributions $F_0(x)$ and $F_1(x)$ are unknown. Even in parametric models, these distributions may depend on unknown parameters, say $\boldsymbol{\omega}_0$ and $\boldsymbol{\omega}_1$, which have to be estimated from the data during the detection processes. In these cases we generally lose the Markovian property of the posterior probability process, and Shiryaev's theory does not hold.

9.2.1 Bayesian Framework

Suppose that F_0 and F_1 depend on (vectors of) parameters $\boldsymbol{\omega}_0$ and $\boldsymbol{\omega}_1$, respectively which belong to a parameter space Ω. The index of shift point θ will assume values in $\mathbb{N} = \{0, 1, 2, \ldots\}$ as before. The observed random variables $X_1, X_2, \ldots$ are conditionally independent given $(\theta, \boldsymbol{\omega}_0, \boldsymbol{\omega}_1)$. Assume that the distributions $F(x; \boldsymbol{\omega})$ have p.d.f.'s $f(x; \boldsymbol{\omega})$. Let $(\boldsymbol{\omega}_0, \boldsymbol{\omega}_1)$ have a prior joint distribution with c.d.f. $H(\boldsymbol{\omega}_0, \boldsymbol{\omega}_1)$. For simplicity of exposition, although it will not necessarily be the case, assume that θ is priorly independent of $(\boldsymbol{\omega}_0, \boldsymbol{\omega}_1)$, having a prior p.d.f. $\pi(\theta)$. It is often reasonable to use the p.d.f. (9.1.5) for $\pi(\theta)$. We continue the exposition with this prior p.d.f. of θ.

According to this setup, the posterior probability of $\{\theta \le n\}$ given $\mathcal{F}_n = \sigma(X_1, X_2, \ldots, X_n)$ is

$$\pi_n(\mathbf{X}_n) = 1 - \frac{(1-p)^n f_H^{(n)}(\mathbf{X}_n)}{D_H^{(n)}(\mathbf{X}_n)}, \tag{9.2.1}$$

where

$$D_H^{(n)}(\mathbf{X}_n) = \frac{\pi}{1-\pi} f_H^{(0)}(\mathbf{X}_n) + p\sum_{j=0}^{n-1}(1-p)^j f_H^{(j)}(\mathbf{X}_n) + (1-p)^n f_H^{(n)}(\mathbf{X}_n) \tag{9.2.2}$$

and where $f_H^{(j)}(\mathbf{x}_n)$, $j = 0, \ldots, n$, are the predictive densities

$$f_H^{(j)}(\mathbf{x}_n) = \int \prod_{i=1}^{j} f(x_i; \boldsymbol{\omega}_0) \prod_{i=j+1}^{n} f(x_i; \boldsymbol{\omega}_1)\, dH(\boldsymbol{\omega}_0, \boldsymbol{\omega}_1). \tag{9.2.3}$$

We understand in (9.2.3) that $\prod_{i=1}^{0} f(x_i; \boldsymbol{\omega}_0) \equiv 1$ and $\prod_{i=n+1}^{n} f(x_i; \boldsymbol{\omega}_1) \equiv 1$. In general, there is no recursive formula for the determination of the predictive densities. For this reason, the sequence $\{\pi_n(\mathbf{X}_n); n \ge 1\}$ is *not* necessarily Markovian. The sequence $\{\pi_n(\mathbf{X}_n), \mathcal{F}_n; n \ge 1\}$ is, however, a *submartingale*. Indeed,

(9.2.4)

$$\begin{aligned} E\{\pi_{n+1}(\mathbf{X}_n, X_{n+1}) \mid \mathcal{F}_n\} \\ &= E\{E\{I\{\tau \le n+1\} \mid \mathcal{F}_{n+1}\} \mid \mathcal{F}_n\} \\ &= E\{E\{I\{\tau \le n\} \mid \mathcal{F}_{n+1}\} \mid \mathcal{F}_n\} + E\{E\{I\{\tau = n+1\} \mid \mathcal{F}_{n+1}\} \mid \mathcal{F}_n\} \\ &= \pi_n(\mathbf{X}_n) + p(1 - \pi_n(\mathbf{X}_n)). \end{aligned}$$

Moreover,

$$E\{\pi_{n+1}(\mathbf{X}_{n+1})\} = (1-p)E\{\pi_n \mathbf{X}_n)\} + p. \tag{9.2.5}$$

Thus, $E\{\pi_{n+1}(\mathbf{X}_{n+1})\} \ge E\{\pi_n(\mathbf{X}_n)\}$ for all $n \ge 1$. From (9.2.1) we obtain that, if the predictive density $f_H^{(n)}(\mathbf{x}_n)$ is uniformly bounded, then

$$\pi_n(\mathbf{X}_n) \to 1 \text{ a.s. as } n \to \infty. \tag{9.2.6}$$

9.2.2 Optimal Stopping Rules

Due to the loss of the Markovian structure, the rule of stopping as soon as $\pi_n(\mathbf{X}_n)$ exceeds a threshold π^* is not necessarily optimal. As before, we assume that the penalty for stopping before the change point is one loss unit and the penalty for delayed stopping after the change point is c loss units per observation. Consider first a truncated stopping rule which must stop after n_0 observations if it has not stopped before. Let $R_n^{(j)}(\mathbf{X}_n)$ denote the minimal posterior risk after n observations when at most j more observations are allowed. Obviously,

$$R_n^{(0)}(\mathbf{X}_n) = 1 - \pi_n(\mathbf{X}_n). \tag{9.2.7}$$

If $j = 1$ and we decide to take that observation, the anticipated risk is

$$\bar{R}_n^{(1)}(\mathbf{X}_n) = c\pi_n(\mathbf{X}_n) + 1 - E\{\pi_{n+1}(X_{n+1}) \mid \mathbf{X}_n\}. \tag{9.2.8}$$

Hence,

$$\begin{aligned} R_n^{(1)}(\mathbf{X}_n) &= \min\{R_n^{(0)}(\mathbf{X}_n), \bar{R}_n^{(1)}(\mathbf{X}_n)\} \\ &= 1 - \pi_n(\mathbf{X}_n) + \min\{0, c\pi_n(\mathbf{X}_n) - p(1 - \pi_n(\mathbf{X}_n))\}. \end{aligned} \tag{9.2.9}$$

Let

$$\pi^* = \frac{p}{c+p}. \tag{9.2.10}$$

It is optimal to stop, when $j = 1$, if $\pi_n(\mathbf{X}_n) \geq \pi^*$.

Define recursively, for $i = 1, 2, \ldots$,

$$\begin{aligned} M_n^{(i)}(\mathbf{X}_n) = E\{&\min\{0, c\pi_{n+1}(\mathbf{X}_{n+1}) - p(1 - \pi_{n+1}(\mathbf{X}_{n+1})) \\ &+ M_{n+1}^{(i-1)}(\mathbf{X}_{n+1})\} \mid \mathbf{X}_n\}, \end{aligned} \tag{9.2.11}$$

where $M_n^{(0)}(\mathbf{X}_n) \equiv 0$ for all n. Applying the backward induction principle of dynamic programming, we obtain, for $j = 1, 2, \ldots$,

$$\begin{aligned} R_n^{(j)}(\mathbf{X}_n) = 1 - \pi_n(\mathbf{X}_n) + \min\{&0, c\pi_n(\mathbf{X}_n) - p(1 - \pi_n(\mathbf{X}_n)) \\ &+ M_n^{(j-1)}(\mathbf{X}_n)\}. \end{aligned} \tag{9.2.12}$$

Define the sequence

$$b_n^{(j)}(\mathbf{X}_n) = \min\left\{\pi^* - \frac{M_n^{(j-1)}(\mathbf{X}_n)}{c+p}, 1\right\}, \quad j \geq 1. \tag{9.2.13}$$

According to (9.2.11),

$$b_n^{(j)}(\mathbf{X}_n) \geq b_n^{(j-1)}(\mathbf{X}_n) \geq \pi^* \ \text{ a.s.}, \quad j = 1, 2, \ldots .$$

Moreover, it is optimal to stop after n observations when only j additional observations are allowed if $\pi_n(\mathbf{X}_n) \geq b_n^{(j)}(\mathbf{X}_n)$. One can prove by induction (see Zacks and Barzily, 1981; Brown and Zacks, 2006) that

$$M_n^{(i)}(\mathbf{X}_n) \leq M_n^{(i-1)}(\mathbf{X}_n) \text{ a.s.,} \quad \text{all } i = 1, 2, \ldots . \tag{9.2.14}$$

It follows that, with probability 1, for each $n \geq 1$,

$$b_n^{(j)}(\mathbf{X}_n) \geq b_n^{(j-1)}(\mathbf{X}_n), \quad j = 1, 2, \ldots . \tag{9.2.15}$$

Hence $\lim_{j\to\infty} b_n^{(j)}(\mathbf{X}_n) \equiv b_n^{(\infty)}(\mathbf{X}_n) \leq 1$. The optimal untruncated stopping rule is: *stop after N observations, where N is the least positive integer n such that $\pi_n(\mathbf{X}_n) \geq b_n^{(\infty)}(\mathbf{X}_n)$.* It is generally difficult to determine the optimal stopping boundaries $b_n^{(\infty)}(\mathbf{X}_n)$ for $n \geq 1$.

9.2.3 Detecting a Change in the Success Probabilities of Binomial Trials: An Example

Zacks and Barzily (1981) considered the problem of detecting a change in the success probability in a sequence of binomial trials. Thus, let $J_n = 0, 1$ and let $\omega_n = P\{J_n = 1\}$. We assume that $J_1, J_2, \ldots$ are *conditionally* independent. Let $\tau = 0, 1, \ldots$ be the index of the random change point. The model is

$$\omega_n = \begin{cases} \omega_0 & \text{if } n < \tau, \\ \omega_1 & \text{if } n \geq \tau. \end{cases} \tag{9.2.16}$$

Both success probabilities (ω_0, ω_1) are unknown. It is assumed that $\omega_0 < \omega_1$. Thus, we consider a uniform prior p.d.f. on the simplex $\Omega^* = \{(\omega_0, \omega_1) : \omega_0 \leq \omega_1\}$ and the prior probability (9.1.3) for θ. Let $T_j = \sum_{i=1}^{j} J_j$ $(j = 1, 2, \ldots)$ and $T_j^{(n)} = \sum_{i=j+1}^{n} J_j = T_n - T_j$. In the present case, from formula (9.2.2) we obtain the expression

$$\begin{aligned} D_H^{(n)}(\mathbf{X}_n) = {} & \left(\frac{\pi}{1-\pi} + p\right) B(T_n + 2, n - T_n + 1) \\ & + p \sum_{j=1}^{n-1} (1-p)^j B(T_{n-j}^{(n)} + 1, n - j - T_{n-j}^{(n)} + 1) \\ & \cdot \sum_{i=0}^{T_{n-j}^{(n)}} \binom{n-j-1}{i} B(T_j + i + 1, n - T_j - i + 2) \\ & + (1-p)^n B(T_n + 1, n - T_n + 2), \end{aligned} \tag{9.2.17}$$

and

$$\pi_n(\mathbf{X}_n) = 1 - \frac{(1-p)^n B(T_n + 1, n - T_n + 2)}{D_H^{(n)}(\mathbf{X}_n)}. \tag{9.2.18}$$

Here $B(\nu_1, \nu_2) = \int_0^1 u^{\nu_1 - 1}(1-u)^{\nu_2 - 1}\, du$ is the beta function.

Zacks and Barzily considered a two-step-ahead suboptimal policy. For that purpose one should derive the boundary $b_n^{(2)}(\mathbf{X}_n)$. The following two results are proven:

1. $\pi_{n+1}(\mathbf{X}_n, 1) > \pi_n(\mathbf{X}_n)$ a.s. for all $n = 1, 2, \ldots$.

2. For all $\mathbf{X}_n$ such that $\pi_n(\mathbf{X}_n) \geq \pi^*$,

(9.2.19)

$$M_n^{(1)}(\mathbf{X}_n) = \left[c\frac{D_H^{(n+1)}(\mathbf{X}_n, 0)}{D_H^{(n)}(\mathbf{X}_n)} - (c+p)(1-p)\bar{\pi}_n(\mathbf{X}_n)\frac{n+2-T_n}{n+3} \right]^-,$$

where $a^- = \min(a, 0)$ and $\bar{\pi}_n(\mathbf{X}_n) = 1 - \pi_n(\mathbf{X}_n)$.

Substituting (9.2.19) in (9.2.13) and specifying $j = 2$, we obtain the function

(9.2.20)

$$B_n(\mathbf{X}_n) = \min\left\{ \pi^* - \left[c\frac{D_H^{(n+1)}(\mathbf{X}_n, 0)}{D_H^{(n)}(\mathbf{X}_n)} \right.\right.$$
$$\left.\left. -(c+p)(1-p)\bar{\pi}_n(\mathbf{X}_n)\frac{n+2-T_n}{n+3} \right]^- \Big/ (c+p), 1 \right\}.$$

Since $\bar{\pi}_n(\mathbf{X}_n) \to 0$ a.s. as $n \to \infty$, the boundary function $B_n(\mathbf{X}_n) \to \pi^*$ as $n \to \infty$. Notice that, for all $\mathbf{X}_n$ such that $\pi(\mathbf{X}_n) \geq \pi^*$, $B_n(\mathbf{X}_n) = b_n^{(2)}(\mathbf{X}_n)$.

In Table 9.2 we present the functions $\pi_n(\mathbf{X}_n)$ and $B_n(\mathbf{X}_n)$ for $\pi = 0.01$, $p = 0.01$, $c = 0.06$. The values of $\mathbf{X}_n$ have been simulated with $\omega_0 = 0.3$, $\omega_1 = 0.7$, and the shift at $\tau = 11$. In the present example $\pi^* = 0.14286$. We see in Table 9.2 that, in run A, $\pi_{14}(\mathbf{X}_{14}) > \pi^*$ but $\pi_{14}(\mathbf{X}_{14}) < B_{14}(\mathbf{X}_{14})$. If we consider the stopping variable

(9.2.21) $$N^* = \text{ least } n \geq 1 \text{ such that } \pi_n(\mathbf{X}_n) \geq B_n(\mathbf{X}_n),$$

then, in run A, $N^* = 18$. The optimal stopping time is $N_{\text{opt}} \geq N^*$ a.s. due to the monotonicity in j of the $b_n^{(j)}(\mathbf{X}_n)$ sequence. Thus, run A illustrates that the stopping rule which stops as soon as $\pi_n(\mathbf{X}_n) \geq \pi^*$ is not optimal.

Table 9.2: Posterior Probabilities and the $B_n(X_n)$ Function for Three Simulation Runs

	Run A			Run B			Run C		
n	T_n	$\pi_n(x_n)$	$B_n(x_n)$	T_n	$\pi_n(x_n)$	$B_n(x_n)$	T_n	$\pi_n(x_n)$	$B_n(x_n)$
2	1	0.01502	0.41039	0	0.00838	0.44057	0	0.00838	0.44057
3	2	0.03919	0.35260	0	0.01091	0.40993	0	0.01091	0.40993
4	2	0.02829	0.34243	0	0.01294	0.38782	1	0.05828	0.34610
5	3	0.05461	0.30473	0	0.01464	0.37105	2	0.13568	0.28698
6	4	0.08681	0.27341	0	0.01612	0.35787	2	0.07454	0.29882
7	4	0.05783	0.27754	0	0.01741	0.34721	3	0.13648	0.25537
8	4	0.04712	0.27790	0	0.01857	0.33839	3	0.09103	0.26649
9	5	0.07394	0.25505	1	0.10809	0.27296	3	0.07097	0.27084
10	5	0.05786	0.25820	1	0.06716	0.28453	3	0.06009	0.27247
11	5	0.05054	0.25939	2	0.18662	0.21179	3	0.05349	0.27283
12	6	0.07775	0.24003	3	0.38013	0.14286	4	0.09568	0.24351
13	7	0.11325	0.22092	3	0.24004	0.16652	4	0.07539	0.24913
14	8	0.15840	0.20194	4	0.40718	0.14286	5	0.12311	0.22068
15	9	0.17397	0.18322	5	0.58537	0.14286	5	0.09587	0.22919
16	9	0.13504	0.19864	6	0.73529	0.14286	6	0.14641	0.20182
17	10	0.17519	0.18267	7	0.84040	0.14286	6	0.11501	0.21205
18	11	0.22231	0.16691	8	0.90617	0.14286	7	0.16692	0.18577
19	12	0.27619	0.15158	8	0.80757	0.14286	8	0.23587	0.15732
20	12	0.19094	0.16777	9	0.87581	0.14286	9	0.32355	0.14286
21	13	0.23261	0.15415	10	0.92056	0.14286	10	0.42758	0.14286
22	14	0.27920	0.14286	11	0.94911	0.14286	11	0.29560	0.14286
23	14	0.20873	0.15506	12	0.96716	0.14286	11	0.37500	0.14286
24	14	0.17030	0.15506	12	0.96716	0.14286	11	0.37500	0.14286
25	15	0.20286	0.15346	14	0.98586	0.14286	12	0.35599	0.14286
26	16	0.23967	0.14286	14	0.96855	0.14286	12	0.28599	0.14286
27	17	0.28088	0.14286	14	0.94183	0.14286	13	0.34813	0.14286
28	18	0.32644	0.14286	15	0.95861	0.14286	14	0.41691	0.14286
29	19	0.37604	0.14286	15	0.93062	0.14286	15	0.49041	0.14286

9.3 CUSUM PROCEDURES FOR SEQUENTIAL DETECTION

9.3.1 Structure of CUSUM Procedures

As before, we consider a sequence of (conditionally) independent r.v.'s $X_1, X_2, \ldots$. We assume that r.v.'s $X_1, \ldots, X_{k-1}$ have the same distribution F_0 and r.v.'s $X_k, X_{k+1}, \ldots$ have the distribution F_1, where $F_0 \not\equiv F_1$; that is, k is a change point. The objective is to detect the change point soon after it occurs with a small number of false alarms. This objective will be formulated rigorously in the next section. Page (1954, 1955, 1957) proposed the so-called cumulative sums (CUSUM) procedure for this problem of detection.

The CUSUM procedure can be considered as a sequence of repeated tests about the change point k. Indeed, if $f_0(x)$ and $f_1(x)$ are the density functions corresponding to F_0 and F_1 with respect to some σ-finite measure μ and if

$$f_{k,n}(\mathbf{x}_n) = \prod_{i=1}^{k-1} f_0(x_i) \prod_{j=k}^{n} f_1(x_j), \quad k = 1, \ldots, n,$$

where $\prod_{i=1}^{0} f_0(x_i) \equiv 1$ and $\mathbf{x}_n = (x_1, \ldots, x_n)$, then one can consider a stopping rule

$$N = \inf\left\{n : n \geq 1, \frac{f_{k,n}(\mathbf{x})}{f_{0,n}(\mathbf{x})} \geq A_k \text{ for some } k = 1, \ldots, n\right\}, \tag{9.3.1}$$

where $f_{0,n}(\mathbf{x}_n) = \prod_{i=1}^{n} f_0(x_i)$ and where $\{A_k\}$ is a properly defined sequence of positive constants. The above stopping rule is equivalent to the stopping rule

$$\begin{aligned} N &= \inf\left\{n \geq 1;\ \max_{1 \leq k \leq n} \sum_{i=k}^{n} \log R(X_i) \geq h\right\} \\ &= \inf\left\{n \geq 1;\ S_n - \min_{0 \leq k \leq n} S_k \geq h\right\}, \end{aligned} \tag{9.3.2}$$

where $S_i = \sum_{j=1}^{i} \log R(X_j)$, $i = 1, 2, \ldots$, and $S_0 \equiv 0$. Properties of this stopping rule were studied in many papers. In the following section we discuss the asymptotic minimaxity of the CUSUM stopping rule.

9.3.2 Asymptotic Minimaxity of CUSUM Procedures

Let $P_k(\mathbf{x}_n)$ be the joint distribution of $\mathbf{X}_n$ when the point of change is at k, $k \geq 1$. Here $P_0(\mathbf{X}_n)$ will denote the joint distribution where all the observations have the c.d.f. $F_0(x)$. We denote by $\mathcal{F}_n$, $n \geq 1$, the σ-field generated by $\mathbf{X}_n$. Lorden (1971) introduced the objective to determine a stopping rule, N, for which

$$\bar{E}_1\{N\} = \sup_{k \geq 1} \text{ esssup } E_k\{(N - k + 1)^+ \mid \mathcal{F}_{k-1}\} \tag{9.3.3}$$

is minimized subject to the constraint

$$E_0\{N\} \geq \gamma^*, \quad 1 < \gamma^* < \infty. \tag{9.3.4}$$

Notice that $E_k\{(N - k + 1)^+ \mid \mathcal{F}_{k-1}\}$ is a random variable, depending on the realizations of $(X_1, \ldots, X_{k-1})$. The symbol essup (essential supremum) denotes the supremum over almost all possible realizations.

Let $T_n = S_n - \min_{0 \leq k \leq n}\{S_i\}$. Notice that T_n can be computed recursively by the formula

$$T_{n+1} = (T_n + \log\ R(X_{n+1}))^+, \quad n = 0, 1, \ldots,$$

where $T_0 \equiv 0$.

Let N^* be the stopping rule which stops as soon as $T_n \geq \gamma$, where $\gamma = \log \gamma^*$. This detection procedure can be considered as a sequence of one-sided Wald SPRTs (see Chapter 10) with boundaries $(0, \gamma)$. Whenever the T_n statistic hits the lower boundary, 0, the SPRT is recycled and all the previous observations can be discarded. On the other hand, for the first time, $T_n \geq \gamma$, the sampling process is stopped. The repeated cycles are *independent* and identically distributed (renewal cycles). Thus, Wald's theory of SPRT can be used to obtain the main results of the present theory.

Let α and β be the error probabilities in each such independent cycle of the Wald SPRT; that is, $\alpha = P_0[T_n \geq \gamma]$ and $\beta = P_1[T_n = 0]$. Let N_1 be the length of a cycle. Then,

$$
\begin{aligned}
E_0\{N^*\} &= \frac{1}{\alpha} E_0\{N_1\}, \\
E_1\{N^*\} &= \frac{1}{1-\beta} E_1\{N_1\}.
\end{aligned}
\tag{9.3.5}
$$

Let $\gamma^* = 1/\alpha$. Then (9.3.5) implies that $E_0\{N^*\} \geq \gamma^*$. Thus, N^* satisfies the constraint (9.3.4). We show now that $\bar{E}_1\{N^*\} = E_1\{N^*\}$. We follow the proof of Lorden (1971). Obviously, $\bar{E}_1\{N^*\} \geq E_1\{N^*\}$.

Let $t_1, t_2, \ldots$ denote the recurrence points of $\{T_n = 0\}$. We assumed that $T_0 \equiv 0$ and set $t_0 \equiv 0$. Let N_k^*, $k = 1, 2, \ldots$, denote the stopping rule (9.3.2) applied to $X_{t_k+1}, X_{t_k+2}, \ldots$. The event $\{T_{t_k} = 0\} \in \mathcal{F}_{t_k}$, and the tail sequence $X_{t_k+1}, X_{t_k+2}, \ldots$ is independent of $\mathcal{F}_{t_k}$. The stopping rule N^* can be written as

$$
N^* = \min_{k \geq 1}\{N_k^* + t_k\}. \tag{9.3.6}
$$

Furthermore, since, at t_k, $T_{t_k} = 0$ and the process has not been stopped before,

$$
\bar{E}_1\{N^*\} = \sup_{k \geq 1} \ \text{esssup} \ E_{t_k}\{N^* - t_k \mid \mathcal{F}_{t_k}\}. \tag{9.3.7}
$$

But, for every $k = 1, 2, \ldots$, since N_k^* is independent of $\mathcal{F}_{t_k}$,

$$
E_{t_k}\{N^* - t_k \mid \mathcal{F}_{t_k}\} \leq E_{t_k}\{N_k^* \mid \mathcal{F}_{t_k}\} = E_1\{N^*\}. \tag{9.3.8}
$$

From (9.3.7) and (9.3.8) we obtain that $\bar{E}_1\{N^*\} \leq E_1\{N^*\}$. This proves the equality.

Applying the well-known results about the expected sample size in Wald's SPRT [see Eq. (10.1.21)], we obtain that

$$
E_1\{N^*\} \sim \frac{|\log \alpha|}{I_1} \quad \text{as } \alpha \to 0, \tag{9.3.9}
$$

where I_1 is the Kullback–Leibler information number for discriminating between $F_0(x)$ and $F_1(x)$, under F_1, that is,

$$I_1 = \int \left(\log \frac{f_1(x)}{f_0(x)} \right) f_1(x)\, d\mu(x). \tag{9.3.10}$$

On the other hand, it is proven by Lorden (1971, Theorem 3) that the right-hand side of (9.3.9) is asymptotically the minimum expected sample size. This shows that Page's CUSUM stopping variable, N^*, is asymptotically minimax.

Pollak (1985) studied the same detection problem and presented a stopping rule N_A^* which satisfies the constraint (9.3.4) and to within a negligible term (as $\gamma^* \to \infty$) minimizes $\sup_{1 \leq k < \infty} E_k\{N - k \mid N \geq k\}$. The stopping rule N_A^* is based on the statistic

$$T_n = \sum_{j=0}^{n-1} \prod_{i=j+1}^{n} R(X_i), \quad n = 1, 2, \ldots, \tag{9.3.11}$$

which can be obtained from expression (9.1.8) of the posterior probability π_n by substituting $\pi = 0$ and letting $p \to 0$. Let N_A^* is the first integer $n \geq 1$ for which $T_n \geq A$. This application of the CUSUM procedure is based on the assumption that the distributions $F_i(x)$ $(i = 0, 1)$ are known. The procedure based on (9.3.11) is also called the *Shiryaev–Roberts procedure.* See Kenett and Zacks (1998, p. 389) for a discussion of the merits of the Shiryaev–Roberts procedure in small samples. For recent results on asymptotic optimality of change-point detection schemes see the prize winning paper of Baron and Tartakovsky (2006).

9.3.3 Exact Distribution of Stopping Variables in CUSUM Procedures

In the present section we present a method of computing the distribution of the stopping variable, N, associated with a CUSUM procedure. We will consider a nonnegative discrete r.v. X having a one-parameter distribution belonging to the exponential family with p.d.f.

$$p(x; \theta) = h(x) \exp\{\theta x + \psi(\theta)\}, \tag{9.3.12}$$

where $\psi(\theta)$ is strictly increasing. Suppose that F_0 and F_1 correspond to these distributions with parameters θ_0, θ_1; $-\infty < \theta_0 < \theta_1 < \infty$. Then, $\log R(X) = (\theta_1 - \theta_0)X + \psi(\theta_1) - \psi(\theta_0)$. Therefore, without loss of generality, we will consider the CUSUM stopping variable

$$N(b_0, b_1) = \inf\{n; n \geq 1, W_n \geq b_0\}, \tag{9.3.13}$$

where

$$W_n = \max_{0 \leq j \leq n-1} \sum_{i=j+1}^{n} Y_i, \quad Y_i = X_i - b_1,$$

and where b_0 and b_1 are positive integers.

Obviously,

(9.3.14)

$$W_{n+1} = \max\left\{\sum_{i=1}^{n} Y_i + Y_{n+1}, \sum_{i=2}^{n} Y_i + Y_{n+1}, \ldots \sum_{i=n}^{n} Y_i + Y_{n+1}, Y_{n+1}\right\}$$
$$= Y_{n+1} + \max\{0, W_n\}, \quad n \geq 0,$$

where $W_0 \equiv 0$. Notice that, since $X_1, X_2, \ldots$ is a sequence of independent r.v.'s, Y_{n+1} is independent of W_n for every $n \geq 0$.

In the following derivations we will denote by $f_i(x)$ and $F_i(x)$ the p.d.f. and c.d.f. of X_i. If the change point is at τ, then

$$f_i(x) = \begin{cases} f_0(x) & \text{if } i \leq \tau - 1, \\ f_1(x) & \text{if } i \geq \tau. \end{cases} \tag{9.3.15}$$

Let $K_n(x)$ designate the defective c.d.f. of W_n under the condition that $N \geq n$. For simplicity of notation, we use N for the stopping variable $N(b_0, b_1)$. Thus,

$$K_n(x) = P\{W_n \leq x, N \geq n\}, \quad n \geq 1. \tag{9.3.16}$$

Since $P\{N \geq 1\} = 1$, $K_1(x) = F_1(x + b_1)$. Let $k_n(x) = K_n(x) - K_n(x-1)$, $x = -b_1, -b_1 + 1, \ldots$. From (9.3.14) and (9.3.16) we obtain

$$\begin{aligned} K_n(x) &= \sum_{j=-b_1}^{b_0-1} P\{Y_n + W_{n-1}^{+} \leq x, W_{n-1} = j, N \geq n-1\} \\ &= \sum_{j=-b_1}^{b_0-1} P\{Y_n + W_{n-1}^{+} \leq x \mid W_{n-1} = j, N \geq n-1\} k_{n-1}(j). \end{aligned} \tag{9.3.17}$$

Moreover, since Y_n is independent of W_{n-1},

(9.3.18)

$$P\{Y_n + W_{n-1}^{+} \leq x \mid W_{n-1} = j, N \geq n-1\} = \begin{cases} F_n(x + b_1) & \text{if } j \leq 0, \\ F_n(x + b_1 - j) & \text{if } j > 0. \end{cases}$$

Therefore, for every $n \geq 2$,

$$K_n(x) = F_n(x + b_1) K_{n-1}(0) + \sum_{j=1}^{b_0-1} F_n(x + b_1 - j) k_{n-1}(j). \tag{9.3.19}$$

The corresponding p.d.f. is

$$k_n(x) = f_n(x + b_1) K_{n-1}(0) + \sum_{j=1}^{b_0-1} f_n(x + b_1 - j) k_{n-1}(j). \tag{9.3.20}$$

Having determined the functions $k_n(x)$ and $K_n(x)$ recursively, one can determine

$$P\{N > n\} = K_n(b_0 - 1). \tag{9.3.21}$$

From (9.3.19) and (9.3.21) we deduce the inequality

$$P\{N > n\} \le F_n(b_0 + b_1 - 1)P\{N > n - 1\}, \quad n \ge 1. \tag{9.3.22}$$

Thus, if $F_n(b_0 + b_1 - 1) \le \rho < 1$ for all $n \ge 1$, $P\{N > n\} \le \rho^{n-1}$. This implies that all moments of N exist. According to (9.3.19) one can evaluate the functions $K_n(j)$ only for $j \in \{0, 1, \ldots, b_0 - 1\}$. This can be done in the following manner. Let $\Psi^{(n)}$ be a $b_0 \times b_0$ matrix whose elements are

$$\Psi_{ij}^{(n)} = \begin{cases} f_n(b_1 + i - j), & j = 1, \ldots, b_0 - 1, \\ F_n(b_1 - b_0 + i), & j = b_0. \end{cases} \tag{9.3.23}$$

Let $\mathbf{K}_n = (K_n(0), \ldots, K_n(b_0 - 1))'$. Then,

$$\mathbf{K}_n = \Psi^{(n)}\mathbf{K}_{n-1} = \left(\prod_{j=2}^{n} \Psi^{(j)}\right)\mathbf{K}_1, \quad n \ge 2, \tag{9.3.24}$$

where

$$\mathbf{K}_1 = (F_1(b_1), \ldots, F_1(b_1 + b_0 - 1))'.$$

Let Ψ_ν $(\nu = 0, 1)$ denote the $b_0 \times b_0$ matrices whose elements are

$$\psi_{ij,\nu} = \begin{cases} f_\nu(b_1 + i - j), & j = 1, \ldots, b_0 - 1, \\ F_\nu(b_1 - b_0 + i), & j = b_0. \end{cases} \tag{9.3.25}$$

Then, if the change point is at k, $k \ge 1$, we obtain from (9.3.24) that

$$\mathbf{K}_n = \begin{cases} \Psi_0^n \mathbf{K}_1 & \text{if } n \le k - 1, \\ \Psi_1^{n-k+1}\Psi_0^{k-1}\mathbf{K}_1 & \text{if } n \ge k, \end{cases} \tag{9.3.26}$$

where $\mathbf{K}_1 = (F_0(b_1), \ldots, F_0(b_1 + b_0 - 1))'$. The vectors $\mathbf{K}_n$ $(n \ge 1)$ can be determined numerically by matrix multiplications. Explicit formulas can be derived by using the theory of Markov chains. For example, if $b_0 = 2$, then, if $n < k$, we obtain

$$P\{N > n\} = f_0^n(b_1) \sum_{i=0}^{n} \binom{n}{i} R^i(\lambda_1^{(i+1)} F_0(b_1) + F_0(b_1 + 1)), \tag{9.3.27}$$

where $R = F_0(b_1 - 1)/F_0(b_1)$ and

$$\begin{aligned} &\lambda_1^{(1)} = 0, \quad \lambda_2^{(1)} = 1, \\ &\lambda_1^{(i)} = \frac{Q}{R}\lambda_2^{(i-1)}, \quad \lambda_2^{(i)} = \lambda_1^{(i-1)} + \lambda_2^{(i-1)}, \quad i \ge 2, \end{aligned} \tag{9.3.28}$$

and $Q = f_0(b_1+1)/f_0(b_1)$.

The *average run length* (ARL) of a CUSUM procedure is defined in the literature as the expected stopping time when all the r.v.'s have the same distribution, P_0 or P_1. Notice that

$$E\{N\} = \sum_{n=1}^{\infty} P\{N \geq n\} = 1 + \sum_{n=1}^{\infty} P\{N > n\} = 1 + \sum_{n=1}^{\infty} K_n(b_0 - 1).$$

Thus, in order to find the ARL under P_ν ($\nu = 0, 1$) define for each $j = 0, \ldots, b_0 - 1$, $G_\nu(j) = \sum_{n=1}^{\infty} K_n^{(\nu)}(j)$, where $K_n^{(\nu)}(j)$ is computed according to the previous formula with the matrix Ψ_ν. Applying the recursive relationship (9.3.19), it is straightforward to obtain the equation

$$\begin{aligned} G_\nu(j) &= F_\nu(b_1 + j) + \sum_{i=0}^{b_0-2} G(i) p_\nu(b_1 + j - i) \\ &\quad + G(b_0 - 1) F_\nu(b_1 - b_0 + j + 1), \quad j = 0, \ldots, b_0 - 1. \end{aligned} \tag{9.3.29}$$

Thus, let $\mathbf{G}_\nu = (G_\nu(0), \ldots, G_\nu(b_0 - 1))'$. Then the vector $\mathbf{G}_\nu$ is given by

$$\mathbf{G}_\nu = (I - \Psi_\nu)^{-1} \mathbf{P}_\nu, \quad \nu = 0, 1, \tag{9.3.30}$$

where $\mathbf{F}_\nu = (F_\nu(b_1), \ldots, F_\nu(b_1 + b_0 - 1))'$. Finally,

$$E_\nu\{N\} = 1 + G_\nu(b_0 - 1). \tag{9.3.31}$$

Returning to the previous example of $b_0 = 2$, we obtain from (9.3.30) and (9.3.31) that the ARL under P_0 is

$$E_0\{N(2, b_1)\} = 1 + \frac{(1 - f(b_1))F_0(b_1 + 1) + f_0(b_1 + 1)F_0(b_1)}{(1 - f_0(b_1))(1 - F_0(b_1) - f_0(b_1 + 1))F_0(b_1 + 1)}. \tag{9.3.32}$$

In Table 9.3 we present the probability distribution function for Poisson distributions with $\lambda_0 = 4$, $\lambda_1 = 9$, and a change point at $k = 10$. The CUSUM procedure is defined with $b_0 = 2$ and $b_1 = 8$.

We see in Table 9.3 that the probability of detecting the change right at $n = 10$, with the $N(2, 8)$ stopping variable, is 0.38 and the probability that we need more than five observations after the change is only 0.03. The probability of false alarm (PFA) is 0.07. The expected value of $N(2, 8)$ when a change from $\lambda_0 = 4$ to $\lambda_1 = 9$ occurs at $k = 10$ is approximately 10.83. The ARL under F_0 is, on the other hand, $E_0\{N(2, 8)\} = 120.3$, with a median of $N_{0.5}(2, 8) = 84$. The value of the ARL was computed using formula (9.3.32). The computation of the median requires the computation of $K_n^{(0)}(b_0 - 1)$ for $n \geq 1$. Indeed, a p-quantile of $N(b_0, b_1)$ according to F_ν is

$$N_p^{(\nu)}(b_0, b_1) = \text{ least } n \geq 1 \text{ such that } K_n^{(\nu)}(b_0 - 1) \geq (1 - p). \tag{9.3.33}$$

For comparison of the efficiency of different CUSUM procedures, one has to compute $E_0\{N(b_0, b_1)\}$, but the value of ARL under P_1 is of no value unless we know that $W_n^+ = 0$ at the point of change. What we need to compute for comparing procedures having a similar $E_0\{N(b_0, b_1)\}$ is the function $E_k\{N(b_0, b_1); \delta\}$, which is the expected stopping time when a change of size δ occurs at $n = k$.

Table 9.3: Distribution of $\mathbf{N(2,8)}$ in the Poisson Case, $\lambda_0 = 4$, $\lambda_1 = 9$, $k = 10$

n	$P\{N = n\}$	$P\{N > n\}$	$\sum_{j=1}^{n} P\{N \geq j\}$
1	0.00813	0.99187	1.99
2	0.00824	0.98362	2.98
3	0.00818	0.97545	3.95
4	0.00811	0.96734	4.92
5	0.00804	0.95930	5.88
6	0.00797	0.95132	6.83
7	0.00791	0.94343	7.77
8	0.00784	0.93557	8.71
9	0.00778	0.92780	9.64
10	0.38446	0.54334	10.18
11	0.24028	0.30305	10.48
12	0.13447	0.16858	10.65
13	0.07482	0.09377	10.74
14	0.04161	0.05215	10.80
15	0.02315	0.02901	10.83

Several authors have used Markov chain techniques to determine the distribution of the run length N of a CUSUM procedure. See Yashchin (1985) for a comprehensive treatment of the run length distribution of two-sided CUSUM procedures and for additional references. R.A. Khan (1978, 1979, 1984) applied the Wald approximations in SPRT to find approximate formulas for the ARL. He also provided asymptotic approximations when $b_1 \to \infty$. Pollak (1987) studied the asymptotic behavior of N_A^* when $A \to \infty$ for a one-parameter exponential family. He proved, under the condition $I_1 < \infty$, that $E_0\{N_A^*\} = O(A)$ as $A \to \infty$.

Zacks (2004a) derived the exact distribution of the run length of a one-sided CUSUM procedure applied on a Poisson process. Vardeman and Ray (1985) derived formulas for the ARL of a one-sided CUSUM when the observations are exponentially distributed. The values of the ARL in the two papers are the same. Zacks, however, derived the actual distribution of the run length and gave explicit formulas for the moments. See also Woodall (1983) and Tartakovsky (1995), who studied the asymptotic properties of the CUSUM and Shiryaev's procedures for detecting a change point in a nonhomogeneous Gaussian process.

9.4 TRACKING ALGORITHMS FOR PROCESSES WITH CHANGE POINTS

9.4.1 General Comments

Tracking and estimation of process levels are the second component of SPC. Such estimates are particularly meaningful when there are specification limits to the variable being tracked. For example, if one tracks the noise level of telecommunication equipment on an X-bar–R-chart, the test results can be used for both process control and acceptance testing. If the decision is that the products do not meet the required specifications, some intervention is required to calibrate or rework the product. Both the 3-sigma control chart and the CUSUM procedure provide crude estimates of the process level and of the points of change. Control charts are sometimes combined with acceptance sampling to form acceptance control charts. Exponentially weighted moving average (EWMA) charts have been suggested as providing both detection and estimation capabilities and their use is gaining popularity. (For details on current approaches to SPC see Stephens et al., 1986.) The problem of tracking quality levels at AT&T led to the quality measurement plan (QMP), which dynamically estimates a quality index distribution using empirical Bayes methods (Hoadley, 1981). The QMP mechanism tracks ratios of observed to expected defects and triggers an alert when the 95th quantile of the index posterior distribution is bigger than 1. The QMP Bayesian framework therefore combines estimation with detection.

Chernoff and Zacks (1964) developed a Bayesian tracking method for a simple normal process which is subjected to changes in the mean at unknown time points. Their fundamental work, which was originally motivated by a radar tracking problem, is the basic reference for this study. Zacks (1991a) reviewed sequential detection procedures for change points and also presented a Bayesian tracking algorithm designed to sequentially estimate parameters of the posterior distributions of a Gaussian process mean under a model of at most one change (AMOC). The details of this algorithm are presented in Kenett and Zacks (1990). In the present chapter we expand the AMOC Bayesian tracking algorithm to accommodate for Poisson and binomial data. These new Bayesian tracking procedures provide both estimators of process levels and diagnostics for suspected epochs of change.

There is a large number of articles in the literature on dynamic estimation of the current process level (filtering) and forecasting (see Harrison and Stevens, 1976; West, Harrison, and Migon, 1985; Migon and Harrison, 1983; Smith and West, 1983; Souza, 1981; West, 1981; Gordon and Smith, 1988; Gamerman, 1992). The models in these papers are based on variations of the dynamic linear model (DLM) and recursive estimation. Gordon and Smith (1988) extended the DLM to include changes of different types at the structures of the error covariance matrices of the random input components. Our modeling, which is based on random change points in the level of the processes, is basically different and somewhat simpler.

In Section 9.4.2 we present a basic model of a dynamic adaptive estimation procedure based on repeated application of an AMOC Bayesian model on moving subsequences (windows) of the data. In Section 9.4.3 we discuss in general terms the structure of our procedures and present the adaptive algorithms. Section 9.4.4 presents the formulas for the special but important cases of Poisson, binomial, and normal random variables. In Section 9.4.5 we illustrate the effectiveness of the procedures on actual data. For the Poisson case we use the celebrated data of coal mining disasters in England (see Cox and Lewis, 1966; Jarrett, 1979; Raftery and Akman, 1986; Carlin, Gelfand, and Smith, 1992). For the binomial case we use data on shorts in wave soldering found in successive batches of printed circuits. Finally, for normal data we use sequences of daily movements of the Dow Jones financial index. These sequences demonstrate nonstationary time series with repeated changes of different type. Nevertheless, it will be shown that our relatively simple model provides a procedure which closely tracks the movements of these time series. All the examples illustrate the effectiveness of the proposed tracking algorithm.

9.4.2 Tracking a Process with Change Points

Let $X_1, X_2, X_3, \ldots$ be a sequence of observable independent random variables. The distribution function of X_t is $F(\cdot; \boldsymbol{\theta}_t)$, where $\boldsymbol{\theta}_t$ is some parametric vector which may change with time. Let

$$\mu_t = E_{\theta_t}\{X_t\} = M(\boldsymbol{\theta}_t), \quad t = 1, 2, \ldots . \tag{9.4.1}$$

The problem is to estimate the current position of the process, μ_t, $t = 1, 2, \ldots$. More specifically, given n observations on $X_1, \ldots, X_n$, the problem is to choose an estimator $\hat{\mu}_n(X_1, \ldots, X_n)$ of μ_n having certain desired properties. There are many different estimation schemes in the literature, known as filters. For example, the well-known class of Kalman filters are best linear estimators when the structural relationships are, for $t = 1, 2, \ldots$,

$$\boldsymbol{\theta}_t = A_t \boldsymbol{\theta}_{t-1} + B_t \mathbf{e}_t \tag{9.4.2}$$

and

$$M(\boldsymbol{\theta}_t) = F_t \boldsymbol{\theta}_t, \tag{9.4.3}$$

where A_t, B_t, and F_t are known matrices and $\mathbf{e}_t$ is a vector of random variables having zero means and known covariance matrix V_t. Equations (9.4.2) and

(9.4.3) represent dynamic linear models of change in the parameters of the distribution. In the present section we are concerned with a different class of change models, similar to that considered by Yao (1984a,b).

Let $I_1, I_2, \ldots$ be a sequence of Bernoulli random variables, that is, $I_1, I_2, \ldots$ are independent and identically distributed with

$$
\begin{aligned}
P\{I_t = 1\} &= p, \quad t = 1, 2, \ldots, \\
P\{I_t = 0\} &= 1 - p, \quad t = 1, 2, \ldots,
\end{aligned}
\tag{9.4.4}
$$

where $0 < p < 1$. If $I_t = 1$, we say that there is a change point between the tth and $(t+1)$st observation epochs. Thus, among n consecutive observations we expect np change points. Moreover, the structural change model we consider is

$$
\boldsymbol{\theta}_t = \boldsymbol{\theta}_1 + \sum_{i=1}^{t} I_i \mathbf{Z}_t, \quad t = 1, 2, \ldots, \tag{9.4.5}
$$

where $\mathbf{Z}_1, \mathbf{Z}_2, \ldots$ is a sequence of i.i.d. random vectors with $E\{Z_i\} = \boldsymbol{\delta}$ and covariance matrix $\boldsymbol{\Sigma}(Z_i) = \mathbf{C}$, $i = 1, 2, \ldots$. Assume $\boldsymbol{\theta}_1$ is a random vector having (a prior) distribution $H(\boldsymbol{\theta})$. The change model (9.4.5) is a dynamic nonlinear one.

We will consider problems in which the probability of change, p, between two consecutive epochs is small. Thus, let $\{X_{t-n_w+1}, \ldots, X_t\}$ be a moving window of n_w observations. The size of the window, n_w, is chosen so that $P\{\sum_{l=1}^{n_w} I_{t-n_w+l} > 1\}$ is small a priori. We construct the estimators of μ_t, $t = 1, 2, \ldots$, on the basis of the observations in the moving windows. The dynamic algorithm that will be developed is based on a Bayesian AMOC model. Although the number of possible change points in every moving window of size n_w could be theoretically greater than 1, the AMOC model provides good approximation when p is a priori small.

9.4.3 Recursive Nonlinear Estimation with Moving Windows

9.4.3.1 Bayes AMOC Estimation Let $X_1, X_2, \ldots, X_n$ be a sequence of n independent random variables having probability density (distribution) functions $f(x; \boldsymbol{\theta}_i)$, $i = 1, \ldots, n$. Let $\mu_i = E_{\boldsymbol{\theta}_i}\{X_i\}$, $i = 1, \ldots, n$.

The AMOC model assumes that

(i) $\sum_{i=1}^{n} I_i \le 1$ (at most one change point) with probability 1

and the epoch of change is at

$$
\text{(ii)} \quad \tau_n = \begin{cases} \min\{i : 1 \le i \le n-1, \ \sum_{j=1}^{i} I_j = 1\} & \text{if } \sum_{i=1}^{n-1} I_j = 1, \\ n & \text{if } \sum_{i=1}^{n-1} I_j = 0. \end{cases}
$$

The event $\{\tau_n = i\}$ corresponds to the case that the epoch of change is between the ith and $(i+1)$st observation, $i = 1, \ldots, n-1$. The event $\{\tau_n = n\}$ corresponds to the case that the first change occurred after the n observations. Accordingly, τ_n has the truncated geometric distribution

$$\begin{aligned} P\{\tau_n = i\} &= p(1-p)^{i-1}, \quad i = 1, \cdots, n-1, \\ &= (1-p)^{n-1}, \quad i = n. \end{aligned} \tag{9.4.6}$$

In the Bayesian AMOC model we use Eq. (9.4.6) for the prior distribution of the epoch of change, τ_n. The AMOC model for $\boldsymbol{\theta}_t$, $t = 1, 2, \ldots, n$, is

$$\boldsymbol{\theta}_t = \begin{cases} \boldsymbol{\theta} & \text{if } t \leq \tau_n, \\ \boldsymbol{\phi} & \text{if } t > \tau_n, \end{cases}$$

where $(\boldsymbol{\theta}, \boldsymbol{\phi})$ are random vectors having a prior distribution $H(\boldsymbol{\theta}, \boldsymbol{\phi})$ with joint p.d.f. $h(\boldsymbol{\theta}, \boldsymbol{\phi})$. Notice that in our model τ_n and $(\boldsymbol{\theta}, \boldsymbol{\phi})$ are priorly independent.

The likelihood function of $(\tau_n, \boldsymbol{\theta}, \boldsymbol{\phi})$ given $\mathbf{X}^{(n)} = (X_1, \cdots, X_n)$ is

$$\begin{aligned} L_n(\tau_n, \boldsymbol{\theta}, \boldsymbol{\phi}) = &\sum_{j=1}^{n-1} I\{\tau_n = j\} \prod_{i=1}^{j} f(X_i; \boldsymbol{\theta}) \prod_{i=j+1}^{n} f(X_i; \boldsymbol{\phi}) \\ &+ I\{\tau_n = n\} \prod_{i=1}^{n} f(X_i; \boldsymbol{\theta}). \end{aligned} \tag{9.4.7}$$

From Eq. (9.4.7) and the prior assumptions on the distributions of τ_n and $(\boldsymbol{\theta}, \boldsymbol{\phi})$ one can get the posterior distributions of these variables given n by employing Bayes's formula. Accordingly, the posterior probability of $\{\tau_n = i\}$, $i = 1, \ldots, n$, given $\mathbf{X}_n$, is

$$\pi_n(i \mid \mathbf{X}^{(n)}) = \frac{P\{\tau_n = i\} \int\int L_n(i, \boldsymbol{\theta}, \boldsymbol{\phi}) h(\boldsymbol{\theta}, \boldsymbol{\phi}) \, d\boldsymbol{\theta} \, d\boldsymbol{\phi}}{\sum_{j=1}^{n} P\{\tau_n = j\} \int\int L_n(j, \boldsymbol{\theta}, \boldsymbol{\phi}) h(\boldsymbol{\theta}, \boldsymbol{\phi}) \, d\boldsymbol{\theta} \, d\boldsymbol{\phi}}. \tag{9.4.8}$$

Similarly, the posterior p.d.f. of $\boldsymbol{\theta}_n$ given $\mathbf{X}^{(n)}$ is
(9.4.9)

$$\begin{aligned} h_n(\boldsymbol{\theta}_n \mid \mathbf{X}^{(n)}) = &\sum_{j=1}^{n-1} P\{\tau_n = j\} \int L_n(j, \boldsymbol{\theta}, \boldsymbol{\theta}_n) \cdot h(\boldsymbol{\theta}, \boldsymbol{\theta}_n) d\boldsymbol{\theta} / D_n(\mathbf{X}^{(n)}) \\ &+ P\{\tau_n = n\} \int L_n(n, \boldsymbol{\theta}_n, \boldsymbol{\phi}) h(\boldsymbol{\theta}_n, \boldsymbol{\phi}) d\boldsymbol{\phi} / D_n(\mathbf{X}^{(n)}), \end{aligned}$$

where

$$D_n(\mathbf{X}^{(n)}) = \sum_{i=1}^{n} P\{\tau_n = i\} \int\int L(i, \boldsymbol{\theta}, \boldsymbol{\phi}) h(\boldsymbol{\theta}, \boldsymbol{\phi}) \, d\boldsymbol{\theta} \, d\boldsymbol{\phi}. \tag{9.4.10}$$

By an appropriate transformation method one can derive the posterior distribution of the current location $\mu_n = M(\boldsymbol{\theta}_n)$. Let $g_n(\mu \mid \mathbf{X}^{(n)})$ denote the posterior p.d.f. of this distribution. Let $\hat{\mu}_{n,p} = G_n^{-1}(p \mid \mathbf{X}^{(n)})$ denote the pth quantile of the posterior distribution of μ_n given $\mathbf{X}^{(n)}$. A Bayes estimator of μ_n for the squared error loss is the mean of the posterior distribution, that is,

$$
\begin{aligned}
\hat{\mu}_n(\mathbf{X}^{(n)}) &= E\{\mu_n \mid \mathbf{X}^{(n)}\} \\
&= \int \mu g_n(\mu \mid \mathbf{X}^{(n)})\, d\mu.
\end{aligned}
\tag{9.4.11}
$$

In problems where the posterior distribution of μ_n is very skewed, it might be more prudent to estimate μ_n by the posterior median $G_n^{-1}(0.5 \mid \mathbf{X}^{(n)})$, which is the Bayes estimator for the absolute deviation loss.

9.4.3.2 Moving Windows AMOC Algorithm The moving windows AMOC algorithm is based on repeated applications of the AMOC estimation model of Section 9.4.3.1 to moving windows of constant size n_w, $n_w \geq 2$. At time t, $t = 2, 3, \ldots$, the data window consists of the observations on $\mathbf{X}_t^{(n)} = (X_{t-n+1}, X_{t-n+2}, \ldots, X_t)'$, where $n = \min\{t, n_w\}$. An iteration of the procedure consists of seven steps, which are listed below. At the end of each iteration the prior of the posterior distribution $H(\boldsymbol{\theta}, \boldsymbol{\phi} \mid \mathbf{X}_{t-n}^{(n)})$ is replaced by $H(\boldsymbol{\theta}, \boldsymbol{\phi} \mid \mathbf{X}_{t-n+1}^{(n)})$ to serve as "prior" for the next iteration. In this manner the algorithm resembles a dynamic recursive estimation procedure (see West et al. 1985). We label this algorithm MW-AMOC. The algorithm is specified in the following sequence of steps:

Step 0: Set $t = 2, 3, \ldots$; $n = \min\{t, n_w\}$; $\mathbf{X}_t^{(n)} = (X_{t-n+1}, \ldots, X_t)$; p; and $H(\boldsymbol{\theta}, \boldsymbol{\phi})$.

Step 1: Compute the posterior probabilities

$$\pi_t(i \mid \mathbf{X}_t^{(n)}), \quad i = 1, \ldots, n.$$

Step 2: Determine the posterior distribution $H(\boldsymbol{\theta}, \boldsymbol{\phi} \mid \mathbf{X}_t^{(n)})$.

Step 3: Determine the posterior distribution $G_t(\mu \mid \mathbf{X}_t^{(n)})$.

Step 4: Estimate μ_t by $G_t^{-1}(0.5 \mid \mathbf{X}_t^{(n)})$ or by $E\{\mu_t \mid \mathbf{X}_t^{(n)}\}$.

Step 5: Find i_t^0 such that $\pi_t(i_t^0 \mid \mathbf{X}_t^{(n)}) = \max_{1 \leq i \leq n} \pi_t(i \mid \mathbf{X}_t^{(n)})$. If $1 \leq i_t^0 \leq n-1$, flag that a change point occurred at $t - n + i_t^0$; else, do not flag a change.

Step 6: Set $H(\boldsymbol{\theta}, \boldsymbol{\phi}) \leftarrow H(\boldsymbol{\theta}, \boldsymbol{\phi} \mid X_{t-n+1}^{(n)})$.

Step 7: Increase $t \leftarrow t + 1$; move the window, $X_t^{(n)} \leftarrow X_{t+1}^{(n)}$; go to step 1.

In the following section we develop specific formulas for three cases.

9.4.4 Specific Cases

9.4.4.1 Case I: Poisson Random Variables Let $X_1, X_2, \ldots, X_n$ be independent random variables having Poisson distributions with means θ_t, $t = 1, 2, \ldots, n$. According to the AMOC model, for $n = 1, 2, \ldots$

$$\mu_t = \begin{cases} \theta & \text{if } t \leq \tau_n, \\ \phi & \text{if } t > \tau_n, \end{cases}$$

conditional on $\{\tau_n = j\}$, $S_j = \sum_{i=1}^{j} X_i$ and $S^*_{n-j} = \sum_{i=j+1}^{n} X_i$ $(j = 1, \ldots, n-1)$ are minimal sufficient statistics for θ and ϕ, and if $\{\tau_n = n\}$, then $S_n = \sum_{i=1}^{n} X_i$ is a minimal sufficient statistic for θ. Accordingly, the joint likelihood function is

(9.4.12)

$$L_n(\tau_n, \theta, \phi) = \sum_{i=1}^{n-1} I\{\tau_n = j\} \frac{\theta^{S_j} \phi^{S^*_{n-j}}}{S_j! S^*_{n-j}!} e^{-j\theta-(n-j)\phi} + I\{\tau_n = n\} \frac{\theta^{S_n} e^{-n\theta}}{S_n!}.$$

We assume that θ and ϕ are priorly independent, having gamma conjugate priors $G(\Lambda_i/\nu_i, \nu_i)$, $i = 1, 2$, respectively. According to the AMOC Bayesian model, the predictive distribution of S_j given $\{\tau_n = j\}$, $j = 1, \ldots, n$, is the negative binomial distribution with probability distribution function

$$g(s; \psi_j, \nu_1) = \frac{\Gamma(s + \nu_1)}{s! \Gamma(\nu_1)} (1 - \psi_j)^{\nu_1} \psi_j^s, \quad s = 0, 1, \ldots, \tag{9.4.13}$$

where

$$\psi_j = \frac{j\Lambda_1}{\nu_1 + j\Lambda_1}. \tag{9.4.14}$$

Similarly, the predictive p.d.f. of S^*_{n-j}, $j = 1, \ldots, n-1$, given $\{\tau_n = j\}$ is

$$g(s; \psi^*_{n-j}, \nu_2) = \frac{\Gamma(s + \nu_2)}{s! \Gamma(\nu_2)} (1 - \psi^*_{n-j})^{\nu_2} (\psi^*_{n-j})^s, \quad s = 0, 1, \ldots, \tag{9.4.15}$$

where

$$\psi^*_{n-j} = \frac{(n-j)\Lambda_2}{\nu_2 + (n-j)\Lambda_2}. \tag{9.4.16}$$

It follows that the posterior probabilities of π_n are

(9.4.17)

$$\begin{aligned} \pi_n(j \mid \mathbf{X}^{(n)}) = \frac{1}{D_n(\mathbf{X}^{(n)})} \{ & I\{j \leq n-1\} \cdot p(1-p)^{j-1} g(S_j; \psi_j, \nu_1) \\ & \cdot\ g(S^*_{n-j}, \psi^*_{n-j}, \nu_2) + I\{j = n\}(1-p)^{n-1} \\ & \cdot\ g(S_n; \psi_n, \nu_1)\}, \end{aligned}$$

where

$$D_n(\mathbf{X}^{(n)}) = p\sum_{j=1}^{n-1}(1-p)^{j-1}g(S_j;\psi_j,\nu_1)g(S^*_{n-j};\psi^*_{n-j},\nu_2) + (1-p)^{n-1}g(S_n;\psi_n,\nu_1). \tag{9.4.18}$$

Since the prior distributions of θ and ϕ are the conjugate gamma distributions, the posterior distributions of θ and ϕ given $\{\tau = j\}$ are the gamma distributions $G(\Lambda_1/(\nu_1 + j\Lambda_1), S_j + \nu_1)$ and $G(\Lambda_2/(\nu_2 + (n-j)\Lambda_2), S^*_{n-j} + \nu_2)$, respectively.

The current position of the process is given by Eq. (9.4.1). To derive it we notice that the posterior distribution of μ_n given $\mathbf{X}^{(n)}$ is a mixture of gamma distributions. Indeed, if $G(x \mid \beta, \nu)$ denotes the c.d.f. of the gamma $G(\beta, \nu)$, then

(9.4.19)

$$G_n(\mu \mid \mathbf{X}^{(n)}) = \sum_{j=1}^{n-1}\pi_n(j \mid \mathbf{X}^{(n)})G(\mu \mid \Lambda_2/(\nu_2 + (n-j)\Lambda_2), S^*_{n-j} + \nu_2) + \pi_n(n \mid \mathbf{X}^{(n)})G(\mu \mid \Lambda_1/(\nu_1 + n\Lambda_1), S_n + \nu_1).$$

The expected value of $G(\mu \mid \mathbf{X}^{(n)})$ is

$$\hat{\mu}_n(\mathbf{X}^{(n)}) = \sum_{j=1}^{n-1}\pi_n(j \mid \mathbf{X}^{(n)})\Lambda_2\frac{S^*_{n-j} + \nu_2}{\nu_2 + (n-j)\Lambda_2} + \pi_n(n \mid \mathbf{X}^{(n)})\Lambda_1\frac{S_n + \nu_1}{\nu_1 + n\Lambda_1}. \tag{9.4.20}$$

Finally, if ν_1 and ν_2 are integers and if $P(j;\lambda)$ is the c.d.f. of the Poisson distribution with mean λ, then the pth quantile of $G_n(\mu \mid \mathbf{X}^{(n)})$ is

$$\xi_p = \inf\left\{\xi; \sum_{j=1}^{n-1}\pi_n(j \mid \mathbf{X}^{(n)})P\left(S^*_{n-j} + \nu_2 - 1; \frac{\nu_2 + (n-j)\Lambda_2}{\Lambda_2}\xi\right) + \pi_n(n \mid \mathbf{X}^{(n)})P\left(S_n + \nu_1 - 1; \frac{\nu_1 + n\Lambda_1}{\Lambda_1}\xi\right) \le 1 - p\right\}. \tag{9.4.21}$$

9.4.4.2 Case II: Binomial Random Variables In the second case the data consist of a sequence of vectors (J_t, N_t), $t = 1, 2, \ldots$, where J_t is a binomial random variable and N_t is the associated number of trials. The basic model is

$$J_t \mid N_t, \theta_t \sim \text{Binom}(N_t, \theta_t),$$

$t = 1, 2, \ldots$. We develop here the formulas for an application which will be discussed in Section 9.4.5.2. In such data, N_t varies with t and is typically large (several thousands) and the angular transformation is normalizing and variance stabilizing. Thus, we define

$$X_t = 2 \cdot \sin^{-1}\left(\sqrt{\frac{J_t + 3/8}{N_t + 3/4}}\right), \quad t = 1, 2, \dots . \tag{9.4.22}$$

It is well known (see Johnson and Kotz, 1969, p. 69) that the distribution of X_t, given N_t, θ_t, is approximately normal with mean $\eta_t = 2 \cdot \sin^{-1}(\sqrt{\theta_t})$ and variance $\sigma_t^2 = 1/N_t$. We base the MW-AMOC algorithm on this normal model. For a given window of n observations, $\{(X_1, N_1), \dots, (X_n, N_n)\}$, we have

$$\eta_t = \begin{cases} \eta_0 & \text{if } t \le \tau_n, \\ \eta^* & \text{if } t > \tau_n. \end{cases}$$

For $j = 1, 2, \dots, n-1$ define

$$\begin{aligned} N^{(j)} &= \sum_{j=1}^{j} N_j, \quad \bar{X}_j = \frac{1}{N^{(j)}} \sum_{j=1}^{j} N_i X_i, \\ N_*^{(n-j)} &= \sum_{i=j+1}^{n} N_i, \quad \bar{X}_{n-j}^* = \frac{1}{N_*^{(n-j)}} \sum_{i=j+1}^{n} N_i X_i, \\ N^{(n)} &= \sum_{i=1}^{n} N_i, \quad \bar{X}_n = \frac{1}{N^{(n)}} \sum_{i=1}^{n} N_i X_i. \end{aligned} \tag{9.4.23}$$

The likelihood function of (τ_n, η_0, η^*) is equivalent (up to a scaling factor) to

$$\begin{aligned} L_n(\tau_n, \eta_0, \eta^*) = & \sum_{j=1}^{n-1} I\{\tau = j\} \exp\left\{-\frac{1}{2}\sum_{i=1}^{j} N_i (X_i - \eta_0)^2 \right. \\ & \left. -\frac{1}{2}\sum_{i=j+1}^{n} N_i (X_i - \eta^*)^2 \right\} \\ & + I\{\tau = n\} \exp\left\{-\frac{1}{2}\sum_{i=1}^{n} N_i (X_i - \eta_0)^2\right\}. \end{aligned} \tag{9.4.24}$$

After some algebraic operations this likelihood function is reduced to (9.4.25)

$$\begin{aligned} L_n(\tau_n, \eta_0, \eta^*) = & \sum_{j=1}^{n-1} I\{\tau_n = j\} \exp\left\{\frac{N^{(j)} N_*^{(n-j)}}{2N^{(n)}} (\bar{X}_j - \bar{X}_{n-j}^*)^2\right\} \\ & \cdot \exp\left\{-\frac{N^{(j)}}{2}(\bar{X}_j - \eta_0)^2 - \frac{N_*^{(n-j)}}{2}(\bar{X}_{n-j}^* - \eta^*)^2\right\} \\ & + I\{\tau_n = n\} \exp\left\{-\frac{N^{(n)}}{2}(\bar{X}_n - \eta_0)^2\right\}. \end{aligned}$$

We consider η_0 and η^* to be priorly independent having normal prior distribution with prior means ζ_1 and ζ_2 and prior variances σ^2 and ν^2, respectively.

Let $L_n^*(\tau_n)$ be the predictive likelihood function of τ_n, which is the expectation of $L_n(\tau_n, \eta_0, \eta^*)$ with respect to the above normal priors of η_0 and η^*. One obtains

(9.4.26)

$$\begin{aligned}
L_n^*(\tau_n) = & \sum_{j=1}^{n-1} I\{\tau_n = j\} \frac{1}{(1+N^{(j)}\sigma^2)^{1/2}(1+N_*^{(n-j)}\nu^2)^{1/2}} \\
& \cdot \exp\left\{\frac{N^{(j)}N_*^{(n-j)}}{2N^{(n)}}(\bar{X}_j - \bar{X}_{n-j}^*)^2\right\} \\
& \cdot \exp\left\{-\frac{N^{(j)}}{2(1+N^{(j)}\sigma^2)}(\bar{X}_j - \zeta_1)^2 \right. \\
& \left. - \frac{N_*^{(n-j)}}{2(1+N_*^{(n-j)}\nu^2)} \cdot (\bar{X}_{n-j}^* - \zeta_2)^2\right\} \\
& + I\{\tau_n = n\}\frac{1}{(1+N^{(n)}\sigma^2)^{1/2}} \exp\left\{-\frac{N^{(n)}}{2(1+N^{(n)}\sigma^2)} \cdot (\bar{X}_n - \zeta_1)^2\right\}.
\end{aligned}$$

Finally, the posterior probabilities of τ_n are

$$\pi_n(j \mid \mathbf{X}^{(n)}) = \frac{\pi_j L_n^*(j)}{\sum_{i=1}^{n} \pi_i L_n^*(i)}, \tag{9.4.27}$$

where $\pi_j = p(1-p)^{j-1}$ if $j \leq n-1$ and $\pi_n = (1-p)^{n-1}$.

The posterior distribution of the current position η_n given $\mathbf{X}^{(n)}$ is the mixture of the posterior distribution of η_n given $\mathbf{X}^{(n)}$ and $\{\tau_n = j\}$. More specifically, according to (9.4.23), for $\{\tau_n \leq n-1\}$ we have to consider the posterior distributions of η^* given $(\bar{X}_{n-j}^*, N_*^{(n-j)})$, and for $\{\tau_n = n\}$ we consider the posterior distribution of η_0 given $(\bar{X}_n, N^{(n)})$. It is straightforward to verify that, for $j = 1, \ldots, n-1$,

$$\eta^* \mid \bar{X}_{n-j}^*, \tau_n = j \sim N(E_{n-j}^*, D_{n-j}^{*2}), \tag{9.4.28}$$

where

$$E_{n-j}^* = \zeta_2 + \frac{N_*^{(n-j)}\nu^2}{1+N^{(n-j)}\nu^2}(\bar{X}_{n-j} - \zeta_2) \tag{9.4.29}$$

and

$$D_{n-j}^{*2} = \frac{\nu^2}{1+N_*^{(n-j)}\nu^2}. \tag{9.4.30}$$

Similarly,

$$\eta_0 \mid \bar{X}_n, \tau_n = n \sim N(E_n, D_n^2), \tag{9.4.31}$$

with

$$E_n = \zeta_1 + \frac{N^{(n)}\sigma^2}{1 + N^{(n)}\sigma^2}(\bar{X}_n - \zeta_1) \tag{9.4.32}$$

and

$$D_n^2 = \frac{\sigma^2}{1 + N^{(n)}\sigma^2}. \tag{9.4.33}$$

Finally, if $G_n(\eta \mid \mathbf{X}^{(n)})$ denotes the posterior c.d.f. of η_n given $\mathbf{X}^{(n)}$, then
(9.4.34)

$$G_n(\eta \mid \mathbf{X}^{(n)}) = \sum_{j=1}^{n-1} \pi_n(j \mid \mathbf{X}^{(n)})\Phi\left(\frac{\eta - E_{n-j}^*}{D_{n-j}^*}\right) + \pi_n(n \mid \mathbf{X}^{(n)})\Phi\left(\frac{\eta - E_n}{D_n}\right),$$

where $\Phi(z)$ is the standard normal integral.

The posterior mean is

$$\hat{\mu}_n(\mathbf{X}^{(n)}) = \sum_{j=1}^{n-1} \pi_n(j \mid \mathbf{X}^{(n)})E_{n-j}^* + \pi_n(n \mid \mathbf{X}^{(n)})E_n. \tag{9.4.35}$$

The pth quantile of $G_n(\eta \mid \mathbf{X}^{(n)})$, $0 < p < 1$, say $\eta_n(p)$, satisfies the equation

$$G_n(\eta_n(p) \mid \mathbf{X}^{(n)}) = p. \tag{9.4.36}$$

One can solve the nonlinear equation (9.4.35) by the Newton–Raphson method, starting with the initial value

$$\eta_n^0(p) = \sum_{j=1}^{n-1} \pi_n(j \mid \mathbf{X}^{(n)}) \cdot (E_{n-j}^* + Z_p D_{n-j}^*) + \pi_n(n \mid \mathbf{X}^{(n)})(E_n + Z_p D_n),$$

where $Z_p = \Phi^{-1}(p)$. Notice that the quantiles $\eta_n(p)$ should be restricted to the interval $(0, \pi/2)$. After obtaining the required quantiles of the posterior distribution of η_n one can immediately obtain those of θ_n by the inverse angular transformation $\theta_n = \sin^2(\eta_n/2)$.

9.4.4.3 Case III: Normal Random Variables Let $X_1, X_2, \ldots, X_n$ be a sequence of independent random variables. Let

$$X_t = \mu_t + \epsilon_t, \quad t = 1, 2, \ldots, n.$$

We assume that the error components $\epsilon_1, \epsilon_2, \ldots$ are i.i.d. random variables having a common normal distribution with mean zero and variance $\sigma_e^2 = 1$ (standardized data). The AMOC model is

$$\mu_t = \begin{cases} \mu_0 & \text{if } t \le \tau_n, \\ \mu_0 + Z & \text{if } t > \tau_n. \end{cases} \tag{9.4.37}$$

We assume that τ_n, μ_0, and Z are priorly independent, $\mu_0 \sim N(\mu_T, \sigma^2)$ and $Z \sim N(\delta, \tau^2)$. For $j = 1, \dots, n-1$, let

$$\bar{X}_j = \frac{1}{j}\sum_{i=1}^{j} X_i, \quad \bar{X}^*_{n-j} = \frac{1}{n-j}\sum_{i=j+1}^{n} X_i, \quad \bar{X}_n = \frac{1}{n}\sum_{i=1}^{n} X_i.$$

Given $\{\tau_n = j\}$, $j = 1, \dots, n-1$, the joint distribution of $(\mu_n, \bar{X}_j, \bar{X}^*_{n-j})$ is trivariate normal with mean vector $(\mu_T + \delta, \mu_T, \mu_T + \delta)$ and covariance matrix

$$\Sigma_j = \begin{bmatrix} \sigma^2 + \tau^2 & \sigma^2 & \sigma^2 + \tau^2 \\ \sigma^2 & \sigma^2 + \dfrac{\sigma_e^2}{j} & \sigma^2 \\ \sigma^2 + \tau^2 & \sigma^2 & \sigma^2 + \tau^2 + \dfrac{\sigma_e^2}{n-j} \end{bmatrix}. \tag{9.4.38}$$

Thus, the posterior distribution of μ_n given $(\bar{X}_j, \bar{X}^*_{n-j})$ and $\{\tau_n = j\}$ is normal with mean $E_{j,n}(\mathbf{X}^{(n)})$ and variance $D^2_{j,n}$. These posterior means are given by

$$E_{j,n}(\mathbf{X}^{(n)}) = w^{(1)}_{j,n}(\mu_T + \delta(1 + j\sigma^2)) + w^{(2)}_{j,n}\bar{X}_j + w^{(3)}_{j,n}\bar{X}^*_{n-j}, \tag{9.4.39}$$

where

$$\begin{aligned} w^{(1)}_{j,n} &= [1 + n\sigma^2 + (n-j)\tau^2(1 + j\sigma^2)]^{-1}, \\ w^{(2)}_{j,n} &= j\sigma^2 w^{(1)}_{j,n}, \\ w^{(3)}_{j,n} &= 1 - w^{(1)}_{j,n} - w^{(2)}_{j,n}. \end{aligned} \tag{9.4.40}$$

The posterior variances are

$$D^2_{j,n} = (\sigma^2 + \tau^2 + \sigma^2\tau^2 j)w^{(1)}_{j,n}. \tag{9.4.41}$$

The posterior distribution of μ_n given $\mathbf{X}^{(n)}$ and $\{\tau_n = n\}$ is normal with mean

$$E_{n,n} = \frac{\mu_T}{1 + n\sigma^2} + \frac{n\sigma^2}{1 + n\sigma^2}\bar{X}_n \tag{9.4.42}$$

and variance

$$D^2_{n,n} = \frac{\sigma^2}{1 + n\sigma^2}. \tag{9.4.43}$$

Accordingly, the posterior c.d.f. of μ_n given $\mathbf{X}^{(n)}$ is

$$G_n(\mu \mid \mathbf{X}^{(n)}) = \sum_{j=1}^{n} \pi_n(j \mid \mathbf{X}^{(n)})\Phi\left(\frac{\mu - E_{j,n}}{D_{j,n}}\right). \tag{9.4.44}$$

In order to determine the posterior probabilities of τ_n, namely $\pi_n(j \mid \mathbf{X}^{(n)})$, we have to derive the predictive likelihood $L_n^*(\tau_n)$. Derivations similar to those of Section 9.4.4.2 yield, for $j = 1, \ldots, n-1$,

$$L_n^*(j) = \exp\left\{j\left(1 - \frac{j}{n}\right)(\bar{X}_j - \bar{X}_{n-j}^*)^2\right\} L_n^{**}(j), \tag{9.4.45}$$

where

$$\begin{aligned} L_n^{**}(j) = {} & \frac{1}{(1 + n\sigma^2 + (n-j)\tau^2(1 + j\sigma^2))^{1/2}} \\ & \cdot \exp\left\{ - \frac{1}{2(1 + n\sigma^2 + (n-j)\tau^2(1 + j\sigma^2))} \right. \\ & \cdot \left[\frac{1 + (n-j)(\sigma^2 + \tau^2)}{n-j}(\bar{X}_j - \mu_T)^2 \right. \\ & - 2\sigma^2(\bar{X}_j - \mu_T)(\bar{X}_{n-j}^* - \mu_T - \delta) \\ & \left.\left. + \frac{1 + j\sigma^2}{j}(\bar{X}_{n-j} - \mu_T - \delta)^2 \right]\right\} \end{aligned} \tag{9.4.46}$$

and

$$L_n^*(n) = \frac{1}{(1 + n\sigma^2)^{1/2}} \exp\left\{ - \frac{n}{2(1 + n\sigma^2)}(\bar{X}_n - \mu_T)^2 \right\}. \tag{9.4.47}$$

The values of $\pi_n(j \mid \mathbf{X}^{(n)})$ are obtained from (9.4.45)–(9.4.47) according to (9.4.27). Similarly, the quantiles of $G_n(\mu \mid \mathbf{X}^{(n)})$ are obtained by solving Eq. (9.4.35) by the Newton–Raphson method. The expected value of $G_n(\mu \mid \mathbf{X}^{(n)})$ is

$$\hat{\mu}_n(\mathbf{X}^{(n)}) = \sum_{j=1}^{n} \pi_n(j \mid \mathbf{X}^{(n)}) E_{j,n}. \tag{9.4.48}$$

9.4.5 Case Studies

9.4.5.1 Case I: Coal Mining Disasters Cox and Lewis (1966, p. 42) used a quadratic regression model to analyze the intervals between successive explosions in coal mines in Great Britain between 1851 and 1962. The same data, with some corrections, was reanalyzed by Carlin, Gelfand, and Smith (1992), Gamerman (1992), Jarrett (1979), Raftery and Akman (1986), and Worsely (1986), among others. The data consist of the number of days between successive disasters. The commonly adopted model is that the disaster epochs follow a nonstationary Poisson process, and the general objective is to detect, by retrospective analysis, the locations of the change points in the disaster rate $\theta(t)$. According to the regression model of Cox and Lewis, the disaster rate became $\theta = 2$ per year at $t = 45.83$ years (in 1896) and dropped to $\theta = 1$

per year at $t = 85.70$ years (in 1936). Worsely (1986) estimates the point of change at the 43rd year, while Carlin, Gelfand, and Smith (1992) estimate it at the 41st year. Gamerman (1992) compares several dynamic estimators of the disaster rate $\theta(t)$.

We have applied to these data the MW-AMOC Bayesian tracking model for Poisson random variables as developed in Section 9.4.4.1. The data on number of days between successive disasters were transformed to number of disasters per year. In applying the MW-AMOC tracking algorithm, we used a window of size $n_w = 20$. The prior expected Poisson means were set at $\Lambda_1 = 3$ disasters per year and $\Lambda_2 = 1$ disaster per year. The shape parameters and probability of shift p were set respectively at $\nu_1 = \nu_2 = 1$ and $p = 0.05$. The posterior distribution of the current mean, θ_t, given the data in each window is based on Eq. (9.4.19) and the moving windows algorithm of Section 9.4.3.2.

Figure 9.1 presents the number of yearly coal mining disasters and the corresponding Bayesian estimate of the current mean according to the MW-AMOC tracking algorithm. The Bayes estimates clearly smooth the data and show that $\theta(t)$ was almost constant around the level of $\theta(t) = 3$ until 1891 ($t = 40$). At that time the disaster rate $\theta(t)$ started falling, and after about 20 years (1911) it reached a stable level of $\theta(t) = 1$ disaster per year. Figure 9.1 clearly demonstrates that the drop in $\theta(t)$ occurred gradually over a period of 20 years.

9.4.5.2 Case II: Wave Soldering of Circuit Boards The manufacturing process of modern electronic systems begins with the preparation of assembled printed circuit boards. The circuit boards are then wave soldered. After soldering all boards are tested in computerized equipment to identify shorts and other defects. The data set analyzed here consists of results obtained from testing 380 consecutive batches of circuit boards. The batches are of varying size, and each batch includes boards of similar design. There were 30 different designs, which had 300–1200 solder points per board. The proportion of defects relative to the number of solder points in a batch is expressed in parts per million (PPM). These proportions are presented in Figure 9.2. As we see in Figure 9.2, there are many batches for which the proportion of defects is close to zero. On the other hand, every so often there are batches with a high level of defects. Here we apply the tracking algorithm to estimate the current position of the mean level of the processes on the sequence $Y_t = 200 \sin^{-1}(\sqrt{p_t})$, where p_t is the proportion of soldering defects of the tth batch. More specifically, we apply the MW-AMOC algorithm based on the formulas of Section 9.4.4.2. Here N_t is the number of solder points in the tth batch (a known parameter) and J_t is the number of shorts in this batch. In the MW-AMOC algorithm we have taken windows of size $n_w = 100$ batches. This reflects a prior opinion that changes in the defect levels among batches do not appear too frequently. The prior parameters used are $\theta_0 = 50 \times 10^{-6}$, $\theta^* = 100 \times 10^{-6}$, $p = 0.05$, $\xi_1 = 1.1$, $\xi_2 = 2.1$, $\sigma_2 = \tau^2 = 0.1$. Figure 9.3 displays the estimated current mean of Y_t.

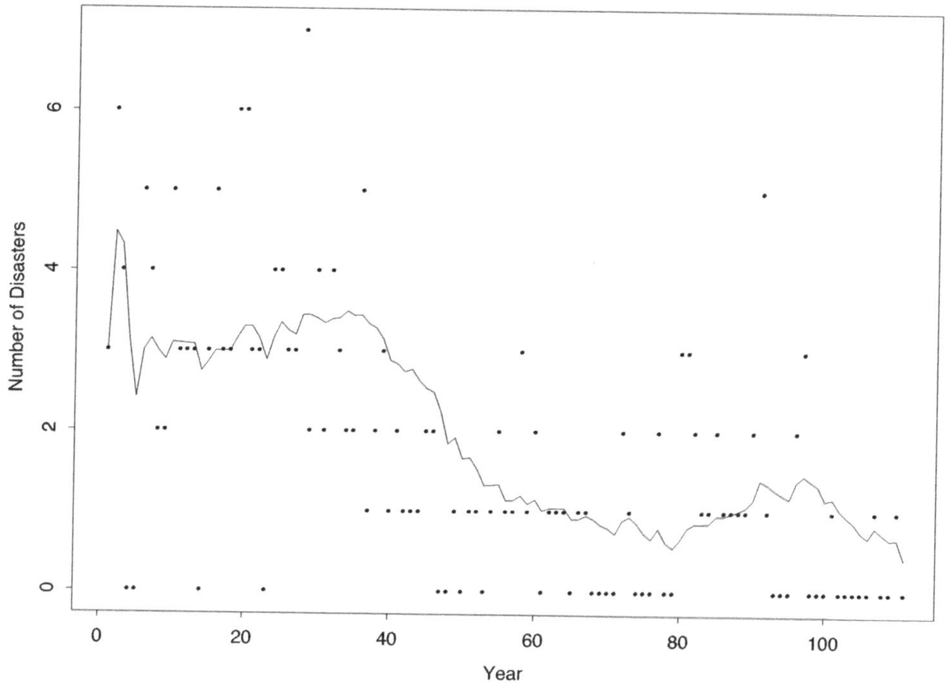

Figure 9.1: Number of coal mine disasters and AMOC tracking.

9.4.5.3 Case 3: The Dow Jones Financial Index For many years both financial economists and statisticians have been concerned with the description of stock market returns. The form of the distribution of stock returns is a crucial assumption for mean–variance portfolio theory and other financial models. In a comparison of different probability structures for stock returns, Kon (1984) proposed a discrete mixture of the normal distribution process as a statistical model for stock returns. He tested his theory empirically on a sample of 30 Dow Jones stocks and concludes that these stocks exhibit a mixture of normals generated by parameter nonstationarity. Since the AMOC tracking procedure, in the normal case, is based on the posterior distribution of the current mean, which is a mixture of normal distributions (see Section 9.4.4.3), we applied it to the Dow Jones financial index in the data set DOW1941.

In Chapter 5 we illustrated several one-day-ahead predictors for the DOW1941 data set. In Figure 9.4 we show the normal AMOC tracking on the same data set. The AMOC Bayesian estimators of the current mean are presented by a

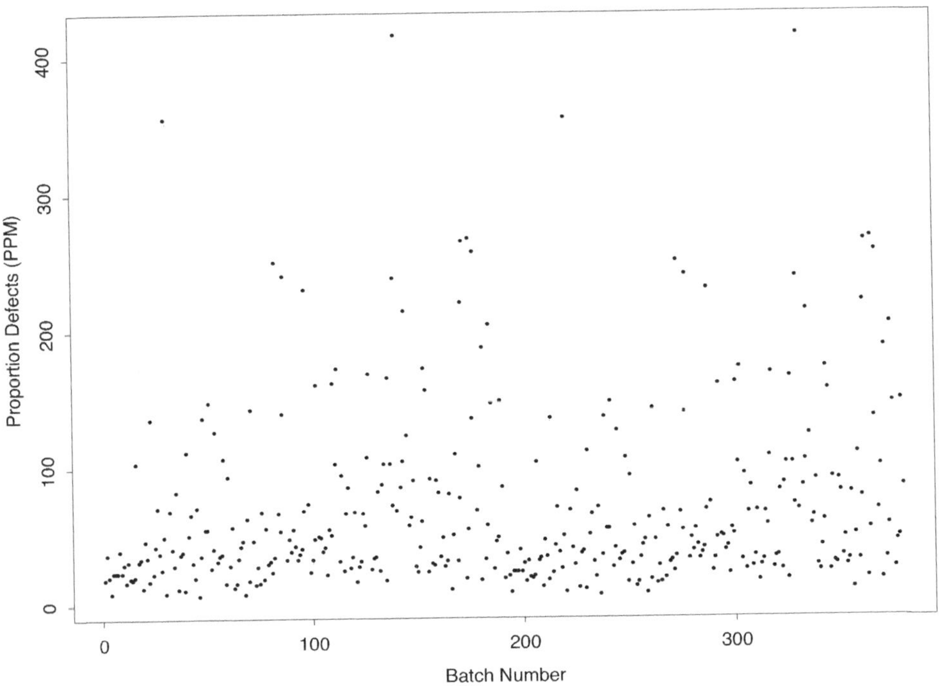

Figure 9.2: Wave soldering defects (PPM).

solid line. These estimates are based on the formulas of Section 9.4.4.3. The parameters used are $n_\omega = 10$, $\zeta_1 = 130$, $\zeta_2 = 115$, $\sigma^2 = \tau^2 = 1$, and $\rho = 0.05$.

9.5 RECURSIVE ESTIMATION WITH CHANGE POINTS

In previous chapters we discussed various recursive procedures, especially in Chapter 5, in the context of forecasting, filtering, and so on. In particular, we developed there the DLMs and the Kalman filter. These are especially important when the time series are not stationary and one wishes to track the trend of the series. In the present section we discuss recursive methods with random change points.

9.5.1 Reaction of Recursive Estimators to Change Points

We illustrate here the ineffectiveness of certain recursive estimators when change points occur.

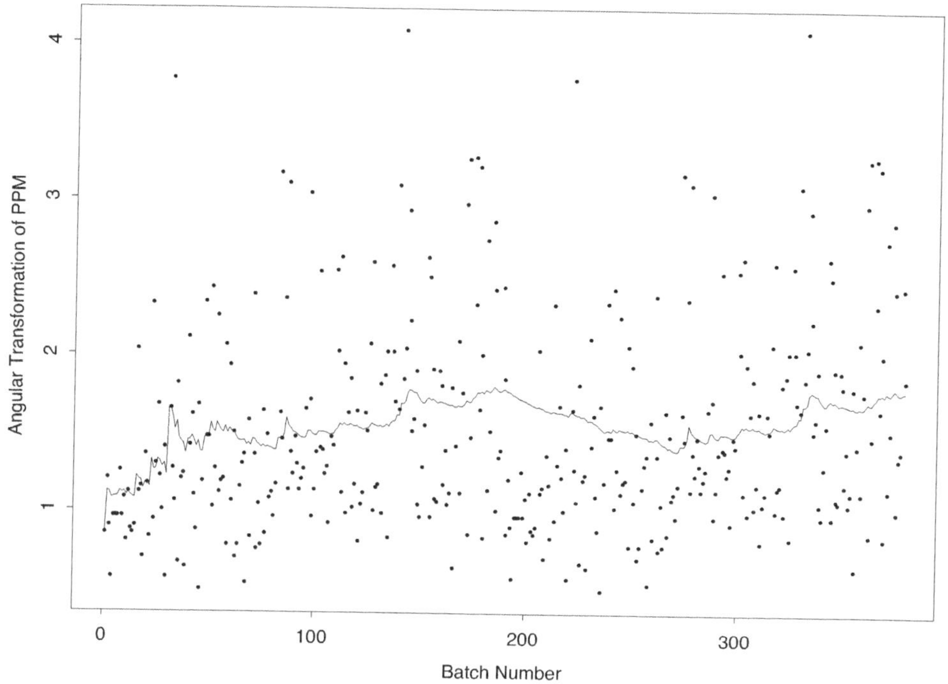

Figure 9.3: Angular transformation of PPM and AMOC tracking.

9.5.1.1 Bayes Estimator of the Mean Consider first the stationary model

$$Y_t = \mu + e_t, \quad t = 1, 2, \ldots, \tag{9.5.1}$$

where μ is an unknown constant and $\{e_t\}$ is a sequence of i.i.d. random variables having a normal distribution $\mathcal{N}(0, \sigma_e^2)$. The Bayes estimator of μ, with respect to a $\mathcal{N}(\mu_0, \tau^2)$ prior distribution, and a squared-error loss function can be written by the recursive formulas

$$\hat{\mu}_{B,t} = B_t \hat{\mu}_{B,t-1} + (1 - B_t) Y_t, \tag{9.5.2}$$

$t = 1, 2, \ldots$, where $\hat{\mu}_{B,0} \equiv \mu_0$, and

$$B_t = \frac{\sigma_e^2}{\sigma_e^2 + w_{t-1}^2}, \quad w_t^2 = w_{t-1}^2 B_t, \quad w_0^2 = \tau^2.$$

The recursive estimator (9.5.2) is a special case of the Kalman filter given in (5.6.30). In order to illustrate the effects of change points on the recursive

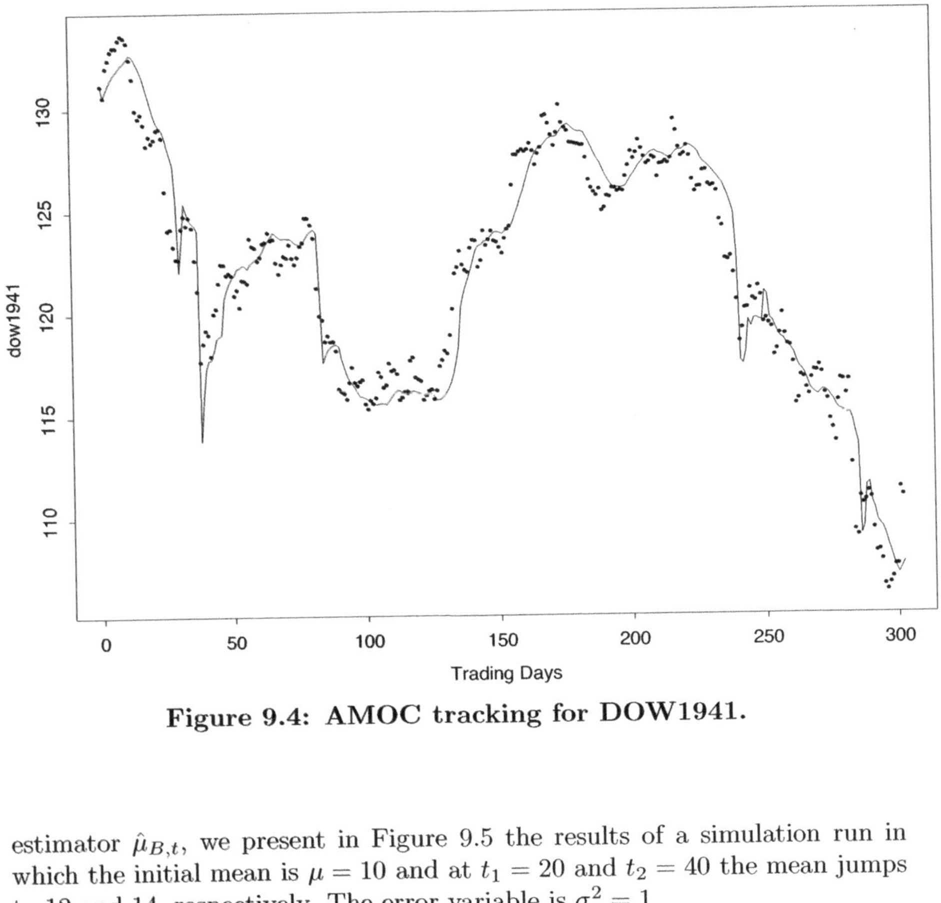

Figure 9.4: AMOC tracking for DOW1941.

estimator $\hat{\mu}_{B,t}$, we present in Figure 9.5 the results of a simulation run in which the initial mean is $\mu = 10$ and at $t_1 = 20$ and $t_2 = 40$ the mean jumps to 12 and 14, respectively. The error variable is $\sigma^2 = 1$.

The recursive estimator with $\mu_0 = 10$ and $\sigma^2 = \tau^2 = 1$ reacts quite fast to the changes in the means. Indeed, if the expected value of Y_t prior to the change point is μ_0 and after the change point it is $\mu_0 + \Delta$ and if the change point occurs right after t_1, then the bias of the Bayes estimator is

$$\text{(9.5.3)} \qquad \text{Bias}(\hat{\mu}_{B,t}; t_1, \Delta) = \begin{cases} 0 & \text{if } t \leq t_1, \\ -\Delta \dfrac{\sigma_e^2 + t_1\tau^2}{\sigma_e^2 + t\tau^2} & \text{if } t > t_1. \end{cases}$$

The magnitude of this bias after the occurrence of a change point diminishes to a quantity smaller than a specified ϵ, $0 < \epsilon < \Delta$, only after $(t_1 + \sigma_e^2/\tau^2)(\Delta/\epsilon - 1)$ units of time. Thus, if the change point t_1 occurs late, it will take a long time until the Bayes estimator will considerably reduce its bias.

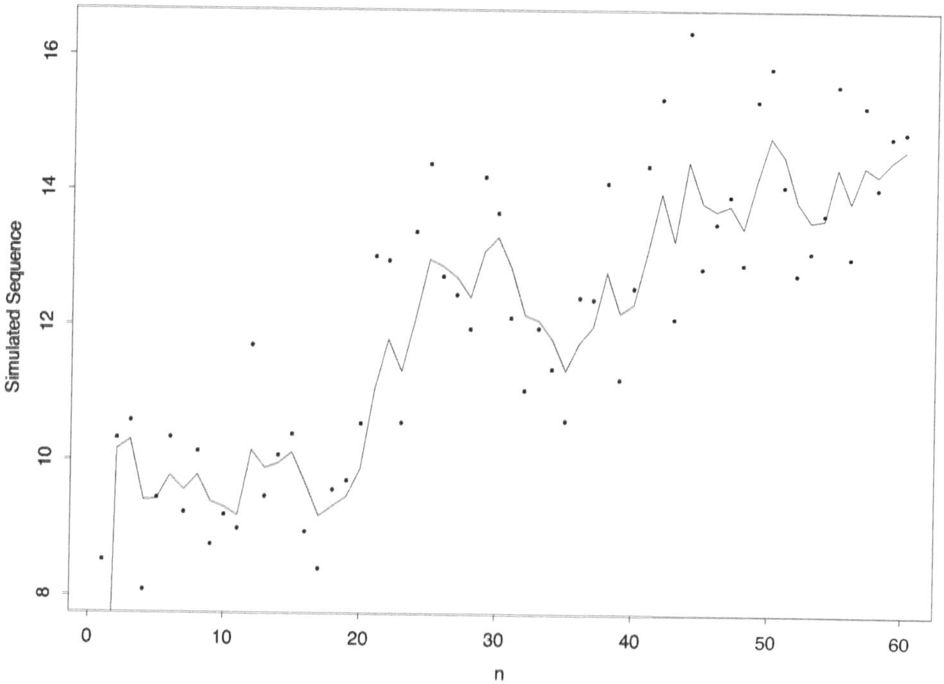

Figure 9.5: Recursive Bayesian tracking.

9.5.1.2 Recursive Least Squares Estimation In the present example we consider a recursive estimator of regression coefficients and apply it on time series data which apparently contain several change points. Consider the linear regression model

$$y_t = \mathbf{h}_t'\boldsymbol{\theta} + e_t, \quad t = 1, 2, \ldots, \tag{9.5.4}$$

where $\mathbf{h}_t' = (h_{t'}, \ldots, h_{t_p})$ is a vector of p covariates at time t, $\boldsymbol{\theta} = (\theta_1, \ldots, \theta_p)'$ is an unknown vector of regression coefficients, and $e_1, e_2, \ldots$ are i.i.d. random variables with mean 0 and variance σ^2.

Let X_k be a $k \times p$ matrix consisting of the first k vectors $\mathbf{h}_1', \ldots, \mathbf{h}_k'$. Assuming that X_k is of full rank ($k > p$), let $P_k = (X_k'X_k)^{-1}$ and let $\hat{\boldsymbol{\theta}}_k$ be the least squares estimator (LSE) given by

$$\hat{\boldsymbol{\theta}}_k = P_k X_k' Y_k, \tag{9.5.5}$$

where $\mathbf{y}_k = (y_1, \ldots, y_k)'$. As new data arrive in a time-ordered fashion, the LSE of $\boldsymbol{\theta}$ can be recursively computed by the formula

$$\hat{\boldsymbol{\theta}}_t = \hat{\boldsymbol{\theta}}_{t-1} + P_t \mathbf{h}_t (y_t - \mathbf{h}_t' \hat{\theta}_{t-1}), \quad t \geq k+1, \tag{9.5.6}$$

where

$$P_t = P_{t-1} - \frac{P_{t-1}\mathbf{h}_t\mathbf{h}_t' P_{t-1}}{\sigma^2 + \mathbf{h}_t' P_{t-1}\mathbf{h}_t}. \tag{9.5.7}$$

Dufour (1982) studied the effect of nonstability of $\boldsymbol{\theta}$ (existence of change points) on the recursive estimator.

In Figure 9.6 we present the Dow Jones index for the 300 business days of 1935 with the recursive regression estimators. We take $\mathbf{h}_t' = (1, t, t^2, t^3)$ with a learning period of size $k = 5$.

The recursive predictor $\hat{y}_t = \mathbf{h}_t' \hat{\boldsymbol{\theta}}_{t-1}$, where $\hat{\boldsymbol{\theta}}_t$ was recursively computed according to (9.5.5) and (9.5.6), is presented in Figure 9.6 as a solid line. We see again that the recursive predictor reacts slowly to changes in the trend after the third change point in the linear trend.

The DLM growth model discussed in Section 5.6 would give better results, as shown in Figure 5.17.

9.5.2 Recursive Estimation with the Kalman Filter

The Kalman filter (KF) was introduced in Chapter 5. We repeat here some basics. The KF is a recursive estimator of the process mean at time t, μ_t, based on the following general DLM.

Let $\boldsymbol{\theta}_t$ be a parametric vector of dimension p, where the current mean μ_t is a function of $\boldsymbol{\theta}_t$, that is, $\mu_t = M(\boldsymbol{\theta}_t)$. Let $\mathbf{Y}_t$ be a random vector which represents the observations at time t. The DLM is given by the following two equations: the system equation

$$\boldsymbol{\theta}_t = G_t \boldsymbol{\theta}_{t-1} + F_t \mathbf{w}_t, \quad t = 1, 2, \ldots, \tag{9.5.8}$$

and the observation equation

$$\mathbf{Y}_t = H_t \boldsymbol{\theta}_t + \mathbf{v}_t, \quad t = 1, 2, \ldots . \tag{9.5.9}$$

We assume that $\{\mathbf{w}_t\}_{t=1}^{\infty}$ is a sequence of i.i.d. random vectors $E\{\mathbf{w}_t\} = \mathbf{0}$ and dispersion matrix $\Sigma(\mathbf{w}_t) = W_t$. Here $\{\mathbf{v}_t\}_{t=1}^{\infty}$ is a sequence of random vectors, $E\{\mathbf{v}_t\} = \mathbf{0}$, and $\Sigma(\mathbf{v}_t) = R_t$; $\boldsymbol{\theta}_0$ is the initial state of the system (random vector with mean $\boldsymbol{\theta}^*$ and dispersion C_0). Moreover $\{\mathbf{w}_t\}$, $\{\mathbf{v}_t\}$, and $\boldsymbol{\theta}_0$ are mutually independent; F_t, G_t, H_t, R_t, and W_t are *known* matrices for all $t = 1, 2, \ldots$. Thus, the DLM can represent phenomena with constantly changing distributions according to *known* linear dynamics. The epochs and intensity of changes are all known and are represented by the known matrices of the model. The KF is a recursive estimator of $\boldsymbol{\theta}_t$ given by

$$\hat{\boldsymbol{\theta}}_t = G_t \hat{\boldsymbol{\theta}}_{t-1} + K_t (\mathbf{Y}_t - H_t G_t \hat{\boldsymbol{\theta}}_{t-1}), \tag{9.5.10}$$

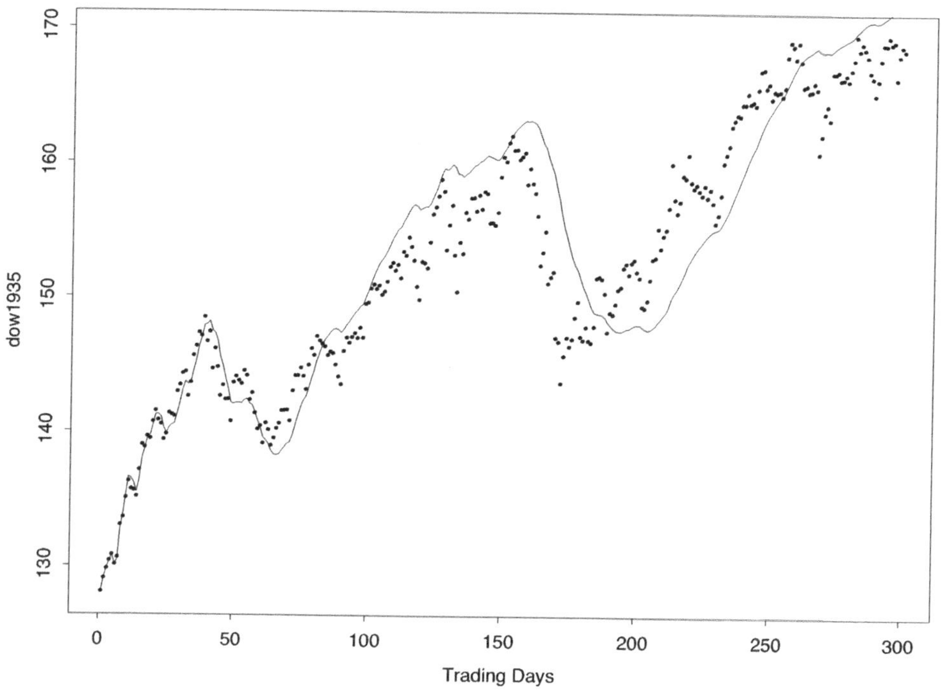

Figure 9.6: DOW1935 with recursive regression tracking.

where $\hat{\boldsymbol{\theta}}_0 \equiv \boldsymbol{\theta}^*$, and the Kalman gain matrix K_t is computed by the recursive equations:

$$
\begin{aligned}
K_t &= (G_t C_{t-1} G_t' + F_t W_t F_t') H_t' D_t^{-1}, \\
D_t &= H_t (G_t C_{t-1} G_t' + F_t W_t F_t') H_t' + R_t, \\
C_t &= G_t C_{t-1} G_t' + F_t W_t F_t' - K_t D_t K_t'.
\end{aligned} \tag{9.5.11}
$$

The dynamic linear growth model is a special case in which

$$
G_t = F_t = \begin{pmatrix} 1 & 1 \\ 0 & 1 \end{pmatrix}, \quad \boldsymbol{\theta}_t = \begin{pmatrix} \mu_t \\ \beta_t \end{pmatrix},
$$

where $H_t = (1, 0)$ and $R_t = \sigma^2$ for $t = 1, 2, \ldots$. The KF presented in Figure 9.7 was computed according to this dynamic growth model, with $\mu_0 = 129$, $\beta_0 = 1.5$, $\sigma^2 = 2.5$, $C_0 = \text{diag}\{1, 0.5\}$ and $W = \text{diag}\{0.5, 0.5\}$. The data are the same as that of Figure 9.6. As seen in Figure 9.7, the Kalman filter tracks the data very well if a proper DLM is applied.

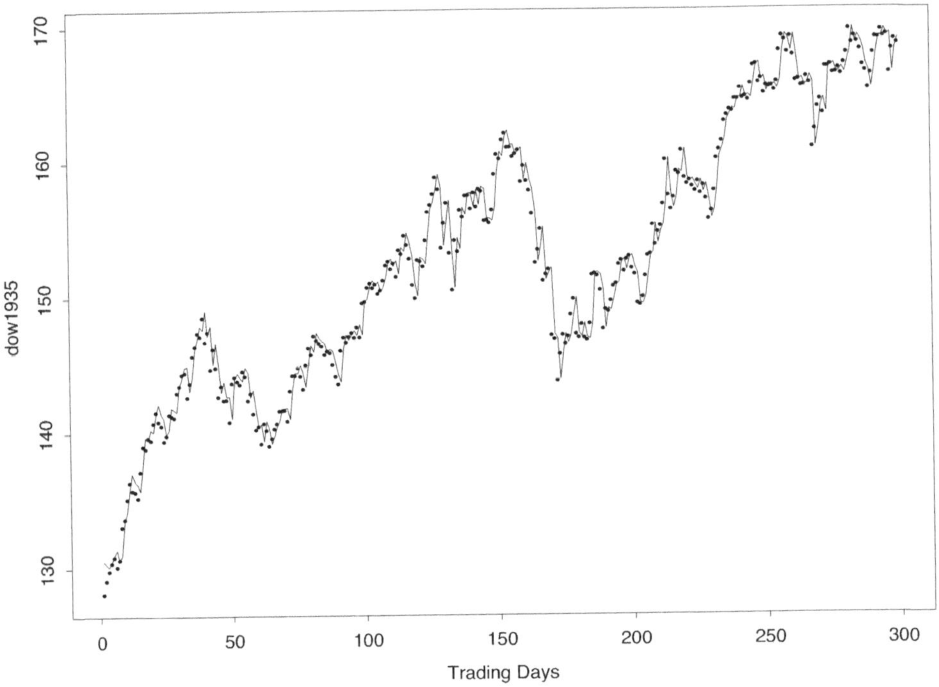

Figure 9.7: DOW 1935 with dynamic linear growth KF.

9.5.3 Detecting Change Points in Recursive Estimation

We say that a DLM is subjected to change points if the structure of the dynamics, as represented by the state equations, changes at unknown time points. The structural change in the DLM might be expressed as changes in the structure of the coefficient matrices F_t, G_t, or H_t or in the covariance matrices W_t or R_t. If change points are not detected and the magnitude of changes is not estimated, the uncorrected KF may become an inefficient estimator, as previously illustrated. The question is how to detect change points while using a recursive procedure and how to compensate the estimator for the changes?

Brown, Durbin, and Evans (1975) suggested to detect change points by performing CUSUM control charts on the recursive residuals $\hat{e}_{t|t-1} = \mathbf{y}_t - H_t G_t \hat{\boldsymbol{\theta}}_{t-1}$ $(t = 1, 2, \ldots)$. More specifically, they considered the recursive regression estimation, which was discussed in Section 9.5.1.2. According to the notation of that section, if $\mathbf{h}_t$ is the regressor (covariate) vector of time t

and $\hat{\boldsymbol{\theta}}_{t-1}$ is the estimator of the regression coefficient from time $t-1$, the innovation $\hat{e}_{t|t-1} = y_t - \mathbf{h}_t'\hat{\boldsymbol{\theta}}_{t-1}$ has zero mean and variance

$$v\{\hat{e}_{t|t-1}\} = \sigma^2(1 + \mathbf{h}_t' P_{t-1}\mathbf{h}_t). \tag{9.5.12}$$

Thus, if there are no change points, the standardized residuals $U_t = \hat{e}_{t|t-1}(1 + \mathbf{h}_t' P_{t-1}\mathbf{h}_t)^{-1/2}$ are independent with zero mean and common standard deviation σ. If a change point occurs, the mean of U_t changes after the change point and the CUSUM procedure should detect it.

West (1986) suggested another recursive procedure for detecting change points. It should be interesting to compare the efficiency of the procedure suggested by West with that of the CUSUM or recursive residuals.

9.5.4 Adjustment of the Kalman Filter for Change Points

9.5.4.1 DLM with Change Points In the present section we assume that the occurrence of change points follows a random process. For simplicity we assume that this is a homogeneous Bernoulli process. Thus, let $I_1, I_2, \ldots$ be a sequence of i.i.d. random variables such that $I_t = 1$ if a change point occurs between y_{t-1} and y_t and $I_t = 0$ otherwise. Moreover, $P[I_t = 1] = p$ for all $t = 1, 2, \ldots$. Let $1 \le t_1 < t_2 < \cdots < t_n < \cdots$ be the random locations of the change points. Letting $t_0 \equiv 0$, we immediately obtain that $t_n - t_{n-1}$ has a prior geometric distribution

$$P\{t_n - t_{n-1} = j\} = p(1-p)^{j-1}, \quad j \ge 1. \tag{9.5.13}$$

Generally, if $t_{n-1} < t < t_n$ $(n = 1, 2, \ldots)$, then the DLM matrices G_t, F_t, W_t, and R_t do not change. At points of change, the change may assume one of several possible types of change. At a change point the above matrices may change their values or a random vector $\boldsymbol{\Delta}_t$ may be added to $\boldsymbol{\theta}_t$. The model can rapidly become very complicated. We will examine it carefully below for the simpler model of AMOC, and at the change point the possible change is at $\boldsymbol{\theta}$. More specifically, we assume that $F_t = F$, $G_t = G$, $W_t = W$, and $R_t = R$ for all $t = 1, 2, \ldots$,

$$\boldsymbol{\theta}_t = \begin{cases} G\boldsymbol{\theta}_{t-1} + F\mathbf{w}_t & \text{if } t \ne t_1, \\ G\boldsymbol{\theta}_{t-1} + F\mathbf{w}_t + \boldsymbol{\Delta} & \text{if } t = t_1, \end{cases} \tag{9.5.14}$$

where t_1 is the epoch of the change point and $\boldsymbol{\Delta}$ is a random vector with mean $\boldsymbol{\delta}$ and covariance matrix D.

9.5.4.2 Likelihood Functions and Posterior Probabilities We develop in this section an expression for the posterior probability $\pi_t = P\{t_1 \le t\}$, that is, that the change point has already occurred. We will assume here that $\mathbf{w}_t$ and $\mathbf{v}_t$ have multivariate normal distributions. According to (9.5.8) and (9.5.9), we can write

$$\boldsymbol{\theta}_t = G^t \boldsymbol{\theta}_0 + \sum_{j=0}^{t-1} G^j \mathbf{z}_{t-j}, \tag{9.5.15}$$

where $\mathbf{z}_t = F_t \mathbf{w}_t$. Moreover $\boldsymbol{\xi}_t = \sum_{j=0}^{t-1} G^j \mathbf{z}_{t-j}$ has a multivariate normal distribution with mean $\mathbf{0}$ and covariance function $\sum_{j=0}^{t-1} G^j F W F'(G^j)'$. Thus, for each $t \le t_1$,

$$\mathbf{y}_t \mid \boldsymbol{\theta}_0, \mathbf{z}_t \sim N(H_t G^t \boldsymbol{\theta}_0 + H_t \mathbf{z}_t, R)$$

and

$$\mathbf{y}_t \mid \boldsymbol{\theta}_0 \sim N(H_t G^t \boldsymbol{\theta}_0, V_t),$$

where $V_t = R + H_t \sum_{j=0}^{t-1} G^j F W F'(G^j)' H_t'$. For $t > t_1$

$$\mathbf{y}_t \mid \boldsymbol{\theta}_0 \sim N(H_t G^{t-t_1}(G^{t_1} \boldsymbol{\theta}_0 + \boldsymbol{\Delta}), V_t).$$

Let $\mathcal{D}_t = (\mathbf{y}_1, \cdots, \mathbf{y}_t)$. Let $L_t(\boldsymbol{\theta}_0, \boldsymbol{\Delta}, t_1)$ denote the likelihood function of $\boldsymbol{\theta}_0$, $\boldsymbol{\Delta}$, and t_1 given $\mathcal{D}_t$, that is,

(9.5.16)

$$\begin{aligned} L_t(\boldsymbol{\theta}_0, \boldsymbol{\Delta}, t_1) = {} & I\{t \le t_1\} \cdot \frac{1}{\prod_{k=1}^t |V_k|^{1/2}} \\ & \cdot \exp\left\{ -\frac{1}{2} \sum_{k=1}^t (\mathbf{y}_k - H_k G^k \boldsymbol{\theta}_0)' V_k^{-1} (\mathbf{y}_k - H_k G^k \boldsymbol{\theta}_0) \right\} \\ & + I\{t > t_1\} \frac{1}{\prod_{k=1}^t |V_k|^{1/2}} \exp\left\{ -\frac{1}{2} \sum_{k=1}^t (\mathbf{y}_k - H_k G^k \boldsymbol{\theta}_0)' V_k^{-1} \right. \\ & \cdot (\mathbf{y}_k - H_k G^k \boldsymbol{\theta}_0) - \boldsymbol{\Delta}' \sum_{k=t_1+1}^t (G^{k-t_1})' H_k' V_k^{-1} (\mathbf{y}_k - H_k G^k \boldsymbol{\theta}_0) \\ & \left. - \frac{1}{2} \boldsymbol{\Delta}' \left(\sum_{k=t_1+1}^t (G^{k-t_1})' H_k' V_k^{-1} H_k G^{k-t_1} \right) \boldsymbol{\Delta} \right\}. \end{aligned}$$

If $\pi(\tau)$ is a prior p.d.f. of the change point t_1, $h(\boldsymbol{\theta}_0, \boldsymbol{\Delta})$ is a joint prior p.d.f. of $\boldsymbol{\theta}_0$ and $\boldsymbol{\Delta}$ assuming that $(\boldsymbol{\theta}_0, \boldsymbol{\Delta})$ is independent of τ, then the joint posterior p.d.f. of $\boldsymbol{\theta}_0$, $\boldsymbol{\Delta}$, τ given $\mathcal{D}_t$ is

$$\psi(\boldsymbol{\theta}_0, \boldsymbol{\Delta}, t_1 \mid \mathcal{D}_t) = \frac{\pi(\tau) h(\boldsymbol{\theta}_0, \boldsymbol{\Delta}) L_t(\boldsymbol{\theta}_0, \boldsymbol{\Delta}, t_1)}{\sum_{j=1}^{\infty} \pi(j) \int \int h(\boldsymbol{\theta}_0, \boldsymbol{\Delta}) L_t(\boldsymbol{\theta}_0, \boldsymbol{\Delta}, j)\, d\boldsymbol{\theta}_0\, d\boldsymbol{\Delta}}. \tag{9.5.17}$$

We will assume now, for simplicity, that both $\boldsymbol{\theta}_0$ and $\boldsymbol{\Delta}$ are *known* and that $\pi(j) = p(1-p)^{j-1}$ for $j = 1, 2, \ldots$. For $j = 1, \ldots, t-1$, define

$$
\begin{aligned}
E_{t,j} = p(1-p)^{j-1} \exp\Bigg\{ \boldsymbol{\Delta}' \sum_{k=j+1}^{t} (G^{k-j})' H_k' V_k^{-1} \mathbf{e}_k \\
- \frac{1}{2} \boldsymbol{\Delta}' \sum_{k=j+1}^{t} (G^{k-j})' H_k' V_k^{-1} H_k G^{k-j} \boldsymbol{\Delta} \Bigg\},
\end{aligned}
\tag{9.5.18}
$$

where $\mathbf{e}_k = \mathbf{y}_k - H_k G^k \boldsymbol{\theta}_0$ and

$$E_{t,t} = (1-p)^{t-1}. \tag{9.5.19}$$

Define also

$$D_t = \sum_{j=1}^{t} E_{t,j} \tag{9.5.20}$$

and

$$
\begin{aligned}
g_{t,j}(\mathbf{y}_t) = \exp\Bigg\{ \boldsymbol{\Delta}' (G^{t-j})' H_t' V_t^{-1} \mathbf{e}_t \\
- \frac{1}{2} \boldsymbol{\Delta}' (G^{t-j})' H_t' V_t^{-1} H_t G^{t-j} \boldsymbol{\Delta} \Bigg\}.
\end{aligned}
\tag{9.5.21}
$$

Then, for each $j = 1, \ldots, t-1$

$$E_{t,j} = E_{t-1,j}\, g_{t,j}(\mathbf{y}_t). \tag{9.5.22}$$

The posterior probabilities of $\{t_1 = j\}$ at epoch t are given by

$$\pi_t(j) = \frac{E_{t,j}}{\sum_{j=1}^{t} E_{t,j}}, \quad j = 1, \ldots, t. \tag{9.5.23}$$

We assume here that the prior probability of $\{t_1 = 0\}$ is zero.

9.5.4.3 Adjustment of the Kalman Filter The Kalman filter estimator of μ_t when $\{t_1 = j\}$ is known is

$$\hat{\mu}_{t,j} = H_t G \hat{\boldsymbol{\theta}}_{t,j}, \tag{9.5.24}$$

where

$$\hat{\theta}_{t,j} = \hat{\boldsymbol{\theta}}_t + I\{t = j\} \boldsymbol{\Delta} \tag{9.5.25}$$

and $\hat{\boldsymbol{\theta}}_t$ is given by the recursive formulas (9.5.10) and (9.5.11).

Since the event $\{t_1 = j\}$ is unknown, the Kalman filter estimator under a change point is

$$\hat{\mu}_t = \sum_{j=1}^{t} \pi_t(j) H_t G \hat{\boldsymbol{\theta}}_{t,j}. \tag{9.5.26}$$

Notice that this estimator is *not recursive.*

9.5.5 Special Case

Consider the special case of a dynamic model in which $W_t = 0$ for all t. More specifically, let $y_t \sim N(\mu_t, 1)$ for $t = 1, 2, \dots$. Assume also that

$$\mu_t = \begin{cases} \mu_0 & \text{if } t \le t_1, \\ \mu_0 + \Delta & \text{if } t > t_1, \end{cases} \tag{9.5.27}$$

where $\mu_0 \sim N(\mu_T, \sigma^2)$ and $\Delta \sim N(\delta, \tau^2)$. For each $j = 1, 2, \dots$ let

$$\bar{Y}_j = \frac{1}{j}\sum_{i=1}^{j} Y_i, \quad \bar{Y}_{t,j}^* = \frac{1}{t-j}\sum_{i=j+1}^{t} Y_i,$$

where $\bar{Y}_0 = \bar{Y}_{t,t}^* = 0$. For this special model, for each $j = 1, 2, \dots, t-1$

$$\hat{\mu}_{t,j} \equiv \hat{\boldsymbol{\theta}}_{t,j} = w_{t,j}^{(1)}(\mu_T + \delta(1 + j\sigma^2)) + w_{t,j}^{(2)}\bar{Y}_j + w_{t,j}^{(3)}\bar{Y}_{t,j}^*, \tag{9.5.28}$$

where

$$\begin{aligned} w_{t,j}^{(1)} &= [1 + t\sigma^2 + (t-j)\tau^2(1 + j\sigma^2)]^{-1}, \\ w_{t,j}^{(2)} &= j\sigma^2 w_{t,j}^{(1)}, \\ w_{t,j}^{(3)} &= 1 - w_{t,j}^{(1)} - w_{t,j}^{(2)}. \end{aligned} \tag{9.5.29}$$

Furthermore

$$\hat{\mu}_{t,t} = \frac{\mu_T}{1 + t\sigma^2} + \frac{t\sigma^2}{1 + t\sigma^2}\bar{Y}_t. \tag{9.5.30}$$

The posterior probabilities $\pi_t(j)$, $j = 1, \dots, t$, are given by the formula

$$\pi_t(j) = \frac{\pi(j) L_t^*(j)}{\sum_{i=1}^{t} \pi(i) L_t^*(i)}, \quad j = 1, \dots, t, \tag{9.5.31}$$

where $\pi(j) = p(1-p)^{j-1}$, $j = 1, \dots, t-1$ and $\pi(t) = (1-p)^{t-1}$. Moreover,

$$L_t^*(j) = \exp\left\{ j\left(1 - \frac{j}{t}\right)(\bar{Y}_j - \bar{Y}_{t,j}^*)^2 \right\} L_t^{**}(j), \tag{9.5.32}$$

and, for $j = 1, \ldots, t-1$

$$
\begin{aligned}
L_t^{**}(j) = {} & \frac{1}{(1 + t\sigma^2 + (t-j)\tau^2(1 + j\sigma^2))^{1/2}} \\
& \cdot \exp\left\{ -\frac{1}{2(1 + t\sigma^2 + (t-j)\tau^2(1 + j\sigma^2))} \right. \\
& \cdot \left[\frac{1 + (t-j)(\sigma^2 + \tau^2)}{t-j} (\bar{Y}_j - \mu_T)^2 \right. \\
& - 2\sigma^2 (\bar{Y}_j - \mu_T)(\bar{Y}_{t,j}^* - \mu_T - \delta) \\
& \left. \left. + \frac{1 + j\sigma^2}{j} (\bar{Y}_{t,j}^* - \mu_T - \delta)^2 \right] \right\}
\end{aligned} \tag{9.5.33}
$$

while

$$
L_t^{**}(t) = \frac{1}{(1 + t\sigma^2)^{1/2}} \exp\left\{ -\frac{t}{2(1 + t\sigma^2)} (\bar{Y}_t - \mu_T)^2 \right\}. \tag{9.5.34}
$$

Finally, the estimator of the current mean is

$$
\hat{\mu}_t = \sum_{j=1}^{t} \pi_t(j) \hat{\mu}_{t,j}. \tag{9.5.35}
$$

In Figure 9.8 we present a graph of the Dow Jones index for 300 business days of 1935. This sequence reflects, apparently, a phenomenon with multiple change points. The Bayes estimator (9.5.35) was computed for this series. Since the estimator (9.5.35) is Bayes for the AMOC model, we modified the formula by applying it on a *moving window* of size $n_w = 10$ and used the parameters $\mu_0 = 130$, $\Delta = 10$, $\sigma^2 = \tau^2 = 1$, $p = 0.05$. The graph of this modified Bayes estimator is presented in Figure 9.8.

9.6 ADDITIONAL THEORETICAL CONTRIBUTIONS

Several papers were published in recent years on efficient change-point detection in hidden Markov models (Fuh, 2003) and efficient likelihood estimation in state space models, (Fuh, 2004). See also Basseville and Nikiforov (1993), Lai (1995), and Yakir (1994). In the DLM, the observed random variable $Y_t = A\theta_t + \epsilon_t$, where $\theta_t = G\theta_{t-1} + \eta_t$ for all t. Thus, the sequence $\{\theta_t\}$ is a Markov sequence, called also a *hidden Markov chain* since it is not directly observable. Recall that ϵ_t and η_t are independent error variables. Estimating $M(\theta_t) = A\theta_t$ is a tracking problem, discussed at length in this chapter.

The joint p.d.f. of $(Y_1, \ldots, Y_n)$ in the case where $A = 1$ and $G = 1$ is

$$
\begin{aligned}
f_n(y_1, \ldots, y_n) = {} & \int_{\theta_0} \cdots \int_{\theta_n} \pi_0(\theta_0) \prod_{t=1}^{n} \pi_t(\theta_{t-1}, \theta_t) f(y_t \mid \theta_t) \\
& \cdot d\lambda(\theta_0) \cdots d\lambda(\theta_n),
\end{aligned} \tag{9.6.1}
$$

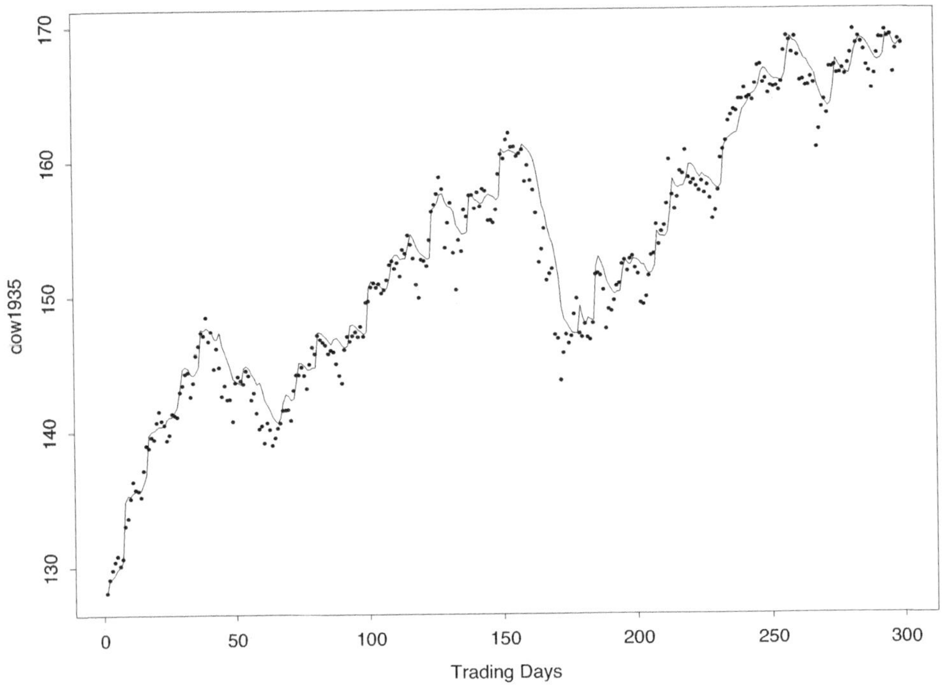

Figure 9.8: DOW1935 with normal AMOC.

where $\pi_t(\theta_{t-1}, \theta_t)$ is a transition kernel of the hidden Markov chain and $f(y_t \mid \theta_t)$ is the conditional density of Y_t. The change-point problem considered by Fuh is that of detecting the unknown epoch τ such that

$$\pi_t(\theta_{t-1}, \theta_t) = \begin{cases} \pi_0(\theta_{t-1}, \theta_t) & \text{if } t < \tau, \\ \pi_1(\theta_{t-1}, \theta_t) & \text{if } t \geq \tau. \end{cases} \tag{9.6.2}$$

Fuh adopts the Shiryaev–Roberts detection scheme and gives conditions under which this procedure is asymptotically optimal.

CHAPTER 10

SEQUENTIAL METHODS IN INDUSTRIAL TESTING, RELIABILITY, AND DESIGN OF EXPERIMENTS

10.1 SEQUENTIAL TESTING (SPRT)

In Section 4.7 we discussed two-stage and sequential sampling from a finite population for the purpose of accepting or rejecting a lot of items. There are in industry other applications of sequential testing connected with the manufacturing processes. For example, consider an insertion machine designed to automatically populate components on a printed circuit board (PCB). The machine is actually a robot controlled by a computer. The robot arm picks a component from a storage place and drops it on the circuit board in a specific location. This is done very fast (4000 components per hour). The standard requires that the proportion of placement errors will not exceed 300 PPM (i.e., 300 $\times 10^{-6}$). After building such a machine it is subjected to a series of tests to verify that its operation is up to the specified standards. How long should it be tested? The statistical test appropriate for this example is to test the hypothesis that the proportion of placement errors p is smaller than $p_0 = 300 \times 10^{-6}$ against the alternative that $p > p_1 = 400 \times 10^{-6}$. A sequential test that both controls probabilities of inference errors and minimizes the expected sample size when $p = p_0$ or $p = p_1$ is the Wald SPRT. We present this procedure here.

10.1.1 Wald Sequential Probability Ratio Test

Let $X_1, X_2, \ldots$ be a sequence of i.i.d. random variables. Consider two simple hypotheses H_0 and H_1 according to which the p.d.f.'s of these random variables are $f_0(x)$ or $f_1(x)$, respectively. Let $R(X_i) = f_1(X_i)/f_0(X_i)$, $i = 1, 2, \ldots$, be the likelihood ratio statistics. The SPRT is specified by two boundary points A, B, $-\infty < A < 0 < B < \infty$, and the stopping rule according to which sampling continues as long as the partial sums $S_n = \sum_{i=1}^{n} \log R(X_i)$, $n = 1, 2, \ldots$, lie between A and B. Accordingly,

$$N(A, B) = \min(n \geq 1 : S_n \leq A \quad \text{or} \quad S_n \geq B). \tag{10.1.1}$$

In the first case H_0 is accepted and in the second case H_1 is accepted. The sample size, N, is a random variable which depends on the past observations. More precisely, the event $\{N \leq n\}$ depends on $\{X_1, \ldots, X_n\}$ but is independent of $\{X_{n+1}, X_{n+2}, \ldots\}$ for all $n = 1, 2, \ldots$. Such a nonnegative integer random variable is called a *stopping variable*. Let $\mathcal{F}_n$ denote the σ-field generated by the random variables $Z_i = \log R(X_i)$, $i = 1, \ldots, n$. A stopping variable N defined with respect to $Z_1, Z_2, \ldots$ is an integer-valued random variable N, $N \geq 1$, such that the event $\{N \geq n\}$ is determined by $Z_1, \ldots, Z_{n-1}$ $(n \geq 2)$. In this case we say that $\{N \geq n\} \in \mathcal{F}_{n-1}$ and $I\{N \geq n\}$ is $\mathcal{F}_{n-1}$ measurable. We will show that for any pair (A, B) the stopping variable N is finite with probability 1. Such a stopping variable is called regular. We will see then how to choose the boundaries (A, B) so that the error probability α and β will be under control. Finally, formulas for the expected sample size will be derived and some optimal properties will be discussed.

In order to prove that the stopping variable $N \equiv N(A, B)$ is finite with probability 1, we have to prove that

$$\lim_{n\to\infty} P_\theta[N > n] = 0 \quad \text{for } \theta = 0, 1.$$

The *Kullback–Leibler information function* to discriminate between f_0 and f_1 is defined as

$$I(f_0, f_1) = E_0\left\{\log \frac{f_0(X)}{f_1(X)}\right\}. \tag{10.1.2}$$

For any $f_0 \neq f_1$ on a set of positive probability, $I(f_0, f_1) > 0$. Similarly $I(f_1, f_0) = E_1\{\log[f_1(X)/f_0(x)]\} > 0$. Notice that $\mu_0 = E_0\{Z\} = -I(f_0, f_1) < 0$ and $\mu_1 = E_1\{Z\} = I(f_1, f_0) > 0$. Accordingly $P_0(\lim_{n\to\infty} S_n = -\infty) = 1$ and $P_1(\lim_{n\to\infty} S_n = \infty) = 1$. It follows that $P_i\{N(A, B) < \infty) = 1$ for all (A, B) and $i = 0, 1$. For $\theta = 0, 1$, let

$$D_\theta^2 = \text{Var}_\theta\{Z\} \tag{10.1.3}$$

and assume that

$$0 < D_\theta^2 < \infty \quad \text{for } \theta = 0, 1. \tag{10.1.4}$$

Thus, from the central limit theorem, for any value of θ the distribution of $S_n = \sum_{i=1}^n Z_i$ is asymptotically normal. Moreover for each $m = 1, 2, \ldots$ and a fixed integer r

(10.1.5)

$$P_\theta[N > mr] \leq P_\theta[A < S_r < B, |S_{2r} - S_r| < C, \ldots, |S_{mr} - S_{r(m-1)}| < C],$$

where $C = |B - A|$.

The variables $S_r, S_{2r} - S_r, \ldots, S_{mr} - S_{(m-1)r}$ are independent and identically distributed. Moreover, by the central limit theorem, if r is sufficiently large

(10.1.6)

$$P_\theta\{|S_r| < C\} \approx \Phi\left(\frac{C}{\sqrt{r}\,D_\theta} + \sqrt{r}\,\frac{\mu_\theta}{D_\theta}\right) + \Phi\left(\frac{C}{\sqrt{r}\,D_\theta} - \sqrt{r}\,\frac{\mu_\theta}{D_\theta}\right) - 1.$$

The r.h.s. of (10.1.6) approaches 0 as $r \to \infty$. Accordingly, for any ρ, $0 < \rho < 1$, if r is sufficiently large, then $P_\theta[|S_r| < C] < \rho$. Finally, since $S_{jr} - S_{(j-1)r}$ is distributed like S_r for all $j = 1, 2, \ldots, r$, if r is sufficiently large, then

$$P_\theta[N > mr] < P_\theta[A < S_r < B]\rho^{m-1}. \tag{10.1.7}$$

This shows that $P_\theta[N > n]$ converges to zero in an exponential rate. This property is called the *exponential boundedness* of the stopping variables $N(A, B)$ (Wijsman, 1971). We prove now a very important result in sequential analysis which is not restricted only to SPRTs.

In Lemma 2.4.1 we have proven:

Wald Lemma. *If N is a stopping variable with finite expectation $E_\theta\{N\}$ and if $X_1, X_2, \ldots$ is a sequence of i.i.d. random variables such that $E_\theta\{|X_1|\} < \infty$, then*

$$E_\theta\left\{\sum_{i=1}^N X_i\right\} = \xi(\theta)E_\theta\{N\}, \tag{10.1.8}$$

where

$$\xi(\theta) = E_\theta\{X_i\}.$$

■

From (10.1.8) we immediately obtain that for $\theta = 0, 1$

$$E_\theta\{N\} = \frac{1}{\mu_\theta}E_\theta\{S_N\}, \tag{10.1.9}$$

where $\mu_1 = E_1\{R(X_1)\} = I(f_1, f_0)$ and $\mu_0 = E_0\{R(X_1)\} = -I(f_0, f_1)$. At stopping $S_N \geq B$ or $S_n \leq A < 0$. Let

$$S_N = (B + R_N^U)I(S_N \geq B) + (A - R_N^D)I(S_N \leq A). \tag{10.1.10}$$

Notice that $R_N^D \geq 0$. Furthermore, let

$$\pi_\theta = P_\theta\{S_N \leq A\}; \tag{10.1.11}$$

then, from (10.1.10)

(10.1.12)

$$E_\theta\{S_N\} = B(1-\pi_\theta) + A\pi_\theta + E_\theta\{R_N^U I(S_n \geq B)\} - E_\theta\{R_N^D I(S_N \leq A)\},$$

where R_N^U and $-R_N^D$ are called the "overshoots" above or below the boundaries B and A. In many cases the expected overshoot is negligible compared to the main term. Accordingly, Wald approximation to $E_\theta\{N\}$ is

$$E_\theta\{N\} \cong \frac{1}{\mu_\theta}[B + (A-B)\pi_\theta]. \tag{10.1.13}$$

The term π_θ will be approximated later.

We remark first that if α and β are the desired error probabilities, we wish to determine the values of A and B so that $\pi_0 = 1-\alpha$ and $\pi_1 = \beta$. Wald suggested to use the values

$$\begin{aligned} A' &= \log\frac{\beta}{1-\alpha}, \\ B' &= \log\frac{1-\beta}{\alpha}. \end{aligned} \tag{10.1.14}$$

Let α' and β' denote the corresponding error probabilities, that is,

$$\alpha' = P_0\left(S_N \geq \log\frac{1-\beta}{\alpha}\right), \quad \beta' = P_1\left\{S_N \leq \log\frac{\beta}{1-\alpha}\right\}.$$

Theorem 10.1.1 *If $0 < \alpha + \beta < 1$, then*

(i) $\alpha' + \beta' \leq \alpha + \beta$

and

(ii) $A' \leq A$, $B' \geq B$.

Proof: For each $n \geq 1$ define the sets

$$\begin{aligned} A_n &= \{\mathbf{x}_n : S_N \leq A', N \geq n\}, \\ R_n &= \{\mathbf{x}_n : S_N \geq B', N \geq n\}, \\ C_n &= \{\mathbf{x}_n : A_n < S_N < B_N, N \geq n\}. \end{aligned}$$

The error probability α' satisfies the inequality

$$\begin{aligned} \alpha' &= \sum_{n=1}^{\infty}\int_{R_n}\prod_{j=1}^{n} dF_0(x_j) \\ &\leq \frac{\alpha}{1-\beta}\sum_{n=1}^{\infty}\int_{R_n}\prod_{j=1}^{n} dF_1(x_j) = \frac{\alpha}{1-\beta}(1-\beta'). \end{aligned} \tag{10.1.15}$$

Similarly,

$$
\begin{aligned}
\beta' &= \sum_{n=1}^{\infty} \int_{A_n} \prod_{j=1}^{n} dF_1(x_j) \\
&\le \frac{\beta}{1-\alpha} \sum_{n=1} \int_{A_n} \prod_{j=1}^{n} dF_0(x_j) = \frac{\beta}{1-\alpha}(1-\alpha').
\end{aligned} \tag{10.1.16}
$$

Thus,

$$
\frac{\alpha'}{1-\beta'} \le \frac{\alpha}{1-\beta}, \quad \frac{\beta'}{1-\alpha'} \le \frac{\beta}{1-\alpha}.
$$

From these inequalities we obtain the first statement of the theorem. To establish (ii) notice that

$$
\begin{aligned}
1-\beta &= \sum_{n=1}^{\infty} \int_{R_n} \prod_{i=1}^{n} dF_1(x_j) \ge e^B \sum_{n=1}^{\infty} \int_{R_n} \prod_{i=1}^{n} dF_0(x_j) \\
&= \alpha e^B.
\end{aligned} \tag{10.1.17}
$$

Hence, $B' = \log[(1-\beta)/\alpha] \ge B$. The other inequality is proven similarly. ■

It is generally difficult to determine the values of A and B to obtain the specified error probabilities α and β. However, according to the theorem, if α and β are small, then, by considering the boundaries A' and B', we obtain a procedure with error probabilities α' and β' close to the specified ones and total test size $\alpha' + \beta'$ is smaller than $\alpha + \beta$. For this reason A' and B' are generally used in applications. For

$$
A' = \log \frac{\beta}{1-\alpha}, \quad B' = \log \frac{1-\beta}{\alpha}
$$

we obtain from (10.1.13)

$$
\begin{aligned}
E_0\{N\} &\cong \frac{(1-\alpha)\log\left(\dfrac{\beta}{1-\alpha}\right) + \alpha \log\left(\dfrac{1-\beta}{\alpha}\right)}{-I(f_0, f_1)} \\
&= \frac{(1-\alpha)\log\left(\dfrac{1-\alpha}{\beta}\right) + \alpha \log\left(\dfrac{\alpha}{1-\beta}\right)}{I(f_0, f_1)}.
\end{aligned} \tag{10.1.18}
$$

Similarly

$$
E_1\{N\} \cong \frac{(1-\beta)\log\left(\dfrac{1-\beta}{\alpha}\right) + \beta \log\left(\dfrac{\beta}{1-\alpha}\right)}{I(f_1, f_0)}. \tag{10.1.19}
$$

Asymptotic versions of these formulas, as α and β go to zero ($A' \to -\infty$ and $B' \to \infty$) are

(10.1.20)
$$E_0\{N\} \approx \frac{|\log \beta|}{I(f_0, f_1)}$$

and

(10.1.21)
$$E_1\{N\} \approx \frac{|\log \alpha|}{I(f_1, f_0)}.$$

We derive now an approximation to the acceptance probability $\pi(\theta)$. This approximation is based on the following important identity:

Theorem 10.1.2 (Wald Fundamental Identity) *Let N be a stopping variable associated with the Wald SPRT and $M_\theta(t)$ the moment generating function (m.g.f.) of Z; then*

(10.1.22)
$$E_\theta\{e^{tS_N}(M_\theta(t))^{-N}\} = 1$$

for all t for which $M_\theta(t)$ exists.

Proof: Let $Y_n = e^{tS_N}(M_\theta(t))^{-n}$, $n \geq 1$. We immediately obtain that $E_\theta\{Y_n \mid \mathcal{B}_{n-1}\} = Y_{n-1}$, $n \geq 2$. Thus, $\{Y_n, \mathcal{B}_n, n \geq 1\}$ is a *martingale sequence* (called the Wald martingale). Notice that $E_\theta\{Y_n\} = 1$ for all $n \geq 1$. Thus, $\{e^{tS_N}(M_\theta(t))^{-n}, n \geq 1\}$ is uniformly integrable. The *optional sampling theorem* for martingales (see Breiman, 1992, p. 84) implies (10.1.22). We can also show it directly. Notice that

(10.1.23)
$$E_\theta\{e^{tS_N}(M_\theta(t))^{-N}\} = \sum_{n=1}^{\infty} E_\theta\{I\{N = n\}e^{tS_n}(M_\theta(t))^{-n}\}$$
$$= \lim_{m\to\infty} \sum_{n=1}^{m} E\{(I\{N \geq n\} - I\{N \geq n+1\})e^{tS_n}(M_\theta(t))^{-n}\}.$$

Moreover, $I\{N \geq n\}$ is $\mathcal{F}_{n-1}$ measurable and therefore, for $n \geq 2$,

(10.1.24)
$$E_\theta\{I\{N \geq n\}e^{tS_n}(M_\theta(t))^{-n}\} = E_\theta\{I\{N \geq n\}e^{tS_{n-1}}(M_\theta(t))^{-(n-1)}\}.$$

Substituting in (10.1.23) we obtain

(10.1.25)
$$E_\theta\{e^{tS_N}(M(t))^{-N}\} = 1 - \lim_{m\to\infty} E\{I\{N \geq m+1\}e^{tS_m}(M(t))^{-m}\}.$$

Finally, since $\{Y_n, n \geq 1\}$ is uniformly integrable and $\lim_{m\to\infty} P_\theta\{N > m\} = 0$,

$$\lim_{m\to\infty} E_\theta\{I\{N \geq m+1\}e^{tS_m}(M_\theta(t))^{-m}\} = 0.$$

■

Choose $\epsilon > 0$ so that

$$P_1 = P_\theta[Z > \epsilon] > 0$$

and

$$P_2 = P_\theta[Z < -\epsilon] > 0;$$

then, for $t > 0$, $M_\theta(t) = E_\theta\{e^{tZ}\} \geq P_1 e^{t\epsilon}$. Similarly, for $t < 0$, $M_\theta(t) \geq P_2 e^{-t\epsilon}$. This proves that $\lim_{|t|\to\infty} M_\theta(t) = \infty$. Moreover, for all t for which $M(t)$ exists

$$\frac{d}{dt}M_\theta(t) = E_\theta\{Ze^{tZ}\}, \quad \frac{d^2}{dt^2}M_\theta(t) = E_\theta\{Z^2 e^{tZ}\} > 0. \tag{10.1.26}$$

Thus, we deduce that the m.g.f. $M_\theta(t)$ is a strictly convex function of t. The expectation μ_θ is $M'_\theta(0)$. Hence, if $\mu_\theta > 0$, then $M_\theta(t)$ attains its unique minimum at a negative value t^* and $M_\theta(t^*) < 1$. Furthermore, there exists a value t_0, $-\infty < t_0 < t^* < 0$, at which $M_\theta(t_0) = 1$. Similarly, if $\mu_\theta < 0$, there exist positive values t^* and t^0, $0 < t^* < t^0 < \infty$, such that $M_\theta(t^*) < 1$ and $M_\theta(t^0) = 1$. In both cases t^* and t_0 are unique.

The fundamental identity can be applied to obtain an approximation for the acceptance probability $\pi(\theta)$ of the SPRT with boundaries A' and B'. According to the fundamental identity

$$\pi(\theta)E_\theta\{e^{t_0(\theta)S_N} \mid S_N \leq A'\} + (1-\pi(\theta))E_\theta\{e^{t_0(\theta)S_N} \mid S_N \geq B'\} = 1, \tag{10.1.27}$$

where $t_0(\theta) \neq 0$ is the point at which $M_\theta(t) = 1$. The approximation for π_θ is obtained by substituting

$$E_\theta\{e^{t_0(\theta)S_N} \mid S_N \leq A'\} \cong e^{t_0(\theta)A'} = \left(\frac{\beta}{1-\alpha}\right)^{t_0(\theta)}$$

and

$$E_\theta\{e^{t_0(\theta)S_N} \mid S_N \geq B'\} \cong \left(\frac{1-\beta}{\alpha}\right)^{t_0(\theta)}.$$

This approximation yields the formula

$$\pi(\theta) \cong \frac{\left(\frac{1-\beta}{\alpha}\right)^{t_0(\theta)} - 1}{\left(\frac{1-\beta}{\alpha}\right)^{t_0(\theta)} - \left(\frac{\beta}{1-\alpha}\right)^{t_0(\theta)}} \tag{10.1.28}$$

for all θ such that $\mu_\theta \neq 0$. If $\mu_{\theta_0} = 0$, then

$$\pi(\theta_0) \cong \frac{\log\frac{1-\beta}{\alpha}}{\log\frac{1-\beta}{\alpha} - \log\frac{\beta}{1-\alpha}}. \tag{10.1.29}$$

The approximation for $E_\theta\{N\}$ given by (10.1.13) is inapplicable at θ_0. However, at θ_0 Wald's lemma yields the result

$$E_{\theta_0}\{S_N^2\} = E_{\theta_0}\{N\}E_{\theta_0}\{Z^2\}. \tag{10.1.30}$$

From this for θ_0 we obtain

$$E_{\theta_0}\{N\} = \frac{\pi(\theta_0)\left(\log\dfrac{\beta}{1-\alpha}\right)^2 + (1-\pi(\theta_0))\left(\log\dfrac{1-\beta}{\alpha}\right)^2}{E_{\theta_0}\{Z^2\}}. \tag{10.1.31}$$

■ EXAMPLE 10.1

Let $X_1, X_2, \ldots$ be a sequence of i.i.d. random variables having a common normal distribution $N(\theta, 1)$, $-\infty < \theta < \infty$. Suppose that for testing the hypothesis $H_0 : \theta \le 0$ against $H_1 : \theta \ge 1$ we construct the Wald SPRT of the two simple hypotheses $H_0^* : \theta = 0$ against $H_1^* : \theta = 1$ with boundaries A' and B' corresponding to $\alpha = 0.05$ and $\beta = 0.05$.

Notice that

$$Z = \log\frac{f_1(X)}{f_0(X)} = -\frac{1}{2}[(X-1)^2 - X^2] = X - \frac{1}{2}.$$

Accordingly

$$\mu_\theta = E_\theta\left\{X - \frac{1}{2}\right\} = \theta - \frac{1}{2}.$$

The m.g.f. of Z at θ is

$$M_\theta(t) = E_\theta\{e^{t(X-1/2)}\} = \exp\left\{\frac{1}{2}t^2 + \left(\theta - \frac{1}{2}\right)t\right\}.$$

Thus, $t_0(\theta) = 1 - 2\theta$, and from (10.1.28) and (10.1.31) the acceptance probabilities are

$$\pi(\theta) \cong \begin{cases} \dfrac{19^{1-2\theta} - 1}{19^{1-2\theta} - 19^{2\theta-1}}, & \theta \ne 0.5, \\ 0.5 & \theta = 0.5. \end{cases}$$

In Table 10.1 we present some of the π_θ and $E_\theta\{N\}$ values determined according to the approximations (10.1.11), (10.1.26), and (10.1.31).

Table 10.1: Operating Characteristics of the SPRT, $\theta_0 = 0$, $\theta_1 = 1$, $\alpha = \beta = 0.05$

θ	$\pi(\theta)$	$E_\theta\{N\}$
−1.00	0.99985	2.0
−0.50	0.99724	2.9
0.00	0.95000	5.3
0.25	0.81339	7.4
0.50	0.50000	8.7
0.75	0.18661	7.4
1.00	0.05000	5.3
1.50	0.00276	2.9

■

In the above example we have illustrated the use of the Wald SPRT for testing two composite hypotheses when the interval Θ_0 corresponding to H_0 is separated from the interval Θ_1 of H_1. We obtained a test procedure with very desirable properties by constructing the SPRT for two simple hypotheses since the family $\mathcal{F}$ of distribution functions under consideration is MLR. For such families we obtain a monotone $\pi(\theta)$ function with acceptance probability greater than $1 - \alpha$ for all $\theta < \theta_0$ and $\pi(\theta) < \beta$ for all $\theta > \theta_1$ (Ghosh, 1970, pp. 100–103). The function $\pi(\theta)$ is called the *operating characteristic* (O.C.) function of the SPRT. The expected sample size function $E_\theta\{N\}$ is increasing to a maximum between θ_0 and θ_1 and then decreases to zero again. At $\theta = \theta_0$ and at $\theta = \theta_1$ the function $E_\theta\{N\}$ assumes the smallest values corresponding to all possible test procedures with error probabilities not exceeding α and β. This is the optimality property of the Wald SPRT. We state this property more precisely in the following theorem.

Theorem 10.1.3 (Wald and Wolfowitz) *Consider any SPRT for testing the two simple hypotheses $H_0 : \theta = \theta_0$ against $H_1 : \theta = \theta_1$ with boundary points (A, B) and error probabilities α and β. Let $E_{\theta_i}\{N\}$, $i = 0, 1$, be the expected sample size. If s is any sampling procedure for testing H_0 against H_1 with error probabilities $\alpha(s)$ and $\beta(s)$ and finite expected sample size $E_{\theta_i}\{N(s)\}$ $(i = 0, 1)$, then, $\alpha(s) \leq \alpha$ and $\beta(s) \leq \beta$ imply that $E_{\theta_i}\{N\} \leq E_{\theta_i}\{N(s)\}$ for $i = 0, 1$.* ■

For the proof of this important theorem see Ghosh (1970, pp. 93–98) and Siegmund (1985, p. 19).

Although the Wald SPRT is optimal at θ_0 and at θ_1 in the above sense, if the actual θ is between θ_0 and θ_1, even in the MLR case, the expected sample size may be quite large. Several papers were written on this subject and more general sequential procedures were investigated in order to obtain procedures with error probabilities not exceeding α and β at θ_0 and θ_1 and expected sample size at $\theta_0 < \theta < \theta_1$ smaller than that of the SPRT. Kiefer and Weiss (1957) studied the problem of determining a sequential test which, subject to the above constraint on the error probabilities, minimizes the maximal expected sample size. They have shown that such a test is a generalized version of an SPRT. The same problem was studied by Lai (1973) for normally distributed random variables using the theory of optimal stopping rules. Lai developed a method of determining the boundaries $\{(A_n, B_n), n \geq 1\}$ of the sequential test which minimizes the maximal expected sample size. We remark in conclusion that many of the results of the present section can be obtained in a more elegant fashion by using the general theory of optimal stopping rules. The reader is referred in particular to the book of Chow, Robbins, and Siegmund (1971). For a comparison of the asymptotic relative efficiency of sequential and nonsequential tests of composite hypotheses see Berk (1973, 1975). A comparison of the asymptotic properties of various sequential tests (on the means of normal distributions) which combines both the Type I error probability and the expected sample size has been provided by Berk (1976). The reader is referred also to the recent review paper of Lai (2001).

10.1.2 Exact Distributions of N in the Exponential Case

Suppose that $X_1, X_2, \ldots$ are i.i.d., having an exponential distribution with mean μ. We construct an SPRT for testing $H_0 : \mu \leq \mu_0$ versus $H_1 : \mu \geq \mu_1$, where $0 < \mu_0 < \mu_1 < \infty$. Let

$$\begin{aligned} Z &= \log \frac{\mu_0 \exp\{-X/\mu_1\}}{\mu_1 \exp\{-X/\mu_0\}} \\ &= \log\left(\frac{\mu_0}{\mu_1}\right) + \left(\frac{1}{\mu_0} - \frac{1}{\mu_1}\right) X. \end{aligned}$$

The SPRT stopping variable is

$$N = \min\{n \geq 1 : S_n \geq a_2 + bn, \quad \text{or} \quad S_n \leq -a_1 + bn\}, \tag{10.1.32}$$

where

$$\begin{aligned} a_1 &= \frac{\mu_0\mu_1 \log\left(\dfrac{1-\alpha}{\beta}\right)}{\mu_1 - \mu_0}, \\ a_2 &= \frac{\mu_0\mu_1 \log\left(\dfrac{1-\beta}{\alpha}\right)}{\mu_1 - \mu_0}, \\ b &= \frac{\mu_0\mu_1 \log\left(\dfrac{\mu_1}{\mu_0}\right)}{\mu_1 - \mu_0}, \end{aligned} \tag{10.1.33}$$

and $S_n = \sum_{i=1}^{n} X_i$.

We develop here the exact distribution of N when the distribution of the X's has mean μ by considering a Poisson process $\{N(t), t \geq 0\}$ with intensity $\lambda = 1/\mu$. The times between jumps (the interarrival times) are i.i.d. exponential with mean μ. For this Poisson process, define the stopping times

$$T_L = \inf\left\{t > 0 : N(t) = -\frac{a_2}{b} + \frac{1}{b}t\right\} \tag{10.1.34}$$

and

$$T_U = \inf\left\{t > 0 : N(t) \geq \frac{a_1}{b} + \frac{1}{b}t\right\}. \tag{10.1.35}$$

Furthermore, let $T = \min\{T_L, T_U\}$. The stopping variable N, given by (10.1.32), is equal to $N(T) + 1$. Notice that

$$\begin{aligned} N(T) &= I\{T = T_L\}\left(-\frac{a_2}{b} + \frac{1}{b}T_L\right) \\ &+ I\{T = T_U\}\left(\left\lfloor \frac{a_1}{b} + \frac{1}{b}T_U\right\rfloor + 1\right), \end{aligned} \tag{10.1.36}$$

where $\lfloor x \rfloor$ designates the largest integer smaller than x. Thus, the distribution of N can be determined from the distribution of T.

Let $t' = t/b$ and $\lambda' = \lambda b$. Let $\{N(t'), t' \geq 0\}$ be a Poisson process with intensity λ'. Let

$$T'_L = \inf\{t' > 0 : N(t') = -\gamma_2 + t'\} \tag{10.1.37}$$

and

$$T'_U = \inf\{t' > 0 : N(t') \geq \gamma_1 + t'\}, \tag{10.1.38}$$

where $\gamma_2 = a_2/b$ and $\gamma_1 = a_1/b$. Accordingly, $T_L = bT'_L$ and $T_U = bT'_U$. Thus, $T = b\min(T'_L, T'_U)$. Zacks (1991b) developed the exact distributions of T'_L and T'_U and of $T' = \min(T'_L, T'_U)$. Here T'_L is a discrete random variable assuming with positive probabilities the values $t'_l = \gamma_2 + l$, $l = 0, 1, \ldots$.

Let $\psi_L(l; \gamma_2) = P\{T'_L = t_l\}$. Obviously, $\psi_L(0; \gamma_2) = e^{-\eta\gamma_2}$, where $\eta = \lambda'$. Moreover, for $l \geq 1$

$$\psi_L(l; \gamma_2) = p(l; \eta t_l) - \sum_{i=0}^{l-1} \psi_L(i; \gamma_2) p(l - i; \eta(l - i)), \tag{10.1.39}$$

where $p(l; \xi)$ is the Poisson p.d.f.

For $|\theta| < 1$, define the generating functions

$$\psi_L^*(\theta; \gamma_2) = \sum_{l=0}^{\infty} \theta^l \psi_L(l; \gamma_2) \tag{10.1.40}$$

and

$$P^*(\theta; \gamma_2) = \sum_{l=0}^{\infty} \theta^l p(l; (\gamma_2 + l)\eta). \tag{10.1.41}$$

From (10.1.39) we obtain the equation

$$\psi_L^*(\theta; \gamma_2) = P^*(\theta; \gamma_2) - \psi_L^*(\theta; \gamma_2) \cdot (P^*(\theta; 0) - 1). \tag{10.1.42}$$

This implies that

$$\psi_L^*(\theta; \gamma_2) = \frac{P^*(\theta; \gamma_2)}{P^*(\theta; 0)}. \tag{10.1.43}$$

Notice that $P^*(\theta; 0) = 1 + p(1; \eta)\theta + p(2; 2\eta)\theta^2 + \cdots$. Accordingly $(P^*(\theta, 0))^{-1} = \sum_{j=0}^{\infty} c_j \theta^j$, where, as shown in Zacks (1991b), $c_0 = 1$ and, for $j \geq 1$,

$$c_j = -\sum_{k=0}^{j-1} c_k p(j-k; (j-k)\eta). \tag{10.1.44}$$

Finally, from (10.1.43) we obtain that

$$\psi_L(l; \gamma_2) = \sum_{j=0}^{l} c_j p(l-j; (l-j+\gamma_2)\eta). \tag{10.1.45}$$

We develop now the distribution of T'_U. Let

$$g(j; t, \gamma_1) = P\{N(t) = j, T'_U > t\}. \tag{10.1.46}$$

Notice that

$$P\{T'_U > t\} = \sum_{j=0}^{\lfloor \gamma_1 + t \rfloor} g(j; t, \gamma - 1). \tag{10.1.47}$$

We derive the function $g(j; t, \gamma_1)$. First, for $j \leq \gamma_1$, $g(j; t, \gamma_1) = p(j; \eta t)$. Moreover, $g(j; t, \gamma_1) = 0$ if $j \geq t + \gamma_1$. For $\gamma_1 < j < \gamma_1 + t$,

(10.1.48)

$$g(j; j-\gamma_1+t, \gamma_1) = p(j; (j-\gamma_1+t)\eta) - \sum_{i=\lfloor \gamma_1 \rfloor + 1}^{j} p(i; (i-\gamma_1)\eta) g(j-i; j-i+t, 0).$$

This equation is obtained by conditioning on the level at which the process enters the region below the upper boundary for the last time. We have to obtain an explicit expression for $g(j; j+t, 0)$. Let $G(\theta; t) = \sum_{j=0}^{\infty} \theta^j g(j; j+t, 0)$ and $P(\theta; t) = \sum_{j=0}^{\infty} \theta^j p(j; (j+t)\eta)$ for $|\theta| < 1$; then by substituting $\gamma_1 = 0$ in (10.1.48) we obtain, after multiplying by θ^j and summing,

$$G(\theta; t) = P(\theta; t) - G(\theta; t)(P(\theta; 0) - 1) \tag{10.1.49}$$

or

(10.1.50)
$$G(\theta; t) = \frac{P(\theta; t)}{P(\theta; 0)}.$$

From this equation we obtain that

(10.1.51)
$$g(j; j+t, 0) = \sum_{i=0}^{j} c_i p(j-i; (j-i+t)\eta)$$

for all $j \geq 0$, where c_i are given in (10.1.44).

Thus, the tail probability of T'_U is

(10.1.52)
$$\begin{aligned} P(T'_U > t) &= \sum_{j=0}^{\lfloor t+\gamma_1 \rfloor} g(j; t, \gamma_1) \\ &= P(\lfloor t+\gamma_1 \rfloor; t\eta) - I(t > 1) \sum_{j=\lfloor \gamma_1 \rfloor+1}^{\lfloor t+\gamma_1 \rfloor} \sum_{i=\lfloor \gamma_1 \rfloor+1}^{j} p(i; (i-\gamma_1)\eta) \\ &\quad \cdot \sum_{l=0}^{j-i} c_l p(j-i-l; (t-i-l+\gamma_1)\cdot\eta), \end{aligned}$$

where $P(\cdot; \cdot)$ designates the c.d.f. of a Poisson distribution. For the distribution of N we need to compute $\psi_U(n; \gamma_1) = P\{n-1-\gamma_1 < T'_U \leq n-\gamma_1\}$. For this, we start, for $n > \gamma_1$, with

(10.1.53)
$$\begin{aligned} P\{T'_U > n-\gamma_1\} &= \sum_{j=0}^{n-1} g(j; n-\gamma_1, \gamma_1) \\ &= P(n-1; (n-\gamma_1)\eta) \\ &\quad - \sum_{j=\lfloor \gamma_1 \rfloor+1}^{n-1} \sum_{i=\lfloor \gamma_1 \rfloor+1}^{j} p(i; (i-\gamma_1)\eta) g(j-i; n-i, 0) \\ &= P(n-1; (n-\gamma_1)\eta) \\ &\quad - \sum_{i=\lfloor \gamma_1 \rfloor+1}^{n-1} p(i; (i-\gamma_1)\eta) \sum_{l=0}^{n-1-i} c_l \sum_{j=0}^{n-1-i-l} p(j; (j+n-i)\eta). \end{aligned}$$

Using this formula we compute, for $n > \gamma_1 + 1$,

(10.1.54)
$$\psi_U(n; \gamma_1) = P(T'_U > n-1-\gamma_1) - P(T'_U > n-\gamma_1).$$

Finally,

(10.1.55)

$$P\{N(T')=n\} = I\{n \le \gamma_1\}\psi_L(n;\gamma_2) + I\{n > \gamma_1\} \cdot [\psi_L(n;\gamma_2) + \psi_U(n;\gamma_1) - \sum_{i=\lfloor\gamma_1\rfloor+1}^{n} \psi_U(i;\gamma_1)g(n-i;\gamma_1+\gamma_2+n-i,0)].$$

For example we consider the following testing problem.

Let $X_1, X_2, \ldots$ be a sequence of i.i.d. random variables having an exponential distribution with mean μ. We have to test $H_0 : \mu \le 1$ versus $H_1 : \mu \ge 2$ with equal error probabilities $\alpha = \beta = 0.05$. Let $S_n = \sum_{i=1}^{n} X_i$. The SPRT boundaries with A' and B' are $\bar{B}_n = a_2 + bn$ and $\underline{B}_n = -a_1 + bn$, where $a_1 = a_2 = 5.889$ and $b = 1.3863$. For the Poisson process we have linear boundaries with intercepts $\gamma_1 = \gamma_2 = a_1/b = 4.248$. The slope of these lines is $1/b = 0.7213$. Thus we consider the stopping times T'_L and T'_U with Poisson intensity $\eta = 1.3863\lambda$, where $\lambda = 1/\mu$. The exact distribution of $N(T') + 1$ was computed according to (10.1.55) (see SPLUS function distNexp). In Table 10.2 we present the c.d.f. of $N(T') + 1$.

Table 10.2: Distribution of $\mathbf{N = N(T') + 1}$ in the Exponential Case with $\boldsymbol{\lambda = 1, \alpha = \beta = 0.05, \mu_0 = 1, \mu_1 = 2}$

n	$P\{N \le n\}$	n	$P\{N \le n\}$
1	0.0028	15	0.6250
2	0.0068	20	0.7715
3	0.0112	25	0.8631
4	0.0155	30	0.9226
5	0.0238	35	0.9620
6	0.0884	40	0.9887
7	0.1637	45	1.0000
8	0.2410	50	1.0000
9	0.3137		
10	0.3801		

Derived with program distNexp.

The expected value of N is $E_1\{N\} = 16.11$. A simulation of 1000 runs yields an empirical distribution very close to the exact distribution with mean $\bar{N} = 15.72 \pm 0.589$. The Wald approximation (10.1.13) is 13.72.

10.2 CHARACTERISTICS OF SEQUENTIAL PROCEDURES IN RELIABILITY ESTIMATION AND TESTING

10.2.1 Reliability Estimation

The material of the present section is based on the article of Zacks (2001). We consider a system whose life distribution is exponential with mean time between failures (MTBF) θ. The reliability function of this system is $R(t;\theta) = \exp(-t/\theta)$. The parameter θ is unknown, and we wish to estimate $R(t;\theta)$ by sequential experiment. Let $\rho(\theta) = R(1;\theta)$ and let $\hat{\rho}_n$ be an estimator of $\rho(\theta)$. For specified values of $0 < \gamma$, $\delta < 1$ we say that $\hat{\rho}_n$ has a *prescribed proportional closeness* (δ, γ) if

$$P_\theta\{|\hat{\rho}_n - \rho(\theta)| < \delta\rho(\theta)\} \geq \gamma \tag{10.2.1}$$

for *all* θ, $0 < \theta < \infty$.

The MLE of $\rho(\theta)$ is $\hat{\rho}_n = \exp(-1/\bar{X}_n)$, where $\bar{X}_n = (1/n)\sum_{i=1}^n X_i$. The asymptotic distribution of this MLE is normal with mean $\rho(\theta)$ and variance $\rho^2(\theta)/\theta^2 n$. Thus, for large values of n, the proportional closeness of the MLE is approximately $2\Phi(\sqrt{n}\ \delta\theta) - 1$. Define

$$n^0(\delta) = \frac{\chi^2_\gamma[1]}{\theta^2\delta^2}. \tag{10.2.2}$$

If $n \geq n^0(\delta)$, for small values of δ, the proportional closeness of $\hat{\rho}_n$ is approximately γ. Equation (10.2.2) leads to the stopping variable

$$N(\delta) = \min\left\{n \geq k : n \geq \frac{\chi^2_\gamma[1]}{\delta^2 \bar{X}^2_n}\right\}. \tag{10.2.3}$$

The asymptotic properties of $N(\delta)$ and of $\hat{\rho}_{N(\delta)}$ are well known. In the present section we derive the exact distribution of $N(\delta)$ and the exact value of the proportional closeness of $\hat{\rho}_{N(\delta)}$. As in the previous section, let $\{N(t), t \geq 0\}$ denote a Poisson process with intensity $\lambda = 1/\theta$. Since S_n represents the time until the nth failure, replacing $\bar{X}^2_n$ by $t^2/N^2(t)$ and n by $N(t)$ in (10.2.3), we obtain the corresponding stopping time

$$T(\delta) = \inf\left\{t \geq t_k : N(t) \leq \frac{\delta^2}{\chi^2_\gamma[1]} t^2\right\}, \tag{10.2.4}$$

where, for $l \geq k$,

$$t_l = \frac{(\chi^2_\gamma[1])^{1/2}}{\delta}\sqrt{l}. \tag{10.2.5}$$

Let $\lambda^* = \lambda(\chi^2_\gamma[1])^{1/2}/\delta$. Then

$$\begin{aligned} P\{N(\delta) = k\} &= P\{T(\delta) = t_k\} \\ &= P\{k; \lambda^*\sqrt{k}\}. \end{aligned} \tag{10.2.6}$$

Let $\psi_T^{(\lambda)}(l) = P_\lambda\{T(\delta) = t_l\}$, $l \geq k$. For $l > k$ we have

$$\psi_T^{(\lambda)}(l) = p(l; x^*\sqrt{l}) - \sum_{j=0}^{k} p(j; \lambda^*\sqrt{k}) p(l-j; \lambda^*(\sqrt{l} - \sqrt{k})) \tag{10.2.7}$$
$$- I(l \geq k+2) \sum_{i=k+1}^{l-1} \psi_T^{(\lambda)}(i) p(l-i; \lambda^*(\sqrt{l} - \sqrt{i})).$$

The values of $\psi_T^{(\lambda)}(l)$, $l \geq k$, are determined from (10.2.6) and (10.2.7) recursively. Notice also that $P_\lambda\{N(\delta) = l\} = \psi_T^{(\lambda)}(l)$, $l \geq k$. Furthermore, moments of $N(\delta)$ are given by

$$M_m(\theta) = \sum_{l=k}^{\infty} l^m \psi_T^{(\lambda)}(l), \quad m \geq 0. \tag{10.2.8}$$

Notice that $P\{N(\delta) < \infty\} = 1$ for all λ since the boundary is parabolic. Hence, $M_0(\theta) = 1$ for all θ.

In Table 10.3 we present some results concerning the distribution of $N(\delta)$. We denote by STD and by Me the standard deviation and the median of $N(\delta)$, respectively.

Table 10.3: Characteristics of $\mathbf{N(\delta)}$, for $\delta = 0.1$, $\gamma = 0.9$

θ	$n^0(\delta)$	k	$E_\theta\{N(\delta)\}$	STD	Me
2	67.65	20	64.01	18.325	66
3	30.06	10	29.02	10.938	29
4	16.91	3	15.64	8.312	15
5	10.82	3	10.04	6.101	9
6	7.52	3	7.26	4.585	3

We see in this table that $E_\theta\{N(\delta)\}$ is generally smaller than the required $n^0(\delta)$. This implies that the proportional closeness of $\hat{\rho}_{N(\delta)}$ when $\theta \leq 4$ is lower than $\gamma = 0.9$. To compute it we remark first that the proportional closeness interval at stopping is

$$\text{PCI} = \left(\frac{\hat{\rho}_{N(\delta)}}{1+\delta}, \frac{\hat{\rho}_{N(\delta)}}{1-\delta} \right). \tag{10.2.9}$$

The proportional closeness probability of this interval is

$$\text{CP}(\delta, \theta) = \sum_{l=k}^{\infty} \psi_T^{(\lambda)}(l) I\{l^*(\theta) < l \leq l^{**}(\theta)\}, \tag{10.2.10}$$

where

$$l^*(\theta) = n^0(\delta)(\max(0, 1 - \theta \log(1+\delta))^2 \tag{10.2.11}$$

and

$$l^{**}(\theta) = n^0(\delta)(1 - \theta\log(1-\delta))^2. \tag{10.2.12}$$

In Table 10.4 we present the values of $\text{CP}(\delta, \theta)$ for the case of Table 10.2.

Table 10.4: Proportional Closeness Probabilities for $\delta = 0.1$, $\gamma = 0.9$

θ	k	$\text{CP}(\delta,\theta)$
2	20	0.8919
3	10	0.8780
4	3	0.8498
5	3	0.9843
6	3	0.9876

One can reduce the expected duration of the trial by having m *independent* systems operate in parallel. Whenever a system fails, it is immediately replaced by an identical system. Let $\{N^{(i)}(t), t \geq 0\}$ be the Poisson counting process for the ith system and $N_m(t) = \sum_{i=1}^{m} N^{(i)}(t)$. The boundary function is defined as

$$B_m(t) = \frac{m^2\delta^2}{\chi^2_\gamma[1]}t^2, \quad t \geq 0. \tag{10.2.13}$$

The corresponding stopping time is

$$T_m(\delta) = \inf\{t \geq t_k^{(m)} : N_m(t) \leq B_m(t)\}, \tag{10.2.14}$$

where

$$t_k^{(m)} = \frac{1}{m}t_k = \frac{\sqrt{\chi^2_\gamma[1]}}{m\delta}\sqrt{k}. \tag{10.2.15}$$

Moreover, $T_m(\delta) = (1/m)T(\delta)$. Let $N^{(m)}(\delta) = N_m(T_m(\delta))$. The estimator of $\rho(\theta)$ at stopping is

$$\hat{\rho}_{N^m(\delta)} = \exp\left(-\frac{N^{(m)}(\delta)}{mT_m(\delta)}\right). \tag{10.2.16}$$

Moreover, for $l \geq k$

$$\begin{aligned} \psi_{T,m}^{(\lambda)}(l) &= P_\lambda(N_m(\delta) = l) \\ &= P_\lambda(N(\delta) = l) \\ &= \psi_T^{(\lambda)}(l). \end{aligned} \tag{10.2.17}$$

If failed systems are not replaced, we can still use the stopping time $T_m(\delta)$. However, the functions $\psi_{T,m}^{(\lambda)}(l)$ have different formulas. Let $b(j;n,p)$ and $B(j;n,p)$ denote, respectively, the p.d.f. and c.d.f. of the binomial distribution $B(n,p)$. We obtain the following recursive equations:

$$\psi_{b,m}^{(\lambda)}(k) = B(k;m,1-e^{-\lambda_m^*\sqrt{k}}), \tag{10.2.18}$$

where $\lambda_m^* = \lambda^*/m$, and for $l > k$,

$$\begin{aligned} \psi_{b,m}^{(\lambda)}(l) &= b(l;m,1-e^{-\lambda_m^*\sqrt{l}}) - \sum_{j=0}^{k} b(j;m,1-e^{-\lambda_m^*\sqrt{k}}) \\ &\quad \cdot b(l-j;m-j,1-e^{-\lambda_m^*(\sqrt{l}-\sqrt{k})}) - I(l \geq k+2) \\ &\quad \cdot \sum_{j=k+1}^{l-1} \psi_{b,m}^{(\lambda)}(j) b(l-j;m-j,1-e^{-\lambda_m^*(\sqrt{l}-\sqrt{j})}). \end{aligned} \tag{10.2.19}$$

Notice that m should be greater than k. In Table 10.5 we present $E_\theta\{T_m(\delta)\}$ and $CP(\delta,\theta)$ when systems are not replaced.

Table 10.5: Expected Value and Coverage Probability of $\mathbf{T_m(\delta)}$, No Replacement, $\boldsymbol{\delta = 0.1}$, $\boldsymbol{\gamma = 0.9}$

θ	k	m	$E_\theta\{T_m(\delta)\}$	CP(δ,θ)
2	20	300	0.401	0.8080
3	10	100	0.767	0.8356
4	3	40	1.323	0.8292
5	2	10	3.512	1.000
6	1	5	5.165	1.000

To achieve high coverage probability one has to pay either by a large number m of system tested or by long duration of the test.

10.2.2 Reliability Testing

Sequential testing is an important procedure in system development and in reliability demonstration. Again, we focus attention on systems whose life distribution is exponential with MTBF θ. The objective is to test systems sequentially to demonstrate that $\theta \geq \theta_1$. Systems with $\theta \leq \theta_0$ are rejected (modified) while systems with $\theta \geq \theta_1$ are accepted. As in Section 10.1.2, consider a Poisson process $\{N(t), t \geq 0\}$ with intensity $\lambda = 1/\theta$. If the number of failures is relatively small, that is, $\lambda \leq 1/\theta_1$, we wish to terminate the test early. Also, if $N(t)$ crosses a constant k_2, we terminate and reject. Thus, the continuation region for $\{N(t), t \geq 0\}$ is bounded by

$$\begin{aligned} B_L(t) &= -k_1 + t, \\ B_U(t) &= k_2. \end{aligned} \tag{10.2.20}$$

The corresponding stopping time is

(10.2.21) $$T = \inf\{t > 0 : N(t) = -k_1(t) \text{ or } N(t) = k_2\}.$$

Notice that $T \le k_1 + k_2$. If $N(T) = -k_1 + T$, then the system is accepted ($H_0 : \lambda \le 1/\theta_1$ is accepted). If $N(T) = k_2$ the system is rejected. For $0 \le l < k_2$, let $\psi_L^{(\lambda)}(l) = P_\lambda\{N(T) = l\}$. The values of $\psi_L^{(\lambda)}(l)$ are obtained according to (10.1.45) with $\eta = \lambda$ and $\gamma_2 = k_1$. Thus, the probability of accepting H_0 is $\pi_\lambda = \sum_{l=0}^{k_2-1} \psi_L^{(\lambda)}(l)$ and $P_\lambda\{N(T) = k_2\} = 1 - \pi_\lambda$. The c.d.f. of T is

(10.2.22)
$$\begin{aligned} P_\lambda(T \le t) &= 1 - P(k_2 - 1; \lambda t) \\ &\quad + I\{t > k_1\} \sum_{j=0}^{[t-k_1]} \psi_L^{(\lambda)}(j) P(k_2 - 1 - j; \lambda(t - k_1 - j)). \end{aligned}$$

From this we get that

(10.2.23)
$$\begin{aligned} E_\lambda\{T\} &= \int_0^{k_1+k_2-1} P_\lambda\{T > t\}\, dt \\ &= \frac{k_2}{\lambda}(1 - P(k_2; \lambda(k_1 + k_2 - 1))) \\ &\quad + \sum_{j=0}^{k_2-1} (k_1 + j)\psi_L^{(\lambda)}(j) P(k_2 - j - 1; \lambda(k_2 - j)) \\ &\quad - \frac{1}{\lambda} \sum_{j=0}^{k_2-1} (k_2 - j)\psi_L^{(\lambda)}(j)(1 - P(k_2 - j; \lambda(k_2 - j))). \end{aligned}$$

In Table 10.6 we present the values of π_λ, $E_\lambda\{T\}$, and the median $T_{0.5}$ for testing $H_0 : \lambda \le 0.8$ versus $H_1 : \lambda \ge 1.6$ with $k_1 = 3$ and $k_2 = 42$. We see that $\alpha = 1 - \pi_{0.8} = 0.0594$ and $\beta = \pi_{1.6} = 0.0459$. Also, $E_{0.8}\{T\} = 11.65$ and $E_{1.6}\{T\} = 25.11$.

Table 10.6: Values of π_λ, $E_\lambda\{T\}$, and $T_{0.5}$ for $k_1 = 3$, $k_2 = 42$

λ	π_λ	$E_\lambda\{T\}$	$T_{0.5}$
0.5	0.9999	6.00	4.50
0.6	0.9989	7.42	5.50
0.7	0.9885	9.31	6.50
0.8	0.9406	11.65	7.50
0.9	0.8237	14.85	12.50
1.0	0.6456	19.10	20.50
1.1	0.4552	23.19	29.50
1.2	0.2974	25.89	30.00
1.3	0.1867	26.95	28.90
1.4	0.1159	26.85	27.60
1.5	0.0725	26.12	26.09
1.6	0.0459	25.11	24.63
1.7	0.0294	24.01	23.26
1.8	0.0192	22.90	22.00
1.9	0.0126	21.83	20.85
2.0	0.0084	20.82	18.80

10.2.3 Total Operating Time of Repairable System

Consider a system that can be repaired after a failure and return it to its original state after repair. Let $T_1, T_2, \ldots$ denote the random operation (life) times of the system. We assume that these are i.i.d. random variables with a common distribution F. Let $R_1, R_2, \ldots$ denote the repair times, which are i.i.d. random variables with distribution G. We have an alternating renewal process.

For $0 < t < \infty$, let $N_F(t)$ denote the number of system failures in the time interval $(0, t]$. This is given by

$$N_F(t) = I\{T_1 < t\} \max(n : n \geq 1 : \sum_{j=0}^{n-1} c_j + T_n < t\}, \tag{10.2.24}$$

where $c_j = T_j + R_j$, $j = 1, 2, \ldots$ and $c_0 \equiv 0$. For $0 < s \leq t$ define the compound process

$$X(s) = s + \sum_{n=0}^{N_F(s)} R_n, \tag{10.2.25}$$

where $R_0 \equiv 0$. Accordingly, the total operation time in $(0, t)$ is

$$W(t) = \inf\{s > 0 : X(s) \geq t\}, \quad t > 0. \tag{10.2.26}$$

Notice that $X(W(t)) = t$ if the system is operating at time t and $X(W(t)) > t$ if the system is being repaired at time t. Obviously, $0 < W(t) \leq t$. The distribution of $W(t)$ has a jump at t, that is,

$$P\{W(t) = t\} = P\{T_1 > t\}. \tag{10.2.27}$$

For $0 < s < t$,

$$P\{W(t) > s\} = \sum_{n=0}^{\infty}(F^{(n)}(s) - F^{(n+1)}(s))G^{(n)}(t-s), \tag{10.2.28}$$

where $F^{(n)}$ and $G^{(n)}$ are the n-fold convolutions of F and G, respectively. In the special case where $F(s) = 1 - e^{-\lambda s}$ and $G(s) = 1 - e^{-\mu s}$, the p.d.f. of $W(t)$ on $(0, t)$ is given by

$$\psi(s;t) = \sum_{n=0}^{\infty} p(n; \mu(t-s))[\mu p(n+1; \lambda s) + \lambda p(n; \lambda s)]. \tag{10.2.29}$$

To verify (10.2.29) substitute in (10.2.28)

$$F^{(n)}(s) - F^{(n+1)}(s) = p(n; \lambda s) \tag{10.2.30}$$

and

$$G^{(n)}(t-s) = 1 - P(n-1; \mu(t-s)). \tag{10.2.31}$$

After that differentiate with respect to s and multiply by -1. Moreover, for $s < t$,

$$P\{W(t) > s\} = \sum_{n=0}^{\infty} p(n; \mu(t-s)) \cdot P(n; \lambda s). \tag{10.2.32}$$

The expected value of $W(t)$ is

$$E\{W(t)\} = \frac{\lambda}{(\lambda+\mu)^2} + \frac{\mu t}{\lambda+\mu} + te^{-\lambda t} - \frac{\lambda}{(\lambda+\mu)^2}e^{-(\lambda+\mu)t}. \tag{10.2.33}$$

Notice that

$$\lim_{t\to\infty} \frac{1}{t} E\{W(t)\} = \frac{\mu}{\lambda+\mu}. \tag{10.2.34}$$

This is a well-known asymptotic result. For more details see Perry, Stadje, and Zacks (1999).

10.3 SOME COMMENTS ON SEQUENTIAL DESIGN OF EXPERIMENTS

In Chapters 3, 6, and 7 we discussed several sequential designs for estimating a quantile of a tolerance distribution. These are designs for generalized linear models. Often the optimal designs depend on unknown parameter(s) and one has to perform stage-wise adaptive or sequential designs to approximate the optimal design. Lindley (1956) suggested the following approach within a Bayesian framework. For a general review of this approach see Chaloner and Verdinelli (1995). We focus attention on a specific recommendation. Let $\mathcal{X}$ be a space of possible design points $\mathbf{x}$ which could be real or vector-valued or even categorical-valued factors. Let $Y_{\mathbf{x}}$ be a response random variable (vector) associated with the design point $\mathbf{x}$. Let $f(y; \boldsymbol{\theta}, \mathbf{x})$ denote the p.d.f. of $Y_{\mathbf{x}}$. This might depend on a parameter $\boldsymbol{\theta}$ belonging to a parameter space Θ. Let $h(\theta)$ be a prior p.d.f. of $\boldsymbol{\theta}$ on Θ, and let

$$h(\boldsymbol{\theta} \mid y, \mathbf{x}) = \frac{f(y; \boldsymbol{\theta}, \mathbf{x}) h(\boldsymbol{\theta})}{\displaystyle\int_{\Theta} f(y; \boldsymbol{\theta}, \mathbf{x}) h(\boldsymbol{\theta}) d\lambda(\boldsymbol{\theta})} \tag{10.3.1}$$

be the posterior p.d.f. of θ given $(\mathbf{x}, Y_{\mathbf{x}})$.

Following Lindley, Stone (1959), DeGroot (1962, 1986), Bernardo (1979), Ben-Gal and Caramanis (2002), and others suggested to choose a design $\mathbf{x}$ which maximizes the predictive expectation of the Kullback–Leibler information to discriminate between $h(\boldsymbol{\theta} \mid y, \mathbf{x})$ and $h(\boldsymbol{\theta})$. More specifically, the Kullback–Leibler information is

$$\int_{\Theta} h(\boldsymbol{\theta} \mid y, \mathbf{x}) \log \frac{h(\boldsymbol{\theta} \mid y, \mathbf{x})}{h(\boldsymbol{\theta})} d\lambda(\boldsymbol{\theta}). \tag{10.3.2}$$

This depends on the observed value of Y_x. The predictive p.d.f. of Y_x is

$$f^*(y \mid \mathbf{x}) = \int_{\Theta} f(y; \boldsymbol{\theta}, \mathbf{x}) h(\boldsymbol{\theta})\, d\lambda(\boldsymbol{\theta}). \tag{10.3.3}$$

Thus, the function to maximize is

$$U(x) = \int_{y} \int_{\Theta} f(y; \boldsymbol{\theta}, \mathbf{x}) h(\boldsymbol{\theta}) \cdot \log \frac{h(\boldsymbol{\theta} \mid y, \mathbf{x})}{h(\boldsymbol{\theta})} d\lambda(\boldsymbol{\theta})\, d\mu\, d(y). \tag{10.3.4}$$

Here $\lambda(\boldsymbol{\theta})$ and $\mu(y)$ are corresponding sigma-finite measures.

As shown by Chaloner and Verdinelli (1995) and others, the criterion to maximize (10.3.4) works well in the normal linear regression case, that is, $\mathbf{Y} \mid \boldsymbol{\beta} \sim N((X)\boldsymbol{\beta}, \sigma^2 I)$, where (X) is an $n \times k$ design matrix of full rank and σ^2 is known. The prior distribution of $\boldsymbol{\beta}$ is normal, $N(\boldsymbol{\beta}_0, \sigma^2 R^{-1})$, where R is a known positive definite matrix. In this case, the posterior distribution of $\boldsymbol{\beta}$ is normal with mean

$$E\{\boldsymbol{\beta} \mid (X), Y\} = (R + (X)'(X))^{-1}(R\boldsymbol{\beta}_0 + (X)'Y) \tag{10.3.5}$$

and covariance matrix

$$\Sigma(\boldsymbol{\beta} \mid (X), Y) = \sigma^2((X)'(X) + R)^{-1}. \tag{10.3.6}$$

The function (10.3.4) becomes

$$U(X) = -\frac{k}{2}\log(2\pi) - \frac{k}{2} + \frac{1}{2}\log(\det((X)'(X) + R)\sigma^{-2}). \tag{10.3.7}$$

The optimal design is one maximizing $|(X)'(X) + R|$. This is known as Bayesian D-optimality. Assume (X) is an orthogonal array such that $(X)'(X) = mI$. Since R is a symmetric positive definite matrix, there exists an orthogonal matrix H such that $HRH' = \text{diag}(\lambda_i, i = 1, \ldots, k)$, where $\lambda_i > 0$ are the eigenvalues of R. Thus if (X) is an orthogonal array, then $|(X)'(X) + R| = \prod_{i=1}^{k}(\lambda_i + m)$. In most linear design problems, Bayesian and non-Bayesian, the optimal sequential design is a fixed nonsequential procedure. A similar result was obtained by Zacks (1968) for the sequential design of fractional replications. If in the above linear design problem σ^2 is unknown, the prior and posterior distributions of $\boldsymbol{\beta}$ are multivariate t and the evaluation of the integrals becomes intractable.

Consider the following nonnormal example. Let $Y_x \sim \text{Pois}(\lambda x)$, where $x \in [a, b]$, $0 < a < b < \infty$, x a design variable. Suppose that one chooses k design points $x_1, \ldots, x_k$ in (a, b). Then $\sum_{i=1}^{k} Y_{x_i} \sim \text{Pois}\left(\lambda \sum_{i=1}^{k} x_i\right)$. Thus, the best unbiased estimator of λ is

$$\hat{\lambda}_k = \frac{\sum_{i=1}^{k} Y_{x_i}}{\sum_{i=1}^{k} x_i}. \tag{10.3.8}$$

The variance of this estimator is

$$V\{\hat{\lambda}_k\} = \frac{\lambda}{\sum_{i=1}^{k} x_i}. \tag{10.3.9}$$

Thus the optimal design to minimize (10.3.9) is to choose all k points at b. This will also maximize the Fisher information on λ. We examine now the criterion of maximizing (10.3.4).

Let λ have a prior gamma distribution $G(\Lambda, \alpha)$, where α is a shape parameter and $E\{\lambda\} = \Lambda^{-1}$. The posterior distribution of λ given (x, Y_x) is $G(\Lambda + x, \alpha + Y_x,)$. Thus

$$\begin{aligned} \log\frac{h(\lambda \mid Y_x, x)}{h(\lambda)} &= \log\left[\frac{\Gamma(\alpha)(\Lambda + x)^{\alpha+Y_x}}{\Gamma(\alpha + Y_x)\Lambda^{\alpha}}\lambda^{Y_x}e^{-\lambda x}\right] \\ &= Y_x \log\lambda - \lambda x + (\alpha + Y_x)\log(\Lambda + x) \\ &\quad + \log\Gamma(\alpha) - \alpha\log\Lambda - \log\Gamma(\alpha + Y_x). \end{aligned} \tag{10.3.10}$$

The Kullback–Liebler information function is

$$\begin{aligned} I(h(\cdot \mid x, Y_x), h(\cdot)) &= Y_x E\{\log(\lambda) \mid x, Y_x\} - x\frac{\alpha + Y_x}{\Lambda + x} \\ &\quad + (\alpha + Y_x)\log(\Lambda + x) \\ &\quad + \log\Gamma(\alpha) - \alpha\log\Lambda - \log\Gamma(\alpha + Y_x). \end{aligned} \tag{10.3.11}$$

Notice that for $a > 0$, $b > 0$

$$\int_0^\infty \log(\lambda)\lambda^a e^{-b\lambda}\, d\lambda = \frac{1}{b^{a+1}}[\Gamma(a) + a\Gamma(a)\psi(a) - a\Gamma(a)\log(b)], \tag{10.3.12}$$

where $\psi(a)$ is the digamma function (see Abramowitz and Stegan, 1968, p. 258)

$$\psi(a) = \frac{\Gamma'(a)}{\Gamma(a)}. \tag{10.3.13}$$

Accordingly, setting $a = \alpha + Y_x - 1$ and $b = \Lambda + x$, we get

$$E\{\log\lambda \mid x, Y_x\} = \psi(\alpha + Y_x - 1) + \frac{1}{\alpha + Y_x - 1} - \log(\Lambda + x). \tag{10.3.14}$$

We now have to substitute (10.3.14) into (10.3.11) and compute the expectation with respect to the predictive distribution of Y_x, which is the negative binomial with parameters $(\alpha, x/(\Lambda + x))$, that is,

$$p\left(y \mid \alpha, \frac{x}{\Lambda + x}\right) = \frac{\Gamma(\alpha + y)}{\Gamma(\alpha)y!}\left(\frac{\Lambda}{\lambda + x}\right)^\alpha \left(\frac{x}{\Lambda + x}\right)^y, \quad y = 0, 1, \ldots. \tag{10.3.15}$$

It is not clear that the result is an increasing function of x. Thus, a very simple design problem becomes obscure and complicated by using Lindley's approach, which is to maximize (10.3.4). We conclude the section with some additional remarks. In the literature there are quite a few sequential or adaptive procedures of experimental designs. The reader is referred to Myers and Montgomery (1995) for stage-wise designs in the exploration of response surfaces. The objective there is to find the region of maximal expected yield. One starts with a series of 2^n factorial experiments. The factor levels change from one stage to another in the direction of the gradient leading to higher expected response. At the region of a maximum a central composite design is executed for estimating the quadratic response surface and its characteristics.

In 1969 Box and Draper developed an evolutionary procedure to improve industrial processes by a sequence of simple factorial experiments, called EVOP. Box (1992) discussed several strategies for designing a second-stage experiment as a result of the observations in the first stage.

10.4 SEQUENTIAL TESTING OF SOFTWARE RELIABILITY

In Chapter 4, Section 4.6, we presented an adaptive procedure for software reliability testing based on estimating the size of a finite population. In the present section we discuss another type of modeling based on the random times it takes for a module containing a fault to be revealed.

10.4.1 Complete Bayesian Model

The time to detect any one of the N faults is a random variable having a Pareto distribution with density

$$f(x;\alpha,\beta)=\frac{\alpha}{\beta}\left(1+\frac{x}{\beta}\right)^{-(\alpha+1)}, \quad 0<x<\infty. \tag{10.4.1}$$

The model stipulates that these random variables $X_1, X_2, \ldots, X_N$ are i.i.d. The observable random variables are the failure times $0<\tau_1<\tau_2<\cdots$. The first n failure times are distributed like the first n-order statistics from a random sample of N Pareto random variables. The likelihood function of N at time t given $0<\tau_1<\cdots<\tau_n<t$ is

$$\begin{aligned} L(N;\tau_1,\ldots,\tau_n,t) &= I\{n<N\}\cdot\frac{N!}{(N-n)!} \\ &\quad\cdot\frac{\alpha^n}{\beta^n}\prod_{j=1}^{n}\left(1+\frac{\tau_j}{\beta}\right)^{-\alpha-1}\left(1+\frac{t}{\beta}\right)^{-\alpha(N-n)}, \\ &\quad n\geq 1. \end{aligned} \tag{10.4.2}$$

If α and β are known, the likelihood statistic is $J(t)$, which is the number of failures in $(0,t)$. If α and β are unknown, then the minimal sufficient statistic is $(J(t),(\tau_1,\cdots,\tau_{J(t)}))$, where α and β are prior parameters. If one knows them, then, assuming that N has a prior Poisson distribution with mean η, the posterior distribution of $N(t)=N-J(t)$ has the p.d.f.

$$P(N(t)=j\mid t,J(t))=p\left(j;\eta\left(1+\frac{t}{\beta}\right)^{-\alpha}\right). \tag{10.4.3}$$

Let

$$C(t,N(t))=\frac{ct}{\beta}+KN(t) \tag{10.4.4}$$

be the cost for stopping the test at time t and leaving $N(t)$ faults in the system. Here C is the cost of testing per unit time and K is the cost of repairing a failed software in the field. The posterior expected cost at time t is

$$C^*(t)=\frac{ct}{\beta}+K\eta\left(1+\frac{t}{\beta}\right)^{-\alpha}. \tag{10.4.5}$$

This function is convex, having a unique minimum at

$$t^0=\beta\left[\left(\frac{K}{c}\eta\alpha\right)^{1/(1+\alpha)}-1\right]. \tag{10.4.6}$$

To minimize the expected cost, one could stop at time t^0. The predictive reliability function of the system at time t^0 is

$$\begin{aligned}\rho_{t^0}(u) &= E\left\{\left(1+\frac{u}{\beta}\right)^{-\alpha N(t_0)}\Bigg| t^0, J(t^0)\right\}\\ &= \exp\left\{-\eta\left(1+\frac{t^0}{\beta}\right)^{-\alpha}\left(1-\left(1+\frac{u}{\beta}\right)^{-\alpha}\right)\right\}.\end{aligned} \tag{10.4.7}$$

Notice that

$$\lim_{u\to\infty}\rho_{t^0}(u) = \exp\left\{-\eta\left(1+\frac{t^0}{\beta}\right)^{-\alpha}\right\}. \tag{10.4.8}$$

This is the predictive probability that, if we stop testing at time t^0, the system will function forever without interruption.

10.4.2 Empirical Bayes: Adaptive Approach When η and α Are Unknown

We still assume that β is known. We estimate η and α from the data.

Let $y_j = \tau_j/\beta$, $j = 1, 2, \ldots$. The predictive (profile) likelihood at time t is

$$\begin{aligned}&L_t^*(\alpha,\eta; J(t) = n, y_1, \ldots, y_n)\\ &\quad = \eta^\alpha\alpha^n\left(\prod_{i=1}^{n}(1+y_j)^{-\alpha}\right)\exp\left(-\eta\left(1-\left(1+\frac{t}{\beta}\right)^{-\alpha}\right)\right).\end{aligned} \tag{10.4.9}$$

The MLEs of α and η at time t, $\hat{\alpha}_t$ and $\hat{\eta}_t$, are values maximizing $L_t^*(\alpha,\eta; J(t), \mathbf{y}_t)$, where $\mathbf{y}_t = (y_1, \ldots, y_{J(t)})$. Let $G(n) = \left(\prod_{i=1}^{n}(1+y_i)\right)^{1/n}$. The MLE of $\hat{\alpha}_t$ and $\hat{\eta}_t$ should satisfy the equations, when $J(t) = n$,

$$\hat{\eta}_t = \frac{n}{1-(1+t/\beta)^{-\hat{\alpha}_t}} \tag{10.4.10}$$

and

$$\frac{1}{\hat{\alpha}_t} - \frac{\log(1+t/\beta)}{(1+t/\beta)^{-\hat{\alpha}_t}-1} = \log G(n). \tag{10.4.11}$$

If $J(t) = 0$, then $\log G(0) = 0$ and $\hat{\alpha}_t$ should satisfy the equation

$$\frac{\hat{\alpha}_t\log(1+t/\beta)}{(1+t/\beta)^{-\hat{\alpha}_t}-1} = 1. \tag{10.4.12}$$

This equation is satisfied only for $\hat{\alpha}_t = 0$. Thus, $\hat{\alpha}_t$ does not exist as long as $J(t) = 0$. From Eq. (10.4.11) we deduce that $\hat{\alpha}_t < 1/\log G(n)$.

We now investigate whether (10.4.11) has a unique positive root. Let $u = t/\beta$. We start with

$$(1+u)^{\alpha} = e^{\alpha \log(1+u)} \tag{10.4.13}$$
$$= \sum_{j=0}^{\infty} \frac{1}{j!}(\alpha \log(1+u))^j.$$

Hence,

$$\frac{\alpha \log(1+u)}{(1+u)^{\alpha}-1} = \frac{\alpha \log(1+u)}{\sum_{j=1}^{\infty} \frac{1}{j!}(\alpha \log(1+u))^j} \tag{10.4.14}$$
$$= \frac{1}{\sum_{j=0}^{\infty} \frac{1}{(j+1)!}(\alpha \log(1+u))^j}.$$

Let

$$D(\alpha, u) = \sum_{j=1}^{\infty} \frac{1}{(j+1)!}(\alpha \log(1+u))^j. \tag{10.4.15}$$

Equation (10.4.11) can be written as

$$\hat{\alpha} = \frac{1}{\log G(n)} \frac{D(\hat{\alpha}, u)}{1 + D(\hat{\alpha}, u)}. \tag{10.4.16}$$

Let

$$V(\alpha) = \frac{1}{\log G(n)} \frac{D(\alpha, u)}{1 + D(\alpha, u)},$$

where $V(\alpha)$ is a concave function of α for a fixed u and $\log G(n)$. If $V'(0) < 1$, there is no MLE of α. One can prove then that $\hat{\alpha}_t$ exists if and only if

$$t > \beta((G(n))^2 - 1). \tag{10.4.17}$$

The proof is based on the fact that

$$\lim_{\alpha \to 0} V'(\alpha) = \frac{1}{2 \log G(n)} \log(1+u).$$

This is greater than 1 if (10.4.17) holds. To obtain the solution of the equation

$$\alpha = V(\alpha), \tag{10.4.18}$$

we can start with an arbitrary $0 < \alpha_0 < 1/\log G(n)$ and define the sequence

$$\alpha_i = V(\alpha_{i-1}), \quad i \geq 1.$$

This sequence converges monotonically to $\hat{\alpha}_t$, where $\hat{\alpha}_t$ is *not* a consistent estimator of α unless $N \to \infty$. Finally, the MLE of η is obtained by substituting $\hat{\alpha}_t$ in (10.4.10). A sequential stopping time can be based on substituting $\hat{\alpha}_t$ and $\hat{\eta}_t$ into (10.4.6). For example, one could use the stopping time

$$T(\beta) = \inf\left\{t > 0 : t > \beta\left[\left(\frac{k}{c}\hat{\eta}_t\hat{\alpha}_t\right)^{1/(1+\hat{\alpha}_t)} - 1\right]\right\}. \tag{10.4.19}$$

The properties of such a stopping time are subject for further research.

Bibliography

Abraham, B. and Ledolter, J. (1983). *Statistical Methods for Forecasting*. Wiley, New York.

Abramowitz, M. and Stegan, I. (1968). *Handbook of Mathematical Functions with Formulas, Graphs and Mathematical Tables*. Dover Publications, New York.

Anbar, D. (1973). On optimal estimation methods using stochastic approximation procedures. *Ann. of Stat.*, **1**, 1175–1184.

Anbar, D. (1977). A modified Robbins-Monro procedure approximating a zero of a regression function from below. *Ann. Stat.*, **5**, 229–234.

Anderson, B. D. O. and Moore, J. B. (1979). *Optimal Filtering*. Prentice-Hall, Englewood Cliffs, NJ.

Anderson, T. W. (1971). *The Statistical Analysis of Time Series*. Wiley, New York.

Anderson, T. W., McCarthy, P. J. and Tukey, J. W. (1946). "Staircase" method of sensitivity testing. In *Naval Ordinance Report*. Princeton Statistical Group, Princeton, NJ, pp. 46–65.

Anscombe, F. J. (1952). Large sample theory of sequential estimation. *Proc. Camb. Philos. Soc.*, **48**, 600–607.

Aoki, M. (1987). *State Space Modelling of Time Series.* Springer-Verlag, New York.

Arbuck, S. G. (1996). Workshop on phase I study design. *Ann. Oncol.*, **7**, 567–573.

Armitage, P. (1975). *Sequential Medical Trials.* Blackwell, Oxford.

Assaf, D. (1988). A dynamic sampling approach for detecting a change in distribution. *Ann. Stat.*, **16**, 236–253.

Atkinson, A. C. (1982). Optimum biased coin designs for sequential clinical trials with prognostic factors. *Biometrika*, **69**, 61–67.

Atkinson, A. C. and Donev, A. N. (1992). *Optimum Experimental Designs.* Clarendon Press, Oxford.

Babb, J. and Rogatko, A. (2001). Patient specific dosing in cancer phase I clinical trials. *Stat. Med.*, **20**, 2079–2090.

Babb, J. and Rogatko, A. (2003). Bayesian methods for Cancer Phase I Clinical Trials. In *Advances in Clinical Trial Biostatistics*, N. L. Geller, Ed. Marcel Dekker, New York, pp. 1–39.

Babb, J., Rogatko, A. and Zacks, S. (1998). Cancer phase I clinical trials: Efficient dose escalation with overdose control. *Stat. Med.*, **17**, 1103–1120.

Bai, Z. D. and Hu, F. (1999). Asymptotic theorem for urn models with nonhomogeneous generating matrices. *Stochast. Proc. Their Appl.*, **80**, 87–101.

Bai, Z. D. and Hu, F. (2005). Asymptotics of randomized urn models. *Ann. Appl. Prob.*, **15**, 914–940.

Barnard, G. A. (1959). Control charts and stochastic processes. *Ann. Math. Stat.* **16**, 236–253.

Baron, M. and Tartakovsky, A. G. (2006). Asymptotic optimality of change-point detection schemes in general continuous-time models. *Sequent. Anal.*, **25**, 257–296 (2007 Abraham Wald Prize in Sequential Analysis).

Bartoff, L. and Lai, T. L. (2008). Efficient adaptive designs with mid-course sample size adjustment in clinical trials. *Stat. Med.*, **27**, 1593–1611.

Basseville, M. and Nikiforov, I. V. (1993). *Detection of Abrupt Changes: Theory and Applications.* Prentice-Hall, Englewood Cliffs, NJ.

Basu, D. (1969). Role of sufficiency and likelihood principles in sample survey theory. *Sankhyā A*, **31**, 441–454.

Bather, J. A. (1963). Control charts and minimization of costs. *J. Roy. Stat. Soc. B*, **25**, 49–80.

Bather, J. A. (1967). On a quickest detection problem. *Ann. Math. Stat.*, **38**, 711–724.

Bather, J. A. (1976). A control chart model and a generalized stopping problem for Brownian motion. *Math. Oper. Res.*, **1**, 209–224.

Bather, J. A. (1981). Randomized allocation of treatments in sequential experiments (with discussion). *J. Roy. Stat. Soc. B*, **43**, 265–292.

Bather, J. A. (1985). On the allocation of treatments in sequential medical trials. *Inst. Stat. Rev.*, **53**, 15–24.

Bather, J. A. and Simons, G. (1985). The minimax risk for clinical trials. *J. Roy. Stat. Soc. B*, **47**, 466–475.

Bauer, P. (1989). Multistage testing with adaptive designs (with discussion). *Biometr. Inform. Med. Biol.*, **20**, 130–148.

Bauer, P. and Einfalt, J. (2006). Application of adaptive design—a review. *Biometr. J.*, **48**, 493–506.

Ben-Gal, I. and Caramanis, M. (2002). Sequential DOE via dynamic programming. *IIE Trans.*, **34**, 1087–1100.

Berk, R. H. (1973). Some asymptotic aspects of sequential analysis. *Ann. Stat.*, **1**, 1126–1138.

Berk, R. H. (1975). Locally most powerful sequential tests. *Ann. Stat.*, **3**, 373–381.

Berk, R. H. (1976). Asymptotic efficiency of sequential tests. *Ann. Stat.*, **4**, 891–900.

Bernardo, J. M. (1979). Expected information as expected utility. *Ann. Stat.*, **7**, 686–690.

Berry, D. A. and Friestedt, B. (1985). *Bandit Problems: Sequential Allocation of Experiments.* Chapman and Hall, New York.

Bertsimas, D. and Nino-Mora, J. (1993). Conservation laws, extended polymatroids and multi-armed bandit problems: A unified approach to indexable systems. DSpace, MIT Libraries, Operatiosn Research Working Papers, http://hdl.handle.net//1721.1/5203.

Bhattacharya, P. K. and Frierson, D. (1981). A nonparametric chart for detecting small disorders. *Ann. Stat.*, **9**, 544–554.

Bickel, P. J. and Yahav, J. A. (1967). Asymptotically pointwise optimal procedures in sequential analysis. In *Proceedings of the Fifth Berkeley Symposium on Mathematical Statistics and Probability*, Vol. 1. University of Berkeley Press, Berkeley, pp. 401–413.

Bickel, P. J. and Yahav, J. A. (1968). Asymptotically optimal Bayes and minimax procedures in sequential estimation. *Ann. Math. Stat.*, **39**, 442–456.

Bickel, P. J. and Yahav, J. A. (1969). On an A.P.O. rule in sequential estimation with quadratic loss. *Ann. Math. Stat.*, **40**, 417–426.

Birkett, M. and Day, S. (1994). Internal pilot studies for estimating sample size. *Stat. Med.*, **13**, 2455–2463.

Blackwell, D. and Hodges, J. L. (1957). Design for the control of selection bias. *Ann. Math. Stat.*, **28**, 449–460.

Bloomfield, P. (1986). *Fourier Analysis of Time Series: An Introduction.* Wiley, New York.

Blum, J. R. (1954). Approximation methods which converge with probability one. *Ann. Math. Stat.*, **25**, 382–386.

Bolfarine, H. and Zacks, S. (1992). *Prediction Theory for Finite Populations.* Springer, New York.

Bose, A. and Mukhopadhyay, N. (1995). Sequential estimation of the mean of an exponential distribution via replicated piecewise stopping number. *Stat. Decisions*, **13**, 351–361.

Box, G. E. P. (1992). Sequential experimentation and sequential assembly of designs. *Qual. Eng.*, **5**, 321–330.

Box, G. E. P. and Draper, N. R. (1969). *Evolutionary Operation: A Statistical Method for Process Improvement.* Wiley, New York.

Box, G. E. P., Jenkins, G. M. and Reinsel, G. L. (1994). *Time Series Analysis Forecasting and Control*, 3rd ed. Prentice-Hall, Englewood Cliffs, NJ.

Braun, T. (2002). The bivariate continual reassessment method: Extending the CRM to phase I trials of two competing outcomes. *Controlled Clin. Trials*, **23**, 240–256.

Breiman, L. (1992). *Probability*, (Classics in Applied Mathematics) SIAM, Philadelphia, PA.

Breslow, N. E. and Day, N. E. (1987). *Statistical Methods in Cancer Research*, Vol. II: *The Design and Analysis of Cohort Studies.* International Agency for Research in Cancer, Lyon.

Brillinger, D. R. (1975). *Time Series Analysis: Data Analysis and Theory.* Holt, Rinehart and Winston, New York.

Brockwell, P. J. and Davis, R. A. (1991). *Time Series: Theory and Methods*, 2nd ed. Springer-Verlag, New York.

Brown, M. and Zacks, S. (2006). A note on optimal stopping for possible change in the intensity of an ordinary Poisson process. *Stat. Prob. Lett.*, **76**, 1417–1425.

Brown, R. L.,Brown, R.L. Durbin, J. and Evans, J. M. (1975). Techniques for testing the constancy of regression relationships over time. *J. Roy. Stat. Soc. Ser B*, **37**, 149–163.

Carlin, B. P., Gelfand, A. E. and Smith, A. F. M. (1992). Hierarchical Bayesian analysis of change-point problems. *Appl. Stat.*, **41**, 389–405.

Cassel, C. M., Särndal, C. E. and Wretman, J. H. (1977). *Foundations of Inference in Survey Sampling.* Wiley, New York.

Chaloner, K. (1987). An approach to design for generalized linear models. In *Model-Oriented Data Analysis*, V. V. Fedorov and H. Läuter, Eds. Springer, Berlin, pp. 3–12.

Chaloner, K. and Larntz, K. (1989). Optimal Bayesian design applied to logistic regression experiments. *J. Stat. Plan. Inf.*, **21**, 191–208.

Chaloner, K. and Verdinelli, I. (1995). Bayesian experimental design: A review. *Stat. Sci.*, **10**, 273–304.

Chatfield, C. (1975). *The Analysis of Time Series: Theory and Practice.* Chapman and Hall, London.

Chatfield, C. (1984). *The Analysis of Time Series: An Introduction*, 3rd ed. Chapman and Hall, London.

Chen, Y-P. (1999). Biased coin design with imbalance intolerance. *Commun. Stat. Stochast. Models*, **15**, 953–975.

Chen, Y-P. (2000). Which design is better? Ehrenfest urn versus biased coin. *Adv. Appl. Prob.*, **32**, 738–749.

Cheng, J. D., Babb, J. S., Langer, S., Aamdal, S., Robert F., Engelhardt, L. P., Ferberg, O., Schiller, J., Forsberg, G., Alpaugh, R. K., Weiner, L. M. and Rogatko, A. (2004). Individualized patient dosing in phase I clinical trials: The role of escalation with overdose control in PNU-214936. *J. Clin. Oncol.*, **22**, 602–609.

Chernoff, H. (1972). *Sequential Analysis and Optimal Design.* Regional Conferences Series in Applied Mathematics, Vol. 8. SIAM, Philadelphia, PA.

Chernoff, H. and Petkau, A. J. (1981). Sequential medical trials involving paired data. *Biometrika*, **68**, 119–132.

Chernoff, H. and Ray, S. N. (1965). A Bayes sequential sampling inspection plan. *Ann. Math. Stat.*, **36**, 1387–1407.

Chernoff, H. and Zacks, S. (1964). Estimating the current mean of a normal distribution which is subjected to changes in time. *Ann. Math. Stat.*, **35**, 999–1018.

Chevret, S. (1993). The continual reassessment method in cancer Phase I clinical trials: A simulation study. *Stat. Med.*, **12**, 1093–1108.

Chow, C-S. and Liu, J-P. (1998). *Design and Analysis of Clinical Trials*. Wiley, New York.

Chow, Y. S. and Robbins, H. (1965). On the asymptotic theory of fixed width sequential confidence intervals for the mean. *Ann. Math. Stat.*, **36**, 457–462.

Chow, Y. S., Robbins, H. and Siegmund, D. (1971). *Great Expectations: The Theory of Optimal Stopping*. Houghton Mifflin, Boston.

Chow, Y. S., Robbins, H. and Siegmund, D. (1971). *The Theory of Optimal Stopping*. Dover Publications, New York.

Cochran, W. G. (1973). Experiments for non-linear functions, R.A. Fisher memorial lecture. *J. Am. Stat. Assoc.*, **68**, 771–781.

Cochran, W. G. (1977). *Sampling Techniques*, 3rd ed. Wiley, New York.

Cox, D. R. and Lewis, P. A. W. (1966). *The Statistical Analysis of Series of Events*. Methuen, London.

Csörgö, M. and Horváth, L. (1987). Detecting changes in a random sequence. *J. Multivar. Anal.*, **23**, 119–130.

Csörgö, M. and Horváth, L. (1988). Nonparametric methods for change-point problems. In *Handbook of Statistics*, Vol. 7, P. R. Krishnaich and C. R. Rao, Eds., Elsevier Science Publishers, New York, pp. 403–423.

Cui, L., Hung, H. M. and Wang, S. J. (1999). Modification of sample size in group sequential clinical trials. *Biometrics*, **55**, 835–857.

Dantzig, G. B. (1940). On the non existence of tests of "Student's" hypothesis having power functions independent of σ^2. *Ann. Math. Stat.*, **11**, 186–192.

Datta, S. and Mukhopadhyay, N. (1995). On fine-tuned bounded risk sequential point estimation of the mean of an exponential distribution. *S. Afr. Stat. J.*, **29**, 9–27.

Davis, M. H. A. and Vinter, R. B. (1985). *Stochastic Modelling and Control*. Chapman and Hall, New York.

DeGroot, M. H. (1962). Uncertainty, information and sequential experiments. *Ann. Math. Stat..*, **33**, 404–419.

DeGroot, M.H. (1986). Concepts of information based on utility. In *Recent Developments in the Foundations of Utility and Risk Theory*. L. Daboni, A. Montesario, and M. Lines, Eds. Reisdel, Dordrecht, pp. 265–275,

Denne, J. S. and Jennison, C. (2000). A group sequential t-test with updating of sample size. *Biometrika*, **87**, 125–134.

Dixon, W. J. (1965). The up-and-down method for small samples. *J. Am. Stat. Assoc.*, **60**, 967–978.

Dixon, W. J. and Mood, A. M. (1948). A method of obtaining and analyzing sensitivity data. *J. Am. Stat. Assoc.*, **43**, 109–126.

Donner, A. (1984). Approaches to sample size estimation in the design of clinical trails—A review. *Stat. Med.*, **3**, 199–214.

Dufour, J.M. (1982). Recursive stability analysis of linear regression relationship. *J. Econometr.*, **19**, 31–76.

Durham, S. D. and Flournoy, N. (1995). Up-and-down designs I: Stationary treatment distributions. *Adapt. Des. IMS Lect. Notes Monogr. Ser.*, **25**, 139–157.

Efron, B. (1971). Forcing a sequential experiment to be balanced. *Biometrika*, **58**, 403–417.

Ehrenfeld, S. (1962). Some experimental design problems in attribute life testing. *J. Am. Stat. Assoc.*, **57**, 668–679.

Eichhorn, B. H. (1973). Sequential search of an optimal dosage. *Naval Res. Logist. Q.*, **20**, 729–736.

Eichhorn, B. H. (1974). Sequential search of an optimal dosage for cases of linear dosage-toxicity regression. *Commun. Stat. Theory Methods*, **3**, 263–271.

Eichhorn, B. H. and Zacks, S. (1973). Sequential search of an optimal dosage, I. *J. Am. Stat. Assoc.*, **68**, 594–598.

Eichhorn, B. H. and Zacks, S. (1981). Bayes sequential search of an optimal dosage: Linear regression with both parameters unknown. *Commun. Stat. Theory Methods*, **10**, 931–953.

Eisele, J. R. and Woodroofe, M. (1995). Central limit theorems for doubly adaptive biased coin designs. *Ann. Stat.*, **23**, 234–254.

Faries, D. (1994). Practical modifications of the continual reassessment method for phase I cancer clinical trials. *J. Biopharm.*, **4**, 147–164.

Fieller, E. C. (1940). The biological standardization of insulin. *Roy. Stat. Soc.*, Suppl. **7**, 1–64.

Finney, D. J. (1964). *Statistical Methods in Biological Assay*, 2nd ed. Griffin, London.

Fisher, L. (1998). Self-designing clinical trials. *Stat. Med.*, **17**, 1551–1562.

Fisher, R.A. (1922). On the mathematical foundations of theoretical statistics. *Philos. Trans. Roy. Soc. Lond. A*, **222**, 309–368.

Flournoy, N. (1993). A clinical experiment in bone marrow transplantation: Estimating a percentage point of a quantal response curve. In *Lecture Notes in Statistics*, C. Gatsonis, J. S. Hodseg, R.E. Kass, and D. Singpurwalla, Eds. Springer-Verlag, New York, pp. 324–336.

Flournoy, N. and Rosenberger, W. F., Editors (1995). *Adaptive Designs: Selected Proceedings of a 1992 Joint AMS-SIAM Summer Conference, IMS Lecture Notes, Monograph Series*, Vol. 25. Hayward, California.

Freeman, P. R. (1972). Sequential estimation of the size of a population. *Biometrika*, **59**, 9–17.

Fuh, C. D. (2003). SPRT and CUSUM in hidden Markov models. *Ann. Stat.*, **31**, 942–977.

Fuh, C. D. (2004). Asymptotic operating characteristics of an optimal change point detection in hidden Markov models. *Ann. Stat.*, **32**, 2305–2339.

Fuller, W. A. (1996). *Introduction to Statistical Time Series*, 2nd ed. Wiley, New York.

Gamerman, D. (1992). A dynamic approach to the statistical analysis of point processes. *Biometrika*, **79**, 39–50.

Gastonis, C. and Greenhouse, J. B. (1992). Bayesian methods for phase I clinical trials. *Stat. Med.*, **11**, 1377–1389.

Ghosh, B. K. (1970). *Sequential Tests of Statistical Hypotheses*. Addison-Wesley, Reading, MA.

Ghosh, M. and Mukhopadhyay, N. (1981). Consistency and asymptotic efficiency of two-stage and sequential estimation procedures. *Sankyha A*, **43**, 220–227.

Ghosh, M., Mukhopadhyay, N., and Sen, P. K. (1997). *Sequential Estimation*. Wiley, New York.

Girshick, M. A. and Rubin, H. (1952). A Bayes approach to a quality control model. *Ann. Math. Stat.*, **23**, 114–125.

Gittins, J. C. (1979). Bandit processes and dynamic allocation indices (with discussion). *J. Roy. Stat. Soc. B*, **41**, 148–177.

Gittins, J. C. (1989). *Multi-Armed Bandit Allocation Indices*. Wiley, New York.

Gittins, J. C. and Jones, D. M. (1974). A dynamic allocation index for the sequential design of experiments. In *Progress in Statistics*. J. Gari, K. Sakadi and I. Vinczo, Eds. North-Holland, Amsterdam, pp. 241–246.

Gittins, J. C. and Jones, D. M. (1979). A dynamic allocation index for the discounted multiarmed bandit problem. *Biometrika*, **66**, 561–565.

Glazebrook, K. D. (1990). Procedures for the evaluation of strategies for resource allocation in a stochastic environment. *J. Appl. Prob.*, **27**, 215–220.

Goodman, S. N., Zahurak, M. L. and Piantadosi, S. (1995). Some practical improvements in the continual reassessment method for phase I studies. *Stat. Med.*, **5**, 1149–1161.

Gordon, K. and Smith, A. F. M. (1988). Modeling and monitoring discontinuous changes in time-series. In *Bayesian Analysis of Time-Series and Dynamic Models*, J. C. Spall, Ed. Marcel Dekker, New York, pp. 359–391.

Gut, A. (1988). *Stopped Random Walks: Limit Theorems and Applications.* Springer-Verlag, New York.

Haldane, J. B. S. (1956). The estimation and significance of the logarithm of a ratio of frequencies. *Ann. Human Genet.*, **20**, 309–311.

Hardwick, J. P. (1995). A modified bandit as an approach to ethical allocation in clinical trials. *Adaptive Des. IMS Lect. Notes Monogr. Ser.*, **25**, 65–87.

Hardwick, J. P. and Stout, Q. F. (1995). Exact computational analysis for adaptive designs. *Adaptive Des. IMS Lect. Notes Monogr. Ser.*, **25**, 223–237.

Harrison, J. and West, M. (1989). *Bayesian Forecasting and Dynamic Models.* Springer-Verlag, New York.

Harrison, J. and Stevens, C. F. (1976). Bayesian forecasting (with discussion). *J. Roy. Stat. Soc. B*, **38**, 205–247.

Hedayat, A. S. and Sinha, B. K. (1991). *Design and Inference in Finite Population Sampling.* Wiley, New York.

Herbert, T. and Jensen, U. (2004). Optimal detection of a change point in a Poisson process for different observation schemes. *Scand. J. Stat.*, **31**, 347–366.

Heyd, J. M. and Carlin, B. P. (1999). Adaptive design improvements in the continual reassessment method for phase I studies. *Stat. Med.*, **18**, 1307–1321.

Hoadley, B. (1981). The quality measurement plan. *Bell Syst. Tech. J.*, **60**, 215–273.

Hu, F. and Rosenberger, W. F. (2006). *The Theory of Response-Adaptive Randomization in Clinical Trials.* Wiley, New York.

Huse, V. R. (1988). On some nonparametric methods for change-point problems. Ph.D. Dissertation, Carleton University, Ottawa, Ontario.

Ivanova, A. (2003). A new dose-finding design for bivariate outcomes, *Biometrics*, **59**, 1001–1007.

Ivanova, A., Montazar-Haghighi, A., Mohanty, S. G. and Durham, S. D. (2003). Improved up-and-down designs for phase I trials. *Stat. Med.*, **22**, 69–82.

Jarrett, R. G. (1979). A note on the interval between coal-mining disasters. *Biometrika*, **66**, 191–193.

Jelinski, Z. and Moranda, P. B. (1972). Software reliability research. In *Statistical Computer Performance Evaluation*, W. Freiberger, Ed. Academic, New York.

Jennison, C. (1987). Efficient group sequential tests with unpredictable group sizes. *Biometrika*, **74**, 155–165.

Jennison, C. and Turnbull, B. W. (2000). *Group Sequential Methods with Applications to Clinical Trials.* Chapman & Hall/CRC, Boca Raton, FL.

Jennison, C. and Turnbull, B. W. (2003). Mid-course sample size modification in clinical trials based on the observed treatment effect. *Stat. Med.*, **22**, 971–993.

Jennison, C. and Turnbull, B. W. (2006). Adaptive and nonadaptive group sequential tests. *Biometrika*, **93**, 1–21.

Johnson, N. L. and Kotz, S. (1969). *Distribution in Statistics: Discrete Distributions.* Houghton Mifflin, Boston.

Johnson, N. L. and Kotz, S. (1970). *Continuous Univariate Distributions 2.* Wiley, New York.

Johnson, N. L. and Kotz, S. (1977). *Urn Models and Their Applications, an Approach to Modern Discrete Probability Theory.* Wiley, New York.

Johnson, N. L. and Leone, F. C. (1962, 1963, 1964). Cumulative sum control charts: Mathematical principles applied to their construction and use, I, II, III. *Ind. Q. Contr.*, **18**, 15–21; **19**, 29–36; **20**, 22–28.

Jones, P. W., Lewis, A. M. and Hartley, R. (1995). Some designs for multi-criteria bandits. *Adapt. Des. IMS Lect. Notes Monogr. Ser.*, **25**, 88–94.

Kadshyap, R. L. (1976). *Dynamic Stochastic Models from Empirical Data.* Academic, New York.

Kao, E. P. C. (1997). *An Introduction to Stochastic Processes.* Duxbury, New York.

Kaspi, H. and Mandelbaum, A. (1995). Levy bandits: Multi-armed bandits driven by Levy processes. *Ann. Appl. Prob.*, **5**, 541–565.

Katehakis, M. N. and Veinott, A. F. Jr. (1987). The multi-armed bandit problem: Decomposition and computation. *Math. Oper. Res.*, **12**, 262–268.

Kedem, B. (1980). *Binary Time Series.* Marcel Dekker, New York.

Keener, R. (1986). Multi-armed bandits with simple arms. *Adv. Appl. Math.*, **7**, 199–204.

Kenett, R. S. and Pollak, M. (1983). On sequential detection of a shift in the probability of a rare event. *J. Am. Stat. Assoc.*, **78**, 389–395.

Kenett, R. S. and Pollak, M. (1991). Data-analytic aspects of the Shiryaev-Roberts control chart: Surveillance of a non-homogeneous Poisson process. Working paper series 91-204. School of Management, SUNY, Binghamton, New York.

Kenett, R. S. and Zacks, S. (1990). Process tracking under random changes in the mean. Working paper series 90-180. School of Management, SUNY, Binghamton, New York.

Kenett, R. S. and Zacks, S. (1998). *Modern Industrial Statistics: Design and Control of Quality and Reliability*. Duxbury, Pacific Grove.

Khan, M. K. (1984). Discrete adaptive design in attribute life testing. *Commun. Stat. Theory Methods*, **13**, 1423–1433.

Khan, M. K. (1988). Optimal Bayesian estimation of the median effective dose. *J. Stat. Plan. Inf.*, **18**, 69–81.

Khan, M. K. and Yazdi, A. A. (1988). On D-optimal designs for binary data. *J. Stat. Plan. Inf.*, **18**, 83–91.

Khan, R. A. (1969). A general method of determining fixed-width confidence intervals. *Ann. Math. Stat.*, **40**, 704–709.

Khan, R. A. (1978). Wald's approximations to the average run length in CUSUM procedures. *J. Stat. Plan. Inf.*, **2**, 63–77.

Khan, R. A. (1979). A sequential detection procedure and the related CUSUM procedure. *Sankhyiā B*, **40**, 146–162.

Khan, R. A. (1984). On cumulative sum procedures and the SPRT with applications. *J. Roy. Stat. Soc. B*, **46**, 79–85.

Khan, R. A. (1985). A stopped Wiener process formula with two barriers. *Sankhyā A*, **47**, 285–290.

Khuri, A. I., Mukherjee, B., Sinha, B. K. and Ghosh, M. (2006). Design issues for generalized linear models: A review. *Stat. Sci.*, **21**, 376–399.

Kiefer, J. and Weiss, L. (1957). Some properties of generalized probability ratio tests. *Ann. Math. Stat.*, **28**, 57–74.

Kon, S. J. (1984). Models of stock returns — A comparison. *J. Finance*, **39**, 147–165.

Kramer, A., Lebecq, A. and Candalh, E. (1999). Continual reassessment methods in phase I trials of the combination of two drugs in oncology. *Stat. Med.*, **18**, 1849–1864.

Kushner, H. G. and Clark, D. S. (1978). *Stochastic Approximations for Constrained and Unconstrained Systems*. Springer-Verlag, New York.

Kushner, H. G. and Yin, G. (1997). *Stochastic Approximation Algorithms and Applications*. Springer-Verlag, New York.

Lachin, J. M. (1981). Introduction to sample size determination and power analysis for clinical trials. *Control. Clin. Trials*, **21**, 167–189.

Lachin, J. M. (1988). Properties of simple randomization in clinical trials. *Control. Clin. Trials*, **9**, 312–326.

Lai, T. L. (1972). Gaussian processes, moving averages and quick detection problems. *Ann. Prob.*, **1**, 825–837.

Lai, T. L. (1973). Optimal stopping and sequential tests which minimize the maximum expected sample size. *Ann. Stat.*, **1**, 659–673.

Lai, T. L. (1974). Control charts based on weighted sums. *Ann. Stat.*, **2**, 134–147.

Lai, T. L. (1987). Adaptive treatment allocation and the multi-armed bandit problem. *Ann. Stat.*, **15**, 1091–1114.

Lai, T. L. (1995). Sequential change point detection in quality control and dynamical systems. *J. Roy. Stat. Soc. B*, **57**, 613–658.

Lai, T. L. and Shih, M. C. (2004). Power, sample size and adaptation considerations in the design of group sequential clinical trials. *Biometrika*, **97**, 507–528.

Lai, T. Z. (2001). Sequential analysis: Some classical problems and new challenges. *Stat. Sinica*, **11**, 303–408.

Lai, T. Z. and Robbins, H. (1979). Adaptive designs and stochastic approximation. *Ann. Stat.*, **7**, 1196–1221.

Lamprecht, E. and Zacks, S. (1998). Two armed bandits with change point in one arm. *J. Stat. Plan. Inf.*, **73**, 47–60.

Lehmann, E. L. (1959). *Testing Statistical Hypotheses*. Wiley, New York.

Lehmann, E. L. and Romano, J. P. (2006). *Testing Statistical Hypothesis*. Springer, New York.

Lindley, D. V. (1956). On the measure of information provided by an experiment. *Ann. Math. Stat.*, **27**, 986–1005.

Ljung, L. (1977). Analysis of recursive stochastic algorithms. *IEEE Trans. Automat. Contr.*, **22**, 551–575.

Lorden, G. (1971). Procedures for reacting to a change in distribution. *Ann. Math. Stat.*, **42**, 1897–1908.

Lorden, G. (1983). Asymptotic efficiency of three-stage hypothesis tests. *Ann. Stat.*, **11**, 129–140.

Lorden, G. and Eisenberger, I. (1973). Detection of failure rate increases. *Technometrics*, **15**, 167–175.

Louv, W. C. (1984). Adaptive filtering. *Technometrics*, **26**, 399–409.

Lucas, J. M. (1985). Counted data CUSUMs. *Technometrics*, **27**, 129–144.

Mathew, T. and Sinha, B. K. (2001). Optimal designs for binary data under logistic regression. *J. Stat. Plan. Inf.*, **93**, 295–307.

Matthews, J. N. S. (2000). *An Introduction to Randomized Controlled Clinical Trials.* Arnold, London.

Melfi, V. F. and Page, C. (2000). Estimation after adaptive allocation. *J. Stat. Plan. Inf.*, **87**, 353–363.

Migon, H. S. and Harrison, J. (1983). An application of non-linear Bayesian forecasting to television advertising. In *Bayesian Statistics*, Vol. 2, J. M. Bernardo et al., Eds. North-Holland, Amsterdam, pp. 681–696.

Montgomery, D. C. and Johnson, L. A. (1976). *Forecasting and Time Series Analysis.* McGraw Hill, New York.

Mukhopadhyay, N. (1988). Sequential estimation problems for negative exponential populations. *Commun. Stat. Theory Methods*, **17**, 2471–2506.

Mukhopadhyay, N. (1991). Parametric sequential point estimation. In *Handbook of Sequential Analysis*, B. K. Ghosh and P. K. Sen, Eds. Marcel Dekker, New York, pp. 245–267.

Mukhopadhyay, N. (1994). Improved sequential estimation of means of exponential distributions. *Ann. Inst. Stat. Math.*, **46**, 509–519.

Mukhopadhyay, N. (1995a). Two-stage and multi-stage estimation. In *The Exponential Distribution*, N. Balakrishnan and A. P. Basu, Eds. Gordon and Breach, Amsterdam, pp. 429–452.

Mukhopadhyay, N. (1995b). Second-order approximations in the time-sequential point estimation methodologies for the mean of an exponential distribution. *Sequential Anal.*, **14**, 133–142.

Mukhopadhyay, N. (1997). Second-order properties of a two-stage fixed-size confidence region for the mean vector of a multivariate normal distribution. Statistical Technical Report No. 97-14. University of Connecticut, Storrs.

Mukhopadhyay, N. and Cicconetti, G. (2004). Estimating reliabilities following purely sequential sampling from exponential populations. In *Advances on Ranking and Selection, Multiple Comparisons and Reliability: Methodology and Applications*, S. Panchapakesan's 70th Birthday Festschrift, N. Balakrishnan, N. Kannan, and H. N. Nagaraja, Eds.; Birkhauser, Boston, pp. 303–332.

Mukhopadhyay, N. and de Silva, B. M. (2005). Two-stage estimation of mean in a negative binomial distribution with applications to Mexican bean beetle data. *Sequential Anal.*, **24**, 99–137.

Mukhopadhyay, N. and Diaz, J. (1985). Two-stage sampling for estimating the mean of a negative binomial distribution. *Sequential Anal.*, **4**, 1–18.

Mukhopadhyay, N. and Duggan, W. T. (1997a). Can a two-stage procedure enjoy second-order properties? *Sankhya Ser. A*, **59**, 435–448.

Mukhopadhyay, N. and Duggan, W. T. (1997b). On a two-stage procedure having second-order properties with applications. Statistical Technical Report. Department of Statistics, University of Connecticut, Storrs, CT.

Mukhopadhyay, N. and Duggan, W. T. (2000). New results on two-stage estimation of the mean of an exponential distribution. In *Perspectives in Statistical Science*, A. K. Basu, J. K. Ghosh, P. K. Sen, and B. K. Sinha, Eds. Oxford University Press, New Delhi, pp. 219–231.

Mukhopadhyay, N. and Pepe, W. (2006). Exact bounded risk estimation when the terminal sample size and estimator are dependent: The exponential case. *Sequential Anal.*, **25**, 85–101.

Mustafi, C.K. (1968). Inference problems about parameters which are subjected to changes over time. *Ann. Math. Stat.*, **39**, 840–854.

Myers, R. H. and Montgomery, D. C. (1995). *Response Surface Methodology: Process and Product Optimization Using Designed Experiments*. Wiley, New York.

Nadler, J. and Robbins, N. B. (1971). Some characteristics of Page's two-sided procedure for detecting changes in a location parameter. *Ann. Math. Stat.*, **42**, 538–551.

Nelson, C. R. (1973). *Applied Time Series Analysis for Managerial Forecasting*. Holden-Day, San Francisco.

Neuhaus, W. (1987). Early warning. *Scand. Actuarial J.*, **87**, 128–156.

Newton, H. J. (1988). *TIMESLAB: A Time Series Analysis Laboratory*. Wadsworth and Brooks/Cole, Pacific Grove, CA.

Ng, H. K. T., Mohanty, S. G. and Balakrishnan, N. (2007). An assessment of the up-and-down designs and associated estimators in phase I trials. In *Advanced Statistical Methods in Health Sciences*, J. L. Auget, N. Balakrishman, and G. Molenberghs, Eds. Burkhäuser, Boston, Chapter 24.

O'Brein, P. C. and Fleming, T. R. (1979). A multiple testing procedure for clinical trials. *Biometrics*, **35**, 549–556.

O'Quigley, J., Pepe, M. and Fisher, L. (1990). Continual reassessment method: A practical design for phase I clinical trials in cancer. *Biometrics*, **46**, 33–48.

O'Quigley, J. and Shen, L. (1996). Continual reassessment method: A likelihood approach. *Biometrics*, **52**, 673–684.

Page, E. S. (1954). Continuous inspection schemes. *Biometrika*, **41**, 100–114.

Page, E. S. (1955). A test for a change in a parameter occurring at an unknown point. *Biometrika*, **42**, 523–527.

Page, E. S. (1957). On problems in which a change in parameter occurs at an unknown point. *Biometrika*, **44**, 248–252.

Perry, D., Stadje, W. and Zacks, S. (1999). First exit times for increasing compound Poisson processes. *Stochast. Models*, **15**, 977–992.

Peskir, G. and Shiryaev, A. N. (2002). Solving the Poisson disorder problem. In *Advances in Finance and Stochastics*. Klaus Sandman and Philip J. Schönbucher, Eds. Springer, New York, pp. 295–312.

Petersen, M. L., Deeks, S. G. and van der Loan, M. J. (2007). Individualized treatment rules: Generating candidate clinical trials. *Stat. Med.*, **26**, 4578–4601.

Phadke, M. S. (1981). Quality audit using adaptive Kalman filtering. *ASCQ Quality Congr. Trans.*, 1045–1052.

Piantadosi, S. and Liu, G. (1996). Improved designs for dose escalation studies using pharmacokinetic measurements. *Stat. Med.*, **15**, 1605–1618.

Pocock, S. J. (1977). Group sequential methods in the design and analysis of clinical trials. *Biometrika*, **64**, 191–199.

Pocock, S. J. (1984). *Clinical Trials: A Practical Approach.* Wiley, New York.

Pollak, M. (1985). Optimal detection of a change in distribution, *Ann. Stat.*, **13**, 206–227.

Pollak, M. (1987). Average run length of an optimal method of detecting a change in distribution. *Ann. Stat.*, **15**, 749–779.

Pollak, M. and Siegmund, D. (1985). A diffusion process and its application to detecting a change in the drift of Brownian motion. *Biometrika*, **72**, 267–280.

Pollock, K. H. and Otto, M. (1983). Robust estimation of population size in closed animal population from capture-recapture experiments. *Biometrics*, **39**, 1035–1049.

Raftery, A. E. and Akman, V. E. (1986). Bayesian analysis of a Poisson process with a change-point. *Biometrika*, **73**, 85–89.

Ray, W. D. (1957). Sequential confidence intervals for the mean of a normal population with unknown variance. *J. Roy. Stat. Soc. Ser. B*, **19**, 133–143.

Reynolds, M. R., Jr. (1975). Approximations to the average run length in cumulative sum control charts. *Technometrics*, **17**, 65–71.

Robbins, H. and Monro, S. (1951). A stochastic approximation method. *Ann. Math. Stat.*, **22**, 400–407.

Robbins, H. and Siegmund, D. (1971). A convergence theorem for nonnegative almost super martingales and some Applications. In *Optimizing Methods in Statistics*, J. S. Rustagi, Ed. Academic Press, New York, pp. 233–257.

Robbins, H. and Siegmund, D. (1974a). Sequential estimation of p in Bernoulli trials. In *Studies in Probab. & Statist., E.J.G. Pitman Volume*, E. J. Williams, Ed. Jerusalem Academic, Jerusalem, pp. 103–107.

Robbins, H. and Siegmund, D. O. (1974b). Sequential tests involving two populations. *J. Am. Stat. Assoc.*, **69**, 132–139.

Roberts, S. W. (1966). A comparison of some control charts procedures. *Technometrics*, **8**, 411–430.

Robinson, J. A. (1978). Sequential choice of an optimal dose: A prediction intervals approach. *Biometrika*, **65**, 75–78.

Rogatko, A. and Babb, J. (1998). Escalation with overdose control. User's guide. Version 1. beta. Available: http://www.fccc.edu/users/rogatko/ewoc.html.

Rosenberger, W. F. and Lachin, J. M. (2002). *Randomization in Clinical Trials, Theory and Practice*. Wiley, New York.

Rosenberger, W. F. and Rukhin, A. L. (2002). Bias properties and nonparametric inference for truncated binomial randomization. *J. Nonparametr. Stat.*, **15**, 455–465.

Ross, S. M. (1983). *Introduction to Stochastic Dynamic Programming*. Academic, New York.

Rukhin, A. L. (2004). Limiting distributions in sequential occupancy problems. *Sequential Anal.*, **23**, 141–158.

Rukhin, A. L. (2006). Gamma distribution order statistics, maximal multinomial frequency and randomization designs. *J. Stat. Plan. Inf.*, **136**, 2213–2226.

Rukhin, A. L. (2007). Randomization with non-uniform allocations: Fulfillment time distributions and bias properties. *Statistics*, **41**, 11–29.

Sacks, J. (1958). Asymptotic distribution of stochastic approximation procedures. *Ann. Math. Stat.*, **29**, 373–405.

Samuel, E. (1968). Sequential maximum likelihood estimation of the size of a population. *Ann. Math. Stat.*, **39**, 1057–1068.

Samuel, E. (1969). Comparison of sequential rules for estimation of the size of a population. *Biometrics*, **25**, 517–527.

Samuel-Chan, E. and Wax, Y. (1986). A sequential test for comparing two infection rates in a randomized clinical trial, and incorporation of data accumulated after stopping. *Biometrics*, **42**, 99–108.

Schmitz, N. (1993). *Optimal Sequentially Planned Decision Procedures*, Vol. 79 of *Lecture Notes in Statistics.* Springer-Verlag, New York.

Seber, G. A. F. (1977). *Linear Regression Analysis.* Wiley, New York.

Seber, G. A. F. (1985). *The Estimation of Animal Abundance*, 2nd ed. Griffin, London.

Sen, P. K. and Singer, J. M. (1993). *Large Sample Methods in Statistics, an Introduction with Applications.* Chapman & Hall, New York.

Shewhart, W. A. (1931). *Economic Control of Quality of Manufactured Product.* Van Nostrand, Princeton, NJ.

Shih, W. J. (1989). Prediction approaches to sequentially searching for an optimal dose. *Biometrics*, **45**, 623–628.

Shiryaev, A. N. (1963a). On optimum methods in quickest detection problem. *Theory Prob. Appl.*, **7**, 22–46.

Shiryaev, A. N. (1963b). On the detection of disorder in a manufacturing process, I, II. *Theory Prob. Appl.*, **8**, 247–264, 402–413.

Shiryaev, A. N. (1973). *Statistical Sequential Analysis: Optimal Stopping Rules.* Translations Math. Monographs, Vol. 38. American Mathematics Society, Providence, RI.

Shiryaev, A. N. (1978). *Optimal Stopping Rules.* Springer-Verlag, New York.

Shiryaev, A. N. (1984). *Probability.* Graduate Text in Mathematics. Springer-Verlag, New York.

Siegmund, D. (1985). *Sequential Analysis: Tests and Confidence Intervals.* Springer-Verlag, New York.

Simon, R. (1989). Optimal two-stage designs for phase II clinical trials. *Control. Clin. Trials*, **10**, 1–10.

Simons, G. (1968). On the cost of not knowing the variance when making a fixed-width confidence interval for the mean. *Ann. Math. Stat.*, **39**, 1946–1952.

Sitter, R. R. and Wu, C.-F. J. (1999). Two-stage design of quantal response studies. *Biometrics*, **55**, 396–402.

Smith, A. F. M. (1975). A Bayesian approach to inference about a change-point in a sequence of random variables. *Biometrika*, **62**, 407–416.

Smith, A. F. M. and West, M. (1983). Monitoring renal transplants: An application of the multi-process Kalman filter. *Biometrics*, **39**, 867–878.

Smith, R. L. (1984). Properties of biased coin designs in sequential clinical trials. *Ann. Stat.*, **12**, 1018–1034.

Sonin, I. M. (1999a). The elimination algorithm for the problem of optimal stopping. *Math. Meth. Oper. Res.*, **4**, 111–123.

Sonin, I. M. (1999b). The state reduction and related algorithms and their applications to the study of Markov chains, graph theory and optimal stopping problems. *Adv. Math.*, **145**, 159–188.

Souza, R. C. (1981). A Bayesian entropy approach to forecasting: the multistate model. In *Time Series Analysis*. Proceedings of The International ... Elsevier Science Publishers, North-Holland, Houston, TX, pp. 535–542.

Spall, J. C. (1988). *Bayesian Analysis of Time Series and Dynamic Models.* Marcel Dekker, New York.

Spall, J. C. (1992). Multivariate stochastic approximation using a simultaneous perturbation gradient approximation. *IEEE Trans. Automated Control.*, **37**, 332 341.

Spall, J. C. and Cristion, J. A. (1994). Nonlinear adaptive control using neural networks: Estimation with a smooth form of simultaneous perturbation gradient approximation. *Stat. Sinica*, **4**, 1–27.

Starr, N. (1966). The performance of a sequential procedure for estimating the mean. *Ann. Math. Stat.*, **36**, 36–50.

Starr, N. and Woodroofe, M. (1972). Further remarks on sequential estimation: The exponential case. *Ann. Math. Stat.*, **43**, 1147–1154.

Stein, C. (1945). A two sample test for a linear hypothesis when power is independent of variance. *Ann. Math. Stat.*, **16**, 243–258.

Stein, C. (1949). Some problems in sequential estimation (abstract). *Econometrika*, **17**, 77–78.

Stenger, H. (1977). Sequential sampling from finite populations. *Sankhyā C*, **39**, 10–20.

Stephens, K. S., Wadsworth, H. M. and Godfrey, A. B. (1986). *Modern Methods for Quality Control and Improvement.* Wiley, New York.

Stone, M. (1959). Application of a measure of information to the design and comparison of regression experiments. *Ann. Math. Stat.*, **30**, 55–70.

Storer, B. (1989). Design and analysis of phase I clinical trials. *Biometrics*, **45**, 925–937.

Stylianou, M. and Flournoy, N. (2002). Dose finding using the biased coin up-and-down design and isotonic regression. *Biometerics*, **58**, 171–177.

Stylianou, M., Proschan, M. and Flournoy, N. (2003). Estimating the probability of toxicity at the target dose following an up-and-down design, *Stat. Med.*, **22**, 535–543.

Tartakovsky, A. (1995). Asymptotic properties of CUSUM and Shiryaev's procedures for detecting a change in a nonhomogeneous Gaussian process. *Math. Methods Stat.*, **4**, 389–404.

Tartakovsky, A. G. and Ivanova, I. A. (1992). Comparison of some sequential rules for detecting changes in distributions. *Prob. Inf. Transmission*, **28**, 117–124.

Telksnys, L. (1986). *Detection of Changes in Random Processes.* Optimization Software, New York.

Thall, P. F. and Cook, J. D. (2004). Dose-finding based on efficacy-toxicity trade-offs. *Biometrics*, **60**, 684–693.

Thall, P. F., Cook, J. D. and Estey, E. H. (2006). Adaptive dose selection using efficacy-toxicity trade-offs: Illustrations and practical considerations. *Jour. Biopharm. Stat.*, **16**, 623–638.

Thall, P. F., Simon, R., Ellenberg, S. S. and Shrager, R. (1988). Optimal two-stage designs for clinical trials with binary response. *Stat. Med.*, **7**, 571–579.

Thompson, S. K. (1990). Adaptive cluster sampling. *Jour. Am. Stat. Assoc.*, **85**, 1050–1059.

Thompson, S. K. (1992). *Sampling.* Wiley, New York.

Thompson, S. K. and Seber, G. A. F. (1996). *Adaptive Sampling.* Wiley, New York.

Tsitsiklis, J. N. (1994). A short proof of the Gittins index theorem, *Ann. Appl. Prob.*, **4**, 194–199.

Tsutakawa, R. K. (1967). Random walk design in bio-assay. *J. Am. Stat. Assoc.*, **62**, 842–856.

Tsutakawa, R. K. (1972). Design of experiment for bioassay. *J. Am. Stat. Assoc.*, **67**, 584–590.

Tsutakawa, R. K. (1975). Bayesian inference for bioassay. Technical Report 5. Mathematical Sciences, University of Missouri, Columbia.

Tsutakawa, R. K. (1980). Selection of dose levels for estimating a percentage point of a logistic response curve. *J. Roy. Stat. Soc. Ser. C Appl. Stat.*, **29**, 25–33.

Vandaele, W. (1983). *Applied Time Series Analysis and Box-Jenkins Models.* Academic, New York.

Vanden Bosh, P. P. J. and vander Klauw, A. C. (1994). *Modeling, Identification and Simulation of Dynamical Systems.* CRC Press, Boca Raton, FL.

van Dobben de Bruyn, C.S. (1968). *Cumulative Sum Tests.* Griffin, London.

Varaiya, P., Warland, J. and Buyukkoc, C. (1985). Extensions of the multi-armed bandit problem: The discounted case. *IEEE Trans. Automatated Control*, **AC-30**, 426–439.

Vardeman, S. and Ray, D. (1985). Average run lengths for CUSUM schemes when observations are exponentially distributed. *Technometrics*, **27**, 145–150.

Wang, Y.-G. (1991). Gittins indices and constrained allocation in clinical trials. *Biometrika*, **78**, 101–111.

Weber, R. (1992). On the Gittins index for multi-armed bandits. *Ann. Appl. Prob.*, **2**, 1024–1035.

Wei, L. J. (1977). A class of designs for sequential clinical trials. *J. Am. Stat. Assoc.*, **72**, 382–386.

Wei, L. J. (1978). The adaptive biased coin design for sequential experiments. *Ann. Stat.*, **6**, 92–100.

Weiss, G. (1988). Branching bandit processes. *Prob. Eng. Inform. Sci.*, **2**, 269–278.

West, M. (1981). Robust sequential approximate Bayes estimation. *J. Roy. Stat. Soc. B*, **43**, 157–166.

West, M. (1986). Bayesian model monitoring. *J. Roy. Stat. Soc. Ser. B*, **48**, 70–78.

West, M., Harrison, J. and Migon, H. S. (1985). Dynamic generalized linear models and Bayesian forecasting. *J. Am. Stat. Assoc.*, **80**, 73–97.

Whitehead, J. (1997). Bayesian decision procedures with application to dose-finding studies. *Int. J. Pharm. Med.*, **11**, 201–208.

Whitehead, J., Whitehead, A., Todd, S., Bollard, K. and Sooriyarachi, M. R. (2001). Mid-trial design reviews for sequential clinical trials. *Stat. Med.*, **20**, 165–176.

Whittle, P. (1980). Multi-armed bandits and the Gittins index, *J. Roy. Stat. Soc. B*, **42**, 143–149.

Wijsman, R. A. (1971). Exponentially bounded stopping time of SPRTs for composite hypotheses. *Ann. Math. Stat.*, **42**, 1859–1869.

Willson, L. J. and Folks, J. L. (1983). Sequential estimation of the mean of the negative binomial distribution. *Sequential Anal.*, **2**, 55–70.

Wittes, J. and Brittain, E. (1990). The role of internal plots in increasing the efficiency of clinical trials. *Stat. Med.*, **9**, 65–72.

Woodall, W. H. (1983). The distribution of the run length of one-sided cusum procedures for continuous random variables. *Technometrics*, **25**, 295–300.

Woodall, W. H. (1984). On the Markov chain approach to the two-sided CUSUM procedure. *Technometrics*, **26**, 41–46.

Woodroofe, M. (1977). Second order approximations for sequential point and interval estimation. *Ann. Stat.*, **5**, 984–995.

Woodroofe, M. (1982). *Nonlinear Renewal Theory in Sequential Analysis.* SIAM, Philadelphia.

Worsely, K. J. (1986). Confidence regions and tests for a change-point in a sequence of exponential family random variables. *Biometrika*, **73**, 91–104.

Wu, C. F. J. (1985). Efficient sequential designs with binary data. *J. Am. Stat. Assoc.*, **80**, 974–984.

Yakir, B. (1994). Optimal detection of a change in distribution when the observations form a Markov chain with a finite state space. In *Change-Point Problems*, E. Carlstein, H. Muller, and D. Siegmund, Eds. Institute of Mathematical Statistics, Hawyard, CA, pp. 346–388.

Yao, Y-C. (1984a). Estimation in the presence of noise of a signal which is flat except for jumps. In *Statistical Signal Processing*, E. J. Wegman and J. G. Smith, Eds. Marcel Dekker, New York, pp. 161–176.

Yao, Y-C. (1984b). Estimation of a noisy discrete-time step function: Bayes and empirical Bayes approaches. *Ann. Stat.*, **12**, 1434–1447.

Yashchin, E. (1985). On a unified approach to the analysis of two-sided cumulative sum control schemes with headstarts. *Adv. Appl. Prob.*, **17**, 562–593.

Young, P. (1984). *Recursive Estimation and Time-Series Analysis, an Introduction.* Springer-Verlag, New York.

Zacks, S. (1968). Bayes sequential design of fractional factorial experiments for the estimation of a subgroup of pre-assigned parameters. *Ann. Math. Stat.*, **39**, 973–982.

Zacks, S. (1969). Bayes sequential design of fixed size samples from finite populations. *J. Am. Stat. Assoc.*, **64**, 1342–1349.

Zacks, S. (1970). Bayesian design for single and double stratified sampling for estimating proportion in finite population. *Technometrics*, **12**, 119–129.

Zacks, S. (1971). *The Theory of Statistical Inference.* Wiley, New York.

Zacks, S. (1973). Sequential estimation of the common mean of two normal distributions, I: The case of one variance known. *J. Am. Stat. Assoc.*, **68**, 422–427.

Zacks, S. (1977). Problems and approaches in design of experiments for estimating and testing in non-linear models. *Jour. of Multivariate Analysis*, Vol. 4. pp. 209–223.

Zacks, S. (1981). The probability distribution and the expected value of a stopping variable associated with one-sided CUSUM procedures for non-negative integer valued random variables. *Commun. Stat. A*, **10**, 2245–2258.

Zacks, S. (1983). A survey of classical and Bayesian approaches to the change-point problem: Fixed sample and sequential procedures of testing and estimation. In *Recent Advances in Statistics*, David Siegmund, Jagdish Rustaigi and G. Gaseb Risvi, Eds. Academic, New York, pp. 245–269.

Zacks, S. (1984). Bayes adaptive estimation of the point of shift to the wear-out phase of reliability systems. *Oper. Res.*, **32**, 741–749.

Zacks, S. (1991a). Detection and change-point problems. In *Handbook of Sequential Analysis*, B. K. Ghosh and P. K. Sen, Eds. Marcel Dekker, New York, Chapter 23.

Zacks, S. (1991b). Distribution of stopping times for Poisson processes with linear boundaries. *Commun. Stat. Stochast. Models*, **7**, 233–242.

Zacks, S. (1996). Adaptive designs for parametric models. In *Handbook of Statistics*, S. Ghosh and C. R. Rao, Eds. Vol. 13, North-Holland, Elsevier, New York, pp. 151–180.

Zacks, S. (2001). The operating characteristics of sequential procedures in reliability. *Handbook Stat.*, **20**, 789–811.

Zacks, S. (2004a). Exact determination of the run length distribution of a one-sided CUSUM procedure applied on an ordinary Poisson process. *Sequential Anal.*, **23**, 159–178.

Zacks, S. (2004b). Some recent results on the distributions of stopping times of compound Poisson processes with linear boundaries. *J. Stat. Plan. Inf.*, **130**, 95–109 (special volume in honor of Herman Chernoff).

Zacks, S. and Barzily, Z. (1981). Bayes procedures for detecting a shift in the probability of success in a series of Bernoulli trials. *J. Stat. Plan. Inf.*, **5**, 107–119.

Zacks, S. and Eichhorn, B. H. (1975). Sequential search of optimal dosages: The linear regression case. In *Survey of Statistical Designs and Linear Models*, J. N. Srivastave, Ed. North-Holland, New York.

Zacks, S. and Mukhopadhyay, N. (2006a). Exact risk of sequential point estimators of the exponential parameter. *Sequential Anal.*, **25**, 203–226.

Zacks, S. and Mukhopadhyay, N. (2006b). Bounded risk estimation of the exponential parameter in a two-stage sampling. *Sequential Anal.*, **25**, 437–452.

Zacks, S. and Mukhopadhyay, N. (2007). Distributions of sequential and two-stage stopping times for fixed-width confidence intervals in Bernoulli trials:

Application in reliability. *Sequential Anal.*, **26**, 425–442 (2008 Abraham Wald Prize in Sequential Anysis).

Zacks, S., Pereira, C. A. and Leite, J. G. (1990). Bayes sequential estimation of the size of a finite population. *J. Stat. Plan. Inf.*, **25**, 363–380.

Zacks, S., Rogatko, A. and Babb, J. (1998). Optimal Bayesian-feasible dose escalation for cancer phase I clinical trials. *Stat. Prob. Lett.*, **38**, 215–220.

Zelen, M. (1974). The randomization and stratification of patients to clinical trials. *J. Chronic Dis.*, **27**, 365–375.

Appendix: SPLUS/R Programs

All computations in the present monograph were performed in SPLUS. The reader can use R instead. All functions given in this appendix can run on either one of these softwares. The objective of the appendix is to explain these various functions. In the book the functions are called programs. All the functions given here were written specifically for the present book. They utilize the functions in the SPLUS library. However, for convenience the following functions were added and are essential for the functions given later. The reader is advised to insert the following functions to his or her collection of objects.

1. ```
   std(x){
   sqrt(var(x))}
   ```

2. ```
   inv(x){
   solve(x)}
   ```

3. ```
   jay(k,m){
   l<-k*m
   a<-c(1:l)/c(1:l)
   res<-matrix(a,nrow=k)
   res}
   ```

4. ```
   psum(x){
   ```

```
n <- length(x)
res <- c(1:n)
res[1] <- x[1]
   for(i in 2:n) {
     res[i] <- res[i - 1] + x[i]
     }
res
}
```

The function std(x) computes the standard deviation of a data set x.
The function inv(x) computes the inverse of a squared matrix x.
The function jay(k,m) computes a $k \times m$ matrix of 1's.
The function psum(x) computes the partial sums of a data set x.

We present now the various functions by the chapter in which they are used. One can copy these functions electronically from the web page mentioned in the Preface, that is, ftp://ftp.wiley.com/public/sci_tech_med/stagewise_designs.

Chapter 2

```
2.1 distNm(alfa, dlt, sigl, sig, Ns)
    {
    m <- floor(qchisq(1 - alfa, 1) * ((sigl/dlt)^2)) + 1
    a <- (dlt/(qt(1 - alfa/2, m - 1) * sig))^2
    res <- c(m:(m + Ns))
    res[1] <- pchisq(m * (m - 1) * a, m - 1)
    for(i in 2:Ns) {
            n <- m + i - 1
            res[i] <- pchisq(n * (m - 1) * a, m - 1) -
                        pchisq((n - 1) * (m - 1) * a, m - 1)
    }
    out <- res[1:(Ns - 1)]
    out
    }
```

This function computes the exact distribution of the stopping variable N_{m^*}, which is plotted in Figure 2.1. The input variables are α, δ (dlt), σ_* (sigl), σ (sig), and Ns. Ns is the upper limit for the argument of the distribution function. The output (out) is the p.d.f. of the distribution. the c.d.f. is obtained by using the function psum() of the output.

```
2.2 Eval(k, A, ck, al, Ms)
    {
    g <- (A/ck)^(1/4)
    tk <- (k/g)^2
    pmk <- 1 - ppois(k - 1, al * tk)
    Ls <- Ms + 1 - k
    Tl <- jay(Ls, 1)
    G <- 0 * jay(Ls + k, Ls)
    Pm <- c(1:Ls)
```

```
Pm[1] <- pmk
Tl[1] <- tk
for(i in 1:k) {
        G[i, 1] <- dpois(i - 1, al * tk)
}
Ex <- (k * (1 - ppois(k, al * tk)))/(al * k)
Ex2 <- ((k + 1) * k * (1 - ppois(k + 1, al * tk
        )))/((al * k)^2)
for(l in 2:Ls) {
        Tl[l] <- ((k + l - 1)/g)^2
        dl <- Tl[l] - Tl[l - 1]
        for(j in 1:(k + l - 1)) {
                G[j, l] <- 0
                for(m in 1:j) {
                        G[j, l] <- G[j, l] + G[
                          m, l - 1] * dpois(j -
                          m, al * dl)
                }
        }
}
for(l in 2:Ls) {
        Pm[l] <- sum(G[, l - 1]) - sum(G[, l])
        cl <- Tl[l - 1]/(k + l - 1)
        cl2 <- 2 * (cl^2)
        dl <- Tl[l] - Tl[l - 1]
        sml <- 0
        sml2 <- 0
        for(j in 1:(k + l - 2)) {
                sml <- sml + G[j, l - 1] * (1 -
                        ppois(k + l - j - 1, al *
                        dl) + ((k + l - j) * (1 -
                        ppois(k + l - j, al *
                        dl)))/(al * Tl[l - 1]))
                sml2 <- sml2 + G[j, l - 1] * ((
                        1 - ppois(k + l - j - 1,
                        al * dl))/2 + ((k + l -
                        j) * (1 - ppois(k + l -
                        j, al * dl)))/(al * Tl[
                        l - 1]) + ((k + l - j) * (
                        k + l - j + 1) * (1 -
                        ppois(k + l - j + 1, al *
                        dl)))/(2 * ((al * Tl[l -
                        1])^2)))
        }
        Ex <- Ex + cl * sml
        Ex2 <- Ex2 + cl2 * sml2
}
Avm <- sum(c(k:Ms) * Pm)
Qvm <- sum((c(k:Ms)^2) * Pm)
svarm <- sqrt(Qvm - Avm^2)
vex <- Ex2 - Ex^2
Rm <- A * (Ex2 - (2 * Ex)/al + 1/(al^2)) + ck *
        Avm
```

```
out <- list(pmk, sum(Pm), Avm, svarm, Ex, Rm)
out
}
```

This function computes the output presented in Table 2.9 under $N(1)$. The input variables are: k, (m), A, ck (c), $\lambda = 1/\beta$ (al), and Ns, where Ns is the number of terms in the (infinite) sums. The output variables are: pmk = probability that the stopping time is at k; sum(Pm) = sum of probabilities of the stopping times. It should be close to 1 if Ns is sufficiently large; avm = expected stopping time; svarm = standard deviation of the stopping time; Ex = expected value of the estimator of beta at stopping; Rm = risk of estimator at stopping. To compute the results for $N(2)$ and $N(3)$, one needs to change the definition of g (γ) in the program.

```
2.3 exmp(p, alfa, delta, N)
    {
    k <- floor((4 * qchisq(1 - alfa, 1))/(delta^2)) +
            1
    res <- k
    for(n in k:(k + N)) {
            up <- (n * (1 + sqrt(1 - k/n)))/2
            dw <- n - up
            if(dw == floor(dw)) {
                    dw <- dw - 1
            }
            res <- res + pbinom(dw, n, p) + pbinom(
                    dw, n, 1 - p)
    }
    res
    }
```

This function computes the expected stopping time of $N(\delta)$ for Tables 2.10 and 2.11. The input variables are: p, α, δ, and N = number of terms in the (infinite) sum in Eq. (2.6.24). The output is the exact value of the expected value of the stopping time.

```
2.4 riskmp(p, alfa, delta, N)
    {
    rho <- p/(1 - p)
    k <- floor((4 * qchisq(1 - alfa, 1))/(delta^2)) +
            1
    me <- dbinom(k/2, k, p)
    mse <- ((1 - rho)^2) * dbinom(k/2, k, p)
    dpu <- c(1:(N + 1))
    dpl <- dpu
    dpu[1] <- 1 - pbinom(floor(k/2) + 1, k, p)
    dpl[1] <- pbinom(floor(k/2), k, p)
    sp <- me
    cp <- 0
    rhodu <- rho * exp(delta)
    rhodl <- rho * exp( - delta)
    if((rhodl <= 1) && (1 <= rhodu)) {
```

```
        cp <- cp + dbinom(k/2, k, p)
}
for(n in (k + 1):(k + N)) {
        ub <- n*(1+sqrt(1-k/n))/2
        lb <- n - ub
        pnl <- pbinom(lb, n, p)
        pnu <- pbinom(lb, n, 1 - p)
        dpu[n - k + 1] <- pnu
        dpl[n - k + 1] <- pnl
        fnu <- dpu[n - k] - pnu
        fnl <- dpl[n - k] - pnl
        fn <- fnl + fnu
        rhol <- (floor(lb) + 1)/(n - 1 - floor(
                     lb))
        rhou <- floor(ub)/(n - floor(ub))
        me <- me + fnu * rhou + fnl * rhol
        mse <- mse + ((rhou - rho)^2) * fnu + ((
                rhol - rho)^2) * fnl
        sp <- sp + fn
        if((rhodl <= rhol) && (rhol <= rhodu))
                {
                cp <- cp + fnl
        }
        if((rhodl <= rhou) && (rhou <= rhodu))
                {
                cp <- cp + fnu
        }
}
res <- list(me, mse, sp, cp)
res
}
```

This function computes the results presented in Table 2.12. The input variables are p, α, δ, N. It is recommended to use $N = 1000$. The output variables are me = expected odds (2.6.31) at stopping; mse = the MSE of the odds estimator (2.6.31); CP = the coverage probability.

Chapter 3

```
3.1 Bayesim2(d1, J, m, M)
    {
    S1 <- 0
    S2 <- 0
    cs1 <- c(1:M)
    cs2 <- c(1:M)
    for(i in 1:M) {
            xi <- rgamma(1, 2)/2
            g1i <- xi * exp(min(100, (d1 * J) * xi)
                    ) * ((1 + exp(d1))/(1 + exp(d1 * (
                    xi))))^m
            g2i <- exp(min(100, (d1 * J) * (xi)) * (
                    (1 + exp(d1))/(1 + exp(d1 * (xi
```

```
                ))))^m
        cs1[i] <- g1i
        cs2[i] <- g2i
}
res <- mean(cs1)/mean(cs2)
res
}
```

The output of this function is displayed in Table 3.3. The input variables are $d_1 = x$ (2.4 for this table); J = number of successes in Bernoulli trials; m = the number of Bernoulli trials; M = number of simulation runs.

```
3.2 bayesnum(w, z, xr)
    {
    n <- length(w)
    S1 <- 0
    S2 <- 0
    J <- 28
    for(i in 1:n) {
            ui <- z[i]
            A1i <- (((1 - ui)/(ui^2))^2) * exp(((-2 +
                    xr * J) * (1 - ui))/ui - 30 *
                    log(1 + exp((xr * (1 - ui))/ui)
                    ))
            A2i <- ((1 - ui)/(ui^3)) * exp(((-2 +
                    xr * J) * (1 - ui))/ui - 30 *
                    log(1 + exp((xr * (1 - ui))/ui)
                    ))
            S1 <- S1 + w[i] * A1i
            S2 <- S2 + w[i] * A2i
    }
    out <- list(S1/S2)
    out
    }
```

This function computes the Bayesian estimator (3.3.8) by Gaussian numerical integration. The input variables w and z should be the sets w and u in the table following (3.3.6). The input variable xr is the value of x (= 2.4). The output is the Bayesian estimator.

```
3.3 adaptiveBS(x1, m, M)
    {
    res <- jay(M, 3)
    xi <- x1
    for(i in 1:2) {
            ji <- rbinom(1, m, logis(0, 1, xi))
            bi <- bayesim2(xi, ji, m, 1000)
            res[i, 1] <- xi
            res[i, 2] <- ji
            res[i, 3] <- bi
            xi <- 2.4/mean(res[1:i, 3])
    }
    for(i in 3:M) {
```

```
                xn <- res[1:i - 1, 1]
                jn <- res[1:i - 1, 2]
                bi <- adaptiveBayes(xn, jn, m, 100)
                res[i, 1] <- xi
                res[i, 2] <- rbinom(1, m, logis(0, 1,
                        xi))
                res[i, 3] <- bi
                xi <- 2.4/bi
        }
        res
        }
```

The present function was employed to compute Table 3.4. It requires the following functions (subroutines) bayesim2, adaptiveBayes, and logis. bayesim2 is given above, and the other functions are given below (3.4 and 3.5). the input variables are x_1 = initial dose; m = number of Bernoulli trials; M = number of iterations.

```
3.4 adaptiveBayes(xn, jn, m, M)
    {
    n <- length(xn)
    Tn <- sum(xn * jn)
    S1 <- 0
    S2 <- 0
    for(j in 1:M) {
            bt <- rgamma(1, 2)/2
            Ln <- 0
            for(i in 1:n) {
                    Ln <- Ln + bt * xn[i] + exp( -
                            bt * xn[i])
            }
            S1 <- S1 + bt * exp(bt * Tn - m * Ln)
            S2 <- S2 + exp(bt * Tn - m * Ln)
    }
    res <- S1/S2
    res
    }

3.5 logis(a, b, x)
    {
    res <- exp(a + b * x)/(1 + exp(a + b * x))
    res
    }
```

Chapter 4

```
4.1 simcp(x, m, delt, Ns)
    {
    al <- qchisq(0.95, 1)/(delt^2)
    res <- jay(Ns, 3)
    for(i in 1:Ns) {
```

```
            xs <- sample(x, m, replace = T)
            sd <- var(xs)
            n <- m
            repeat {
                    rx <- al * sd
                    if(n > rx)
                            break
                    ys <- sample(x, 1, replace = T)
                    xs <- c(xs, ys)
                    sd <- var(xs)
                    n <- n + 1
            }
            res[i, 1] <- n
            res[i, 2] <- mean(xs) - delt
            res[i, 3] <- mean(xs) + delt
    }
    res
```

This function is designed for Table 4.1. The input variables are x = set of 1000 random variates from $G(5, 2)$; m = size of samples; delta = δ; Ns = number of iterations. The output variables are the stopping time, N; lower and upper confidence limits for the mean.

```
4.2 simts2(x, m, delt, Ns)
    {
    N <- length(x)
    cal <- qchisq(0.95, 1)
    res <- jay(Ns, 3)
    for(i in 1:Ns) {
            x2 <- x
            sp <- sample(N, m)
            xs <- x2[sp]
            sd <- var(xs)
            n <- (N * (cal * sd))/(N * (delt^2) +
                    cal * sd)
            n <- floor(n) + 1
            for(j in 1:m) {
                    x2[sp[j]] <- 0
            }
            x2s <- sort(x2)
            x22 <- x2s[(m + 1):N]
            if(n > m) {
                    xs2 <- sample(x22, n - m)
                    xs <- c(xs, xs2)
            }
            res[i, 1] <- n
            res[i, 2] <- mean(xs) - delt
            res[i, 3] <- mean(xs) + delt
    }
    out <- res
    out
    }
```

The present function computes the simulation estimates for Table 4.3 for the nonstratified sampling. The input variables are x = original sample from $G(5, 2)$; m = initial sample size; $\delta = \delta$; Ns = number of simulation runs. The output is a matrix of Ns rows and three columns. Columns 1 gives the total sample size of the two-stage procedure; columns 2 and 3 give the lower and upper confidence limits of the population mean. From this output we have to compute the estimates of the expected total sample and the coverage probabilities.

```
4.3 simtsst(x, m, w, delt, Ns)
    {
    N <- length(x)
    cal <- qchisq(0.95, 1)
    res <- jay(Ns, 3)
    N1 <- w[1] * N
    N2 <- w[2] * N
    N3 <- w[3] * N
    x1 <- x[1:N1]
    x2 <- x[(N1 + 1):(N1 + N2)]
    x3 <- x[(N1 + N2 + 1):N]
    m1 <- w[1] * m
    m2 <- w[2] * m
    m3 <- w[3] * m
    for(i in 1:Ns) {
            x21 <- x1
            sp1 <- sample(N1, m1)
            xs1 <- x21[sp1]
            sd1 <- var(xs1)
            x22 <- x2
            sp2 <- sample(N2, m2)
            xs2 <- x22[sp2]
            sd2 <- var(xs2)
            x23 <- x3
            sp3 <- sample(N3, m3)
            xs3 <- x23[sp3]
            sd3 <- var(xs3)
            td <- w[1] * sd1 + w[2] * sd2 + w[3] *
                    sd3
            nm <- (N * (cal * td))/(N * (delt^2) +
                    cal * td)
            nm <- floor(nm) + 1
            for(j in 1:m1) {
                    x21[sp1[j]] <- 0
            }
            x2s1 <- sort(x21)
            x221 <- x2s1[(m1 + 1):N1]
            for(j in 1:m2) {
                    x22[sp2[j]] <- 0
            }
            x2s2 <- sort(x22)
            x222 <- x2s2[(m2 + 1):N2]
            for(j in 1:m3) {
                    x23[sp3[j]] <- 0
```

```
                }
                x2s3 <- sort(x23)
                x223 <- x2s3[(m3 + 1):N3]
                if(nm > m) {
                        nmm <- nm - m
                        r1 <- w[1] * sqrt(sd1)
                        r2 <- w[2] * sqrt(sd2)
                        r3 <- w[3] * sqrt(sd3)
                        nmm1 <- min(max(1, floor((nmm * r1)/
                                (r1 + r2 + r3))),x221)
                        nmm2 <- min(max(1, floor((nmm * r2)/
                                (r1 + r2 + r3))),x222)
                        nmm3 <- min(max(1, floor((nmm * r3)/
                                (r1 + r2 + r3))),x223)
                        xs21 <- sample(x221, nmm1)
                        xs22 <- sample(x222, nmm2)
                        xs23 <- sample(x223, nmm3)
                        xs1 <- c(xs1, xs21)
                        xs2 <- c(xs2, xs22)
                        xs3 <- c(xs3, xs23)
                        as <- w[1] * mean(xs1) + w[2] *
                                mean(xs2) + w[3] * mean(
                                xs3)
                }
                res[i, 1] <- nm
                res[i, 2] <- as - delt
                res[i, 3] <- as + delt
        }
        out <- res
        out
        }
```

This function computes the values in Table 4.3 for the stratified two-stage sampling. The input variables are x = the population of random variates from $G(5, 2)$; m = total sample size in the first stage; w = vector of strata weights; dlt = δ; Ns = number of iterations. The output is a matrix of Ns rows and three columns.

```
    4.4 seqsim(x, g, kc, K, M)
        {
        res <- c(1:M)
        N <- length(x)
        for(i in 1:M) {
                k <- 951
                xs <- x[k:N]
                n <- length(xs)
                y <- c(1:n)
                for(j in 1:n) {
                        y[j] <- rbinom(1, 1, exp( - g/xs[j]))
                }
                sy <- sum(y)
                if((sy > 0) && (sy < n)) {
                        gm <- gmle(xs, y, runif(1))
```

```
            }
            else {
                    gm <- g
            }
            fi <- 0
            for(j in 1:n) {
                    fi <- fi + exp( - gm/xs[j])/((xs[j]^2) *
                            (1 - exp( - gm/xs[j])))
            }
            gml <- gm - 1.65 * sqrt(1/fi)
            if(K * exp( - gml/min(x)) > kc) {
                    res[i] <- N
            }
            else {
                    repeat {
                            crit <- K * exp( - gml/x[k - 1])
                            if((crit < kc) || (n == 999))
                              break
                            k <- k - 1
                            n <- n + 1
                            xs <- c(xs, x[k])
                            y <- c(y, rbinom(1, 1, exp( - g/x[k])))
                            sy <- sum(y)
                            if((sy > 0) && (sy < n)) {
                              gm <- gmle(xs, y, runif(1))
                            }
                            else {
                              gm <- g
                            }
                            fi <- fi + exp( - gm/xs[n])/((xs[n]^2)
                              (1 - exp( - gm/xs[n])))
                            gml <- gm - 1.65 * sqrt(1/fi)
                    }
                    res[i] <- n
            }
    }
    res
    }
```

This function computes the simulated values of $M*$ which are required for Table 4.7. The input variables are x = set of covariates; g = gamma coefficient; kc = cost c; K = cost of field inspection; M = number of iterations. The output is a set of M simulated values of $M*$.

```
4.5 gmle(x, y, g1)
    {
    n <- length(x)
    repeat {
            s0 <- 0
            for(j in 1:n) {
                    s0 <- s0 + (y[j] - exp( - g1/x[j]))/(x[j] *
                         (1 - exp( - g1/x[j])))
            }
```

```
        if(s0 > 0)
                break
        g1 <- g1 + 1
}
out <- g1 - 1/2
out
}
```

This function is needed for seqsim above (4.4). It computes the MLE of the coefficient gamma.

```
4.6 seqfsim(N, M0, M1, M, m, alf, bet, Ns)
    {
    res <- c(1:Ns)
    for(i in 1:Ns) {
            res[i] <- seqfp2(N, M0, M1, M, m, alf,
                    bet)
    }
    res
    }
```

This function computes the simulated values of the stopping variable N_m (4.7.7). The sequential procedure is designed to test the hypothesis H_0 : $p \leq p_0$ against $H_1 : p \geq p_1$. The input variables are the population size N; $M_0 = [N * p_0]$; $M_1 = [N * p_1]$; M = actual number of defectives; m is the initial sample size; alf = α and bet = β.

```
4.7 seqfp2(N, M0, M1, M, m, alf, bet)
    {
    R1 <- log(1 - bet) - log(alf)
    R0 <- log(bet/(1 - alf))
    U <- c(1:N)
    indx <- sample(U, m)
    jx <- 0
    for(i in 1:m) {
            if(indx[i] <= M) {
                    jx <- jx + 1
            }
    }
    Ur <- U[(jx + 1):(N - m + jx)]
    Nr <- N - m
    n <- m
    repeat {
            llr <- log(dhyper(jx, M1, N - M1, n)) -
                    log(dhyper(jx, M0, N - M0, n))
            if((llr < R0) || (llr > R1))
                    break
            n <- n + 1
            indx2 <- sample(Ur, 1)
            if(indx2 <= M) {
                    jx <- jx + 1
                    Ur <- Ur[2:Nr]
            }
```

```
            else {
                    Ur <- Ur[1:(Nr - 1)]
            }
            Nr <- Nr - 1
    }
    out <- n
    out
    }
```

This function is required for 4.6 above.

Chapter 5

```
5.1 simulacfma(ns,n,iq,a){
    res<-jay(ns,iq)
    for(i in 1:ns){
            u<-rnorm(n)
            x<-u
            for(j in (iq+1):n){
            for(l in 1:iq){
                x[j]<-x[j]+a[l]*u[j-l]}
                }
            ak<-acf(x,iq,plot=F)
            res[i,]<-ak$acf[2:(iq+1)]
            }
            res
    }
```

This function simulates the estimates of the autocorrelations for an MA(q). The input variables are ns = number of iterations; n = sample size; iq = order of the MA(q); a = vector of coefficients. The output is a matrix of ns rows with iq columns.

```
5.2 toeplitz<-function(a){
    n<-length(a)
    res<-jay(n,n)
    res[1,]<-a
        for(i in 2:n){
            res[i,(i:n)]<-a[1:(n-i+1)]
                    for(j in 1:(i-1)){
                    res[i,j]<-res[j,i]
                    }
            }
            res
            }
```

This function computes the Toeplitz matrix for a set of n numbers.

```
5.3 pred1<-function(x,n){
        ns<-length(x)
        res<-c(1:ns)
```

```
res[1:n]<-x[1:n]
  for(i in (n+1):ns){
  xs<-x[1:i]
  ak<-acf(xs,10,plot=F)
  a<-ak$acf[1:9]
  R<-toeplitz(a)
  r<-ak$acf[2:10]
  b<-inv(R)%*%r
  res[i]<-sum(x[(i-1):(i-9)]*b)
  }
  res
  }
```

This function determines the ad hoc predictor with simulated acf coefficients for an MA(q) series(see Figure 5.3).

```
5.4 pred.poly<-function(x,n,s){
    ns<-length(x)
    res<-c(1:ns)
    res[1:(n+s)]<-x[1:(n+s)]
    for(i in (n+1):(ns-s)){
          xs<-x[i:(i-n+1)]
          tx<-c(0:-(n-1))
          z<-cbind(tx^0,tx,tx^2)
          b<-inv(t(z)%*%z)%*%t(z)%*%xs
          ts<-c(1,s,s^2)
          pred<-b[1,1]+s*b[2,1]+b[3,1]*s^2
          res[i+s]<-pred
          }
          res
    }
```

This function determines the quadratic moving LSE. The input variables are x = time series; n = length of the moving window; s = prediction lag. The result at time t is the predictor of the value at time $t+s$.

```
5.5 pred1<-function(x,n){
    ns<-length(x)
    res<-c(1:ns)
    res[1:n]<-x[1:n]
    for(i in (n+1):ns){
          xs<-x[1:i]
          ak<-acf(xs,10,plot=F)
          a<-ak$acf[1:9]
          R<-toeplitz(a)
          r<-ak$acf[2:10]
          b<-inv(R)%*%r
          res[i]<-sum(x[(i-1):(i-9)]*b)
          }
          res
    }
```

A function for determining the QMLSE predictor. The input variables are x = time series; n = length of initial learning sample.

```
5.6 mas.pred1<-function(x,m,s){
    n<-length(x)
    k<-2*m+s
    res<-c(1:n)
    res[1:k]<-x[1:k]
          for( i in (m+1):(n-m-s)){
          xtm<-x[(i-m):(i+m)]
          b0m<-mean(xtm)
          am<-c(1:m)
          amm<-c(-m:-1)
          wm<-c(amm,0,am)
          b1m<-(3*sum(wm*xtm))/(m*(m+1)*(2*m+1))
          res[i+m+s]<-b0m+(m+s)*b1m
    }
    res
    }
```

This function computes the linear MAS(m) predictor. The input variables are x = time series; m = length of window on each side of t; s = prediction lag.

```
5.7 season(x, alfa, beta, gamma, m, l, is)
    {
    n <- length(x)
    xs <- x[1:(m * l)]
    aver <- c(1:m)
       for(i in 1:m) {
       aver[i] <- mean(xs[((i - 1) * l + 1):(i * l)])
       }
    b1 <- (aver[m] - aver[1])/((m - 1) * l)
    b0 <- aver[m] + (l * b1)/2
    c0 <- c(1:(l * m))
       for(i in 1:m) {
       for(j in 1:l) {
          k <- j + (i - 1) * l
          c0[k] <- xs[k]/(aver[i] - ((l + 1)/2 - j) * b1)
       }
       }
    seasf <- c(1:l)
       for(i in 1:l) {
       seasf[i] <- mean(xs[seq(i, (l * m), l)])
       }
    seasf <- (seasf * l)/sum(seasf)
       for(i in 1:m) {
       for(j in 1:l) {
          k <- j + (i - 1) * l
          c0[k] <- seasf[j]
          }
       }
    c1 <- c(1:n)
    c1[1:(l * m)] <- c0
    xpred <- c(1:n)
    xpred[1:(l * m)] <- xs
       for(i in (l * m + 1):(n - is)) {
```

```
            b0n <- (alfa * x[i])/c1[i - l] + (1 - alfa) * (b0 + b1)
            b1 <- beta * (b0n - b0) + (1 - beta) * b1
            b0 <- b0n
            c1[i] <- (gamma * x[i])/b0 + (1 - gamma) * c1[i - l]
            xpred[i + is] <- (b0 + b1 * is) * c1[i + is - l]
            cr <- i/l
            icr <- floor(cr)
            if(cr == icr) {
            a <- c((i - l + 1):i)
            seasfl <- (l * c1[a])/sum(c1[a])
            c1[a] <- seasfl
            }
        }
    a <- c((l * m + 1):(l * m + is))
    xpred[a] <- x[a]
    xpred
    }
```

The present function computes the predictor according to Winter's seasonal model. The input variables are x = time series; alfa, beta, gamma = coefficients; l = number of seasons (month) in the year; m = number of years; is = s is the prediction lag.

```
5.8 dlm1.int(x,v,w,it,tau,z){
    n<-length(x)
    mt<-c(1:n)
    sct<-c(1:n)
    mt[1]<-x[1]
    sct[1]<-w
    for(i in 1:(it-1)){
       sct[i]<-v*(sct[i-1]+w)/(sct[i-1]+v+w)
       mt[i]<-mt[i-1]+sct[i]*(x[i]-mt[i-1])/v
    }
    sct[it]<-v*(sct[it-1]+w+tau^2)/(sct[it-1]+w+v+tau^2)
    mt[it]<-mt[it-1]+z+sct[it]*(x[it]-mt[it-1]-z)/v
    for(i in (it+1):n){
       sct[i]<-v*(sct[i-1]+w)/(sct[i-1]+v+w)
       mt[i]<-mt[i-1]+sct[i]*(x[i]-mt[i-1])/v
    }
    mt
    }
```

A DLM model with intervention. Input variables: x = time series; v, w = variance components; it = location of change point; z = mean of the r.v. Z; τ = STD of Z.

```
5.9 dlm.lg(x,C0,v,W,M0){
    n<-length(x)
    pred<-c(1:n)
    for(i in 1:n){
       at<-as.vector(c(1,i))
       pred[i]<-t(at)%*%M0
       ut<-v+t(at)%*%(C0+W)%*%at
```

```
    ei<-(x[i]-t(at)%*%M0)
    ev<-as.vector(c(ei/ut,(i*ei)/ut))
    M0<-M0+(C0+W)%*%ev
    B<-jay(2,2)
    B[1,1]<-1/ut
    B[1,2]<-i/ut
    B[2,1]<-i/ut
    B[2,2]<-(i^2)/ut
    C0<-(C0+W)-(C0+W)%*%B%*%(C0+W)
  }
  pred
  }
```

DLM model with linear growth. Input variables: x = time series; C_0, M_0 = the initial covariance and initial mean; V, W = covariance matrices.

```
5.10 dlm.reg(y,x,C0,v,W,M0){
     n<-length(y)
     x<-cbind(jay(n,1),x)
     k<-ncol(x)
     pred<-c(1:n)
     for(i in 1:n){
     at<-as.vector(x[i,])
     pred[i]<-at%*%M0
     att<-jay(5,1)
     att[,1]<-at
     ut<-v+at%*%(C0+W)%*%att
     ei<-(y[i]-at%*%M0)
     ev<-jay(k,1)
     ev1<-jay(k,1)
        for(j in 1:k){
        ev[j,1]<-(x[i,j]*ei)/ut
        ev1[j,1]<-(x[i,j])/ut
        }
     M0<-M0+(C0+W)%*%ev
     B<-ev1%*%at
     C0<-(C0+W)-(C0+W)%*%B%*%(C0+W)
     }
     pred
     }
```

DLM regression. Input variables: y = time series for forecasting; x = matrix of covariates; C_0, M_0 = initial covariance and mean; V, W = covariance matrices.

```
5.11 rec.ricatti(S,A,D,FX,n){
     b1<-t(D)%*%D
     b2<-t(FX)%*%FX
     b3<-t(D)%*%FX
     for(i in 1:n){
     S<-(b1+t(A)%*%S%*%A)-(t(A)%*%S%*%B+b3)%*%
     inv(b2+t(B)%*%S%*%B)%*%(t(b3)+t(B)%*%S%*%A)
     }
```

```
S
}
```

Recursive function for solving the algebraic Riccati equation.

Chapter 6

```
6.1 ud1(xd, Qd, Ns){
    mtd <- xd[3]
    res <- jay(Ns, 3)
    for(i in 1:Ns) {
    j <- 1
    k <- 0
    x1 <- xd[j]
    q1 <- Qd[j]
    n <- 3
    N <- n
    repeat {
            j1 <- rbinom(1, n, q1)
                if(j1 == 1) {
                    j1 <- j1 + rbinom(1, n,
                      q1)
                    N <- N + n
                       if(x1 > mtd) {
                          k <- k + n
                       }
                    }
                if(x1 > mtd) {
                    k <- k + n
                }
                if((j1 > 1) || (j == 6))
                   break
                   j <- j + 1
                   x1 <- xd[j]
                   q1 <- Qd[j]
                   N <- N + n
                }
    mtdh <- x1
    res[i, 1] <- mtdh
    res[i, 2] <- N
    res[i, 3] <- k/N
    }
    bias <- mean(res[, 1]) - mtd
    mse <- mean(res[, 1]^2) - 2 * mean(res[, 1]) *
    mtd + mtd^2
    avn <- mean(res[, 2])
    prop <- mean(res[, 3])
    out <- list(bias, mse, avn, prop, quantile(res[,
         1], prob = c(0.25, 0.5, 0.75, 0.9)))
    out
    }
```

Function for the simulation of the estimators of the MTD under UD1. Input variables: xd = vector of doses; qd = vector of $Q(x)$ values corresponding to xd; Ns = number of simulation runs.

```
6.2 ud2(xd, Qd, N, Ns){
    mtd <- xd[3]
    res <- jay(Ns, 2)
    for(i in 1:Ns) {
    j <- 1
    k <- 0
    x1 <- xd[j]
    q1 <- Qd[j]
    n <- 3
    Nt <- n
    ji <- 1
    repeat {
            j1 <- rbinom(1, n, q1)
            if(j1 == 1) {
                j <- j
                Nt <- Nt + n
            }
            if((j1 > 1) && (j > 1)) {
                j <- j - 1
                Nt <- Nt + n
            }
            if((j1 == 0) && (j < 6)) {
                j <- j + 1
                Nt <- Nt + n
            }
            if(x1 > mtd) {
                k <- k + n
            }
            if(Nt == N)
               break
               ji <- ji + 1
               x1 <- xd[j]
               q1 <- Qd[j]
            }
     mtdh <- x1
     res[i, 1] <- mtdh
     res[i, 2] <- k/N
     }
     bias <- mean(res[, 1]) - mtd
     mse <- mean(res[, 1]^2) - 2 * mean(res[, 1]) *
     mtd + mtd^2
     prop <- mean(res[, 2])
     out <- list(bias, mse, prop)
     out
     }
```

Function to simulate the MTD values under UD2. Input variables: xd, qd as above; N = number of patients; Ns as above.

```
6.3 ud3(xd, Qd, N, Ns){
```

```
        mtd <- xd[3]
        res <- jay(Ns, 2)
        for(i in 1:Ns) {
            j <- 1
            k <- 0
            x1 <- xd[j]
            q1 <- Qd[j]
            n <- 1
            Nt <- n
            ji <- 0
            repeat {
                    j1 <- rbinom(1, n, q1)
                    if((j1 > 0) && (j > 1)) {
                            j <- j - 1
                            Nt <- Nt + n
                    }
                    if((j1 == 0) && (ji == 1)) {
                        if(j < 6) {
                           j <- j + 1
                        }
                        ji <- ji + 1
                        Nt <- Nt + n
                    }
                    if((j1 == 0) && (ji == 0)) {
                        ji <- ji + 1
                        j <- j
                        Nt <- Nt + 1
                    }
                    if(x1 > mtd) {
                        k <- k + n
                    }
                    if(Nt == N)
                        break
                        if(ji == 2) {
                            ji <- 0
                        }
                        x1 <- xd[j]
                        q1 <- Qd[j]
                    }
           mtdh <- x1
           res[i, 1] <- mtdh
           res[i, 2] <- k/N
           }
           bias <- mean(res[, 1]) - mtd
           mse <- mean(res[, 1]^2) - 2 * mean(res[, 1]) *
           mtd + mtd^2
           prop <- mean(res[, 2])
           out <- list(bias, mse, prop)
           out
           }
```

Function for UD3. Variables as above.

```
6.4 ud4(xd, Qd, N, Ns){
```

```
mtd <- xd[3]
res <- jay(Ns, 2)
for(i in 1:Ns) {
j <- 1
k <- 0
x1 <- xd[j]
q1 <- Qd[j]
n <- 1
Nt <- n
ji <- 0
jt <- 0
repeat {
        j1 <- rbinom(1, n, q1)
        jt <- jt + j1
        if(jt <- 0) {
             if(j < 6) {
                j <- j + 1
                Nt <- Nt + n
             }
        }
        else {
              if((j1 > 0) && (j > 1)
                 ) {
                 j <- j - 1
                 Nt <- Nt + n
              }
              if((j1 == 0) && (ji ==
                 1)) {
                 if(j < 6) {
                    j <- j + 1
                 }
                 ji <- ji + 1
                 Nt <- Nt + n
              }
              if((j1 == 0) && (ji ==
                 0)) {
                 ji <- ji + 1
                 j <- j
                 Nt <- Nt + 1
              }
        }
        if(x1 > mtd) {
              k <- k + n
        }
        if(Nt == N)
            break
            if(ji == 2) {
                ji <- 0
            }
            x1 <- xd[j]
            q1 <- Qd[j]
        }
  mtdh <- x1
  res[i, 1] <- mtdh
```

```
res[i, 2] <- k/N
}
bias <- mean(res[, 1]) - mtd
mse <- mean(res[, 1]^2) - 2 * mean(res[, 1]) *
mtd + mtd^2
prop <- mean(res[, 2])
out <- list(bias, mse, prop)
out
}
```

Function for UD4. Variables as above.

```
6.5 bcd(xd, Qd, N, Ns){
    mtd <- xd[3]
    res <- jay(Ns, 2)
    pod<-0
    for(i in 1:Ns) {
    j <- 1
    k <- 0
    x1 <- xd[j]
    q1 <- Qd[j]
    n <- 1
    Nt <- n
    ji <- 0
    repeat {
            bx <- q1/(1 - q1)
            j1 <- rbinom(1, n, q1)
            if((j1 > 0) && (j > 1)) {
                 j <- j - 1
                 Nt <- Nt + n
            }
            u <- runif(1)
            if((j1 == 0) && (u < bx)) {
                if(j < 6) {
                   j <- j + 1
                }
                Nt <- Nt + n
            }
            if(x1 > mtd) {
                k <- k + n
            }
            if(Nt == N)
                break
                x1 <- xd[j]
                q1 <- Qd[j]
            }
   mtdh <- x1
   if(mtdh>mtd){pod<-pod+1/Ns}
            res[i, 1] <- mtdh
            res[i, 2] <- k/N
   }
   bias <- mean(res[, 1]) - mtd
   mse <- mean(res[, 1]^2) - 2 * mean(res[, 1]) *
   mtd + mtd^2
```

```
prop <- mean(res[, 2])
out <- list(bias, mse,pod, prop)
out
}
```

Function bcd for simulation estimates of the MTD under procedure BCD1. Variables as above.

```
6.6 bayesim3(g, p1, xs, xt, n, M){
    bet0 <- -3.569
    bet1 <- 0.549
    res <- c(1:(n + 1))
    yr <- c(1:n)
    res[1] <- xs
    w1 <- p1/(1 - p1)
    for(i in 1:n) {
        Tn <- 0
        Td <- 0
        xi <- res[i]
        qi <- exp(bet0 + bet1 * xi)
        qi <- qi/(1 + qi)
        yi <- rbinom(1, 1, qi)
        yr[i] <- yi
        for(l in 1:M) {
            bl <- rgamma(1, 1/2)
            Lj <- 0
            for(j in 1:i) {
                xj <- res[j]
                yj <- yr[j]
                Lj <- Lj + log(1 + w1 *
                exp(bl * (xj - xs))) -
                bl * yj * (xj - xs)
            }
            Ls <- exp( - Lj)
            Tn <- Tn + Ls/bl
            Td <- Td + Ls
        }
        xgh <- xs + ((log(g/(1 - g)) - log(w1)) *
            Tn)/Td
        xgh <- min(xt, xgh)
        res[i + 1] <- xgh
    }
    res
    }
```

Function for simulating the MTD in the CRM procedure shown in Table 6.5. The input variables are: $g = \gamma$; p_1; xs $= x*$; xt $=$ upper bound for dosages; $n =$ number of patients; $M =$ number of iterations for the simulated estimates of the integrals.

```
6.7 bayesim4(g, p1, xs, xt, n, M, al){
    bet0 <- -3.569
    bet1 <- 0.549
```

```
res <- c(1:(n + 1))
yr <- c(1:n)
res[1] <- xs
w1 <- p1/(1 - p1)
for(i in 1:n) {
    Tn <- 0
    Td <- 0
    Tb <- 0
    Tq <- 0
    xi <- res[i]
    qi <- exp(bet0 + bet1 * xi)
    qi <- qi/(1 + qi)
    yi <- rbinom(1, 1, qi)
    yr[i] <- yi
    for(l in 1:M) {
        bl <- rgamma(1, 1/2)
        Lj <- 0
        for(j in 1:i) {
            xj <- res[j]
            yj <- yr[j]
            Lj <- Lj + log(1 + w1 *
            exp(bl * (xj - xs))) -
            bl * yj * (xj - xs)
        }
        Ls <- exp( - Lj)
        Tn <- Tn + Ls/bl
        Td <- Td + Ls
        Tb <- Tb + bl * Ls
        Tq <- Tq + Ls * (bl^2)
    }
    Eb <- Tb/Td
    Sb <- sqrt(Tq/Td - Eb^2)
    xgh <- xs + (log(g/(1 - g)) - log(w1))/(
       Eb + al * Sb)
       xgh <- min(xt, xgh)
       res[i + 1] <- xgh
}
res
}
```

Function for estimating the EWOC MTD by simulations. The input variables are as in 6.6 and al = λ.

```
6.8 bayesim5(g, p1, xs, xt, n, M, al, Ns){
    res <- jay(Ns, 2)
    for(i in 1:Ns) {
    bsimres <- bayesim4(g, p1, xs, xt, n, M,
        al)
    f1 <- 0
    f2 <- 0
    for(j in 1:n) {
        if(bsimres[j] < 5.24) {
            f1 <- f1 + 1/n
            f2 <- f2 + ((5.24 -
```

```
            bsimres[j])/n)
        }
    }
    res[i, 1] <- f1
    res[i, 2] <- f2
    }
    res
    }
```

Function for estimating POD and AVS of Table 6.6. Input variables are as in 6.7; Ns = number of runs.

Chapter 7

```
7.1 distm(N)
    {
    M <- N/2
    res <- c(1:M)
    a <- c(M:(N - 1))
    res[1] <- 2/comb(N, M)
    for(i in 2:M) {
    j <- i - 1
    res[i] <- (2 * comb(M + j - 1, j))/comb(
        N, M)
    }
    out <- list(res, sum(res), sum(a * res))
    out
    }
```

Function to compute the distribution of the stopping variable (7.2.5). The input variable is the total number of patients, N.

```
7.2 distm2(N)
    {
    M <- N/2
    res <- c(1:M)
    res[1] <- (1/2)^(M - 1)
    for(i in 2:M) {
    j <- i - 1
    res[i] <- dbinom(j, M + j - 1, 1/2)
    }
    out <- list(res, sum(res))
    out
    }
```

Function to compute the distribution of (7.2.9). The input variable is the total number of patients.

```
7.3 exbnk(alfa, dlt, k, pk)
    {
    ns <- qchisq(1 - alfa, 1)/(4 * (dlt^2))
```

```
nf <- floor(ns)
M <- nf - k + 1
js <- jay(M, 2)
gf <- jay(M, 2)
pl <- c(1:M)
for(n in 1:M) {
nk <- k + n - 1
js[n, 1] <- floor((nk * (1 - sqrt(1 -
     nk/ns)))/2) + 1
js[n, 2] <- floor((nk * (1 + sqrt(1 -
      nk/ns)))/2)
}
gf[1, 1] <- 0
for(i in 2:M) {
ii <- i - 1
gf[i, 1] <- 0
if((ii >= js[1, 1]) && (ii <= js[1, 2])
      ) {
      gf[i, 1] <- dbinom(ii, k, pk)
}
}
pl[1] <- sum(gf[, 1])
for(n in 1:(M - 1)) {
gf[1, 2] <- 0
for(i in 2:M) {
ii <- i - 1
gf[i, 2] <- 0
if((ii >= js[n + 1, 1]) && (ii <=
      js[n + 1, 2])) {
      gf[i, 2] <- pk * gf[i -
           1, 1] + (1 - pk) * gf[
            i, 1]
}
pl[n + 1] <- sum(gf[, 2])
}
gf[, 1] <- gf[, 2]
}
res <- k + sum(pl)
res
}
```

Function for computing the expected value of (7.3.7). The input variables are α, δ, k, and p.

```
7.4 exbnks(alfa, dlt, k, pk, Ns)
    {
    ns <- qchisq(1 - alfa, 1)/(4 * (dlt^2))
    nf <- floor(ns)
    M <- nf - k + 1
    cp <- 0
    Nkd <- c(1:Ns)
    Bn <- jay(M, 2)
    for(i in 1:M) {
    ni <- i + k - 1
```

```
Bn[i, 1] <- (ni * (1 - sqrt(1 - ni/nf))
    )/2
Bn[i, 2] <- (ni * (1 + sqrt(1 - ni/nf))
    )/2
}
for(j in 1:Ns) {
xn <- rbinom(1, k, pk)
m <- 1
repeat {
        if((xn <= Bn[m, 1]) || (xn >=
            Bn[m, 2]))
            break
            m <- m + 1
            xn <- xn + rbinom(1, 1, pk)
}
pj <- xn/(m + k - 1)
Nkd[j] <- m + k - 1
if(((pk - dlt) <= pj) && ((pk + dlt) >=
     pj)) {
     cp <- cp + 1/Ns
}
}
out <- list(mean(Nkd), 2 * sqrt(var(Nkd)/Ns),
cp, 2 * sqrt((cp * (1 - cp))/Ns))
out
}
```

Function to simulate their expected value of (7.3.7) and the coverage probability. The input variables are as in 7.3 above; Ns is the number of simulation runs.

```
7.5 expros(alfa, al, k, p, MS)
    {
    gsa <- qchisq(1 - alfa, 1)/(al^2)
    M <- MS - k + 1
    Bs <- c(1:M)
    stm <- c(1:MS)
    cp <- 0
    for(n in 1:M) {
    nk <- n + k - 1
    Bs[n] <- floor(gsa/(1 + gsa/(nk)))
    }
    for(i in 1:MS) {
    n <- k
    xn <- rbinom(1, k, p)
    repeat {
            if(xn > Bs[n - k + 1])
                break
                n <- n + 1
                xn <- xn + rbinom(1, 1, p)
            }
    stm[i] <- n
    pn <- xn/n
    if(((1 - al) * p <= pn) && ((1 + al) *
```

```
p >= pn)) {
        cp <- cp + 1/MS
    }
    }
    out <- list(mean(stm), 2 * sqrt(var(stm)/MS),
    cp, 2 * sqrt((cp * (1 - cp))/MS))
    out
    }
```

Function to compute simulation estimates of the expected value and coverage probability of the stopping variable (7.4.4). The input variables are α, λ, k, p, Ms = number of simulation runs.

```
7.6 dexbnks(alfa, dlt, k, p1, p2, Ns)
    {
    cr <- qchisq(1 - alfa, 1)/(dlt^2)
    Nbk <- c(1:Ns)
    cp <- 0
    md <- c(1:Ns)
    for(i in 1:Ns) {
    xn <- rbinom(1, k, p1)
    yn <- rbinom(1, k, p2)
    n <- k
    repeat {
            pn1 <- xn/n
            pn2 <- yn/n
            if(n >= (cr * (pn1 * (1 - pn1) +
                pn2 * (1 - pn2))))
                break
                n <- n + 1
                xn <- xn + rbinom(1, 1, p1)
                yn <- yn + rbinom(1, 1, p2)
    }
    Nbk[i] <- n
    D <- pn1 - pn2
    md[i] <- D
    Da <- p1 - p2
    if(abs(D - Da) < dlt) {
        cp <- cp + 1/Ns
    }
    }
    out <- list(mean(Nbk), 2 * sqrt(var(Nbk)/Ns),
    cp, 2 * sqrt((cp * (1 - cp))/Ns), mean(
        md), 2 * sqrt(var(md)/Ns))
    out
    }
```

Function to compute simulation estimates of the expected value of (7.5.4) and the coverage probability. The input variables are α, δ, k, p_1, p_2, Ns = number of simulation runs.

```
7.7 exgs(alfa, K, p1, p2, m, zb, Ns)
    {
```

```
st <- c(1:Ns)
sty <- c(1:Ns)
sl1 <- 0
sl2 <- 0
for(i in 1:Ns) {
xn <- rbinom(1, m, p1)
yn <- rbinom(1, m, p2)
pa <- xn/m
pb <- yn/m
wa <- 2 * asin(sqrt(pa))
wb <- 2 * asin(sqrt(pb))
dt <- wa - wb
pc <- (xn + yn)/(2 * m)
k <- 1
repeat {
        cr <- (abs(pa - pb) * sqrt(m *
        k))/sqrt(2 * pc * (1 -
        pc))
        if((cr > zb * sqrt(K/k)) || k ==
        K)
        break
        k <- k + 1
        xn <- xn + rbinom(1, m, p1)
        yn <- yn + rbinom(1, m, p2)
        pa <- xn/(m * k)
        pb <- yn/(m * k)
        pc <- (xn + yn)/(2 * m * k)
}
st[i] <- k
if((k < K) || (cr > zb)) {
        sl1 <- sl1 + 1/Ns
}
k <- 1
repeat {
        cr <- sqrt((m * k)/2) * abs(dt)
        if(cr > zb * sqrt(K/k) || (k ==
        K))
        break
        k <- k + 1
        xn <- rbinom(1, m, p1)
        yn <- rbinom(1, m, p2)
        wa <- (wa * (k - 1) + 2 * asin(
        sqrt(xn/m)))/k
        wb <- (wb * (k - 1) + 2 * asin(
        sqrt(yn/m)))/k
        dt <- wa - wb
}
sty[i] <- k
if((k < K) || (cr > zb)) {
        sl2 <- sl2 + 1/Ns
}
}
out <- list(mean(st), 2 * sqrt(var(st)/Ns), sl1,
2 * sqrt((sl1 * (1 - sl1))/Ns), mean(
```

```
sty), 2 * sqrt(var(sty)/Ns), sl2, 2 *
sqrt((sl2 * (1 - sl2))/Ns))
out
}
```

Function to compute simulated estimates of the expected value of stopping times and significance level for two types of standard variables. The input variables are α, K = maximal number of groups; p_1, p_2, m = size of each group; zb = coefficient $\gamma\ \alpha_K$; Ns = number of simulation runs.

```
7.8 Octs(p0, p, m, M, alfa, beta)
    {
    alfap <- alfa
    N1 <- m
    q1 <- qbinom(1 - alfap, N1, p0)
    res <- pbinom(q1 - 1, N1, p)
    exn <- N1 * res
    exk <- res
    for(j in q1:N1) {
    N2j <- min(M, floor(Npower(p0, j/N1,
              alfap, beta)) + 1)
    q2j <- qbinom(1 - alfap, N2j, p0)
    if(N2j <= N1) {
              exn <- exn + dbinom(j, N1, p) *
                        N1
              exk <- exk + dbinom(j, N1, p)
    }
    if(N2j > N1) {
              res <- res + dbinom(j, N1, p) *
                        pbinom(q2j - 1 - j, N2j -
                        N1, p)
              exn <- exn + N2j * dbinom(j, N1,
                        p) * pbinom(q2j - 1 - j,
                        N2j - N1, p)
              exk <- exk + 2 * dbinom(j, N1,
                        p) * pbinom(q2j - 1 - j,
                        N2j - N1, p)
              for(k in q2j:N2j) {
                        N3jk <- min(M, floor(
                          Npower(p0, k/N2j,
                          alfap, beta)) + 1)
                        q3jk <- qbinom(1 -
                          alfap, N3jk, p0)
                        if(N3jk <= N2j) {
                          exn <- exn + dbinom(j,
                            N1, p) * dbinom(k -
                            j, N2j - N1, p) *
                            N2j
                          exk <- exk + 2 *
                            dbinom(j, N1, p) *
                            dbinom(k - j, N2j -
                            N1, p)
                        }
```

```
                    if(N3jk > N2j) {
                      res <- res + dbinom(j,
                        N1, p) * dbinom(k -
                        j, N2j - N1, p) *
                        pbinom(q3jk - 1 - j -
                        k, N3jk - N2j, p)
                      exn <- exn + dbinom(j,
                        N1, p) * dbinom(k -
                        j, N2j - N1, p) *
                        N3jk
                      exk <- exk + 3 *
                        dbinom(j, N1, p) *
                        dbinom(k - j, N2j -
                        N1, p)
                    }
            }
            }
            }
            out <- list(1 - res, exn, exk)
            out
            }
```

Program to compute the values for Table 7.8. The input variables are those defined in that table.

Chapter 8

```
8.1 ropt(N, al)
    {
    M <- (N * (N + 3))/2
    rhom <- c(1:M)
    j <- N
    for(i in 1:(j + 1)) {
    ji <- ((j - 1) * (j + 2))/2 + i
    rhom[ji] <- max(al, i/(N + 1))
    }
    for(n in 1:(N - 1)) {
    j <- N - n
    for(i in 1:(j + 1)) {
    ji <- ((j - 1) * (j + 2))/2 + i
    rhom[ji] <- max((n + 1) * al, i/
        (N + 1 - n) + (i/(N + 1 -
        n)) * rhom[ji + N + 1 -
        n + 1] + ((N + 1 - n -
        i)/(N + 1 - n)) * rhom[
        ji + N + 1 - n])
    }
    }
    out <- rhom
    out
    }
```

Function to compute the optimal $\lambda(N, X)$ criterion. Input variables: N = number of trials, al = λ.

```
8.2  simsr1(alpha, p1, p2, k, N, Ns)
     {
     res2 <- c(1:Ns)
     for(i in 1:Ns) {
     res2[i] <- sr1(alpha, p1, p2, k, N)
     }
     res2
     }
```

Function for simulation of the truncated stopping time (8.1.13). The input variables are α; p_1, p_2; k = initial sample size; N = number of trials; Ns = number of simulation runs. This program requires the following function 8.3.

```
8.3  sr1(alpha, p1, p2, k, N)
     {
     n <- k
     x <- rbinom(1, k, p1)
     a <- x + 1
     b <- k + 1 - x
     repeat {
             if((qbeta(1 - alpha, a, b) <= p2) || (n >=
                 N))
             break
             j <- rbinom(1, 1, p1)
             a <- a + j
             b <- b + 1 - j
             n <- n + 1
     }
     n
     }
```

Subfunction for 8.2. Same input variables.

```
8.4 gindx(r, al, a, b)
    {
    s1 <- 0
    s2 <- 0
    for(i in 0:(r - 1)) {
    s1 <- s1 + (al^i) * beta(a + i, b + 1)
    s2 <- s2 + (al^i) * beta(a + i + 1, b +
        1)
    }
    b1 <- beta(a + r, b + 1)
    b2 <- beta(a + r + 1, b + 1)
    indx1 <- (s2 + (b2 * (al^r))/(1 - al))
    indx2 <- (s1 + (b1 * (al^r))/(1 - al))
    res <- indx1/indx2
    res
    }
```

This function computes the index (8.2.7). The input variables are r; al = coefficient α in (8.2.7); a, b = parameters of the beta prior. This function requires the function beta given below.

```
beta(a,b){
gamma(a)*gamma(b)/gamma(a+b)}

8.5 gittlb(al, a, b)
    {
    r <- 1
    h1 <- gindx(r, al, a, b)
    repeat {
            r <- r + 1
            h2 <- gindx(r, al, a, b)
            if(h2 < h1)
               break
            h1 <- h2
    }
    out <- h1
    out
    }
```

This function computes a lower bound for the Gittins index. The input is as in Table 8.3.

```
8.6 simpgr(p1, p2, al1, al2, k, N, Ns)
    {
    res <- jay(Ns, 2)
    for(i in 1:Ns) {
    n <- k
    n1 <- n/2
    n2 <- n/2
    x1 <- rbinom(1, n1, p1)
    x2 <- rbinom(1, n2, p2)
    a1 <- x1 + 1
    b1 <- n1 - x1 + 1
    a2 <- x2 + 1
    b2 <- n2 - x2 + 1
    ps <- pgr(a1, b1, a2, b2)
    repeat {
            if((ps > (1 - al1)) || (ps <
                al2))
                break
                n1 <- n1 + 1
                n2 <- n2 + 1
                x1 <- x1 + rbinom(1, 1, p1)
                x2 <- x2 + rbinom(1, 1, p2)
                a1 <- x1 + 1
                b1 <- n1 - x1 + 1
                a2 <- x2 + 1
                b2 <- n2 - x2 + 1
                ps <- pgr(a1, b1, a2, b2)
     }
```

```
M <- n1 + n2
if(ps > (1 - al1)) {
        flag <- 2
}
if(ps < al2) {
        flag <- 1
}
res[i, 1] <- flag
res[i, 2] <- max(N - M, 0)
}
res
}
```

This function computes the simulated stopping time (8.3.6). The input variables are p_1, p_2, al1$= \alpha_1$, al2 $= \alpha_2$; k = initial sample size; N = number of trials; Ns = number of simulation runs. This function requires the functions pgr and awr given below.

```
pgr(a1, b1, a2, b2)
{
s1 <- a1 + b1
s2 <- a2 + b2
tot <- 0
for(j in a1:(s1 - 1)) {
tot <- tot + (comb(s1 - 1, j) * beta(a2 +
     j, s1 + b2 - 1 - j))/beta(a2,
     b2)
}
res <- tot
res
}
```

```
awr(x, N)
{
Ns <- length(x[, 1])
N1 <- 0
cp <- 0
for(i in 1:Ns) {
a <- x[i, 1]
b <- x[i, 2]
if(a == 1) {
    N1 <- N1 + (N - b)/2 + b
    cp <- cp + 1/Ns
}
if(a == 2) {
    N1 <- N1 + (N - b)/2
}
}
res <- list(N1/Ns, 1 - cp)
res
}
```

Chapter 9

```
9.1 amocbinom(x, nw, z1, z2, sigs, tausq, p)
    {
    Ns <- length(x)
    res <- c(1:Ns)
    res[1] <- x[1]
    for(it in 2:Ns) {
    n <- min(it, nw)
    itn <- it - n + 1
    xn <- x[itn:it]
    xbn <- mean(xn)
    pst <- 0 * c(1:n)
    for(j in 1:(n - 1)) {
        xbj <- mean(xn[1:j])
        xbnj <- mean(xn[(j + 1):n])
        fj <- sqrt((1 + j * sigs) * (1 + (n - j) * tausq))
        gj <- exp((j * (n - j) * ((xbj - xbnj)^2))/(2 * n))
        hj <- exp(( - j * ((xbj - z1)^2))/(2 * (1 + j * sigs)) - ((n - j) * (
             (xbnj - z2)^2))/(2 * (1 + (n - j) * tausq)))
        pst[j] <- (p * ((1 - p)^(j - 1)) * gj * hj)/fj
    }
    fn <- sqrt(1 + n * sigs)
    pst[n] <- (((1 - p)^(n - 1)) * exp(( - n * ((xbn - z1)^2))/(2 * (1 + n *
        sigs))))/fn
    poster <- pst/sum(pst)
    mut <- 0
    for(j in 1:(n - 1)) {
        xbnj <- mean(xn[(j + 1):n])
        mut <- mut + poster[j] * (z2 + ((n - j) * tausq * (xbnj - z2))/(1 + (
            n - j) * tausq))
    }
    mut <- mut + poster[n] * (z1 + (n * sigs * (xbn - z1))/(1 + n * sigs))
    res[it] <- mut
    }
    out <- res
    out
    }
```

This is a function for the MW-AMOC binomial algorithm. The input variables are X = time series sequence; nw = number of observations in a moving window; z_1, z_2 = the prior parameters ζ_1 and ζ_2; sigs = σ^2; tausq = τ^2; p = prior probability of a change between any two consecutive observations.

```
9.2 amocnorm(x, nw, z1, z2, sigs, tausq, p)
    {
    Ns <- length(x)
    res <- c(1:Ns)
    res[1] <- x[1]
    for(it in 2:Ns) {
    n <- min(it, nw)
    itn <- it - n + 1
    xn <- x[itn:it]
```

```
xbn <- mean(xn)
pst <- 0 * c(1:n)
for(j in 1:(n - 1)) {
    xbj <- mean(xn[1:j])
    xbnj <- mean(xn[(j + 1):n])
    fj <- sqrt((1 + j * sigs) * (1 + (n - j) * tausq))
    gj <- exp((j * (n - j) * ((xbj - xbnj)^2))/(2 * n))
    hj <- exp(( - j * ((xbj - z1)^2))/(2 * (1 + j * sigs)) - ((n - j) * (
        (xbnj - z2)^2))/(2 * (1 + (n - j) * tausq)))
    pst[j] <- (p * ((1 - p)^(j - 1)) * gj * hj)/fj
}
fn <- sqrt(1 + n * sigs)
pst[n] <- (((1 - p)^(n - 1)) * exp(( - n * ((xbn - z1)^2))/(2 * (1 + n *
    sigs))))/fn
poster <- pst/sum(pst)
mut <- 0
for(j in 1:(n - 1)) {
    xbj <- mean(xn[1:j])
    xbnj <- mean(xn[(j + 1):n])
    wj1 <- 1/(1 + n * sigs + (n - j) * tausq * (1 + j * sigs))
    wj2 <- j * sigs * wj1
    wj3 <- 1 - wj1 - wj2
    mut <- mut + poster[j] * (wj1 * (z1 + (z2 - z1) * (1 + j * sigs)) +
        wj2 * xbj + wj3 * xbnj)
}
mut <- mut + poster[n] * (z1/(1 + n * sigs) + (n * sigs * xbn)/(1 + n *
        sigs))
res[it] <- mut
}
out <- res
out
}
```

Function to compute the MW-AMOC normal algorithm. Input variables as in 9.1.

```
9.3 amocpois(x, nw, al1, al2, v1, v2, p)
    {
    Ns <- length(x)
    res <- c(1:Ns)
    res[1] <- x[1]
    for(it in 2:Ns) {
    n <- min(it, nw)
    itn <- it - n + 1
    xn <- x[itn:it]
    sn <- sum(xn)
    pst <- 0 * c(1:n)
    for(j in 1:(n - 1)) {
        sj <- sum(xn[1:j])
        snj <- sn - sj
        fj <- (j * al1)/(v1 + j * al1)
        gj <- nb(sj, fj, v1)
        fnj <- ((n - j) * al2)/(v2 + (n - j) * al2)
        gnj <- nb(snj, fnj, v2)
```

```
    pst[j] <- p * ((1 - p)^(j - 1)) * gj * gnj
}
fn <- (n * al1)/(v1 + n * al1)
pst[n] <- ((1 - p)^(n - 1)) * nb(sn, fn, v1)
poster <- pst/sum(pst)
mut <- 0
for(j in 1:(n - 1)) {
    sj <- sum(xn[1:j])
    snj <- sn - sj
    mut <- mut + (poster[j] * al2 * (snj + v2))/(v2 + (n - j) * al2)
}
mut <- mut + (poster[n] * al1 * (v1 + sn))/(v1 + n * al1)
res[it] <- mut
}
res
}
```

Function to compute MW-AMOC Poisson algorithm. Input variables are x = time series; nw = size of moving window; al1, al2, v_1, v_2 = prior parameters of the corresponding gamma distributions; p = probability of a change between any two consecutive observations.

```
9.4 recurfilter(x, k, sigs)
    {
    Ns <- length(x)
    res <- c(1:Ns)
    res[1:k] <- x[1:k]
    yk <- jay(k, 1)
    yk[, 1] <- x[1:k]
    A <- jay(k, 3)
    A[, 2] <- c(1:k)
    A[, 3] <- c(1:k)^2
    Pk <- inv(t(A) %*% A)
    Bk <- Pk %*% t(A) %*% yk
    for(it in (k + 1):Ns) {
    ht <- jay(3, 1)
    ht[2, 1] <- it
    ht[3, 1] <- it^2
    cf <- 1/(sigs + t(ht) %*% Pk %*% ht)
    Ck <- (Pk %*% ht) %*% t(Pk %*% ht)
    Dk <- 0 * jay(3, 3)
    Dk[1, 1] <- cf
    Dk[2, 2] <- cf
    Dk[3, 3] <- cf
    Pk <- Pk - Dk %*% Ck
    Ek <- (x[it] - t(ht) %*% Bk)
    Fk <- 0 * jay(3, 3)
    Fk[1, 1] <- Ek
    Fk[2, 2] <- Ek
    Fk[3, 3] <- Ek
    Bk <- Bk + Fk %*% (Pk %*% ht)
    res[it] <- t(Bk) %*% ht
    }
```

```
out <- res
out
}
```

This function computes a recursive filter. The input variables are x = time series; k = size of initial learning sample; sigs = prior parameter σ^2.

Chapter 10

```
10.1 distNexp(g1, g2, al, Ns)
     {
     dlt <- g1 + g2
     cq <- c(1:Ns)
     fsl <- c(1:Ns)
     fsu <- c(1:Ns)
     fnu <- c(1:Ns)
     fn <- c(1:Ns)
     G0 <- c(1:Ns)
     kg1 <- floor(g1)
     cq[1] <- 1
     for(i in 1:(Ns - 1)) {
     si <- 0
     for(j in 0:(i - 1)) {
          si <- si + cq[j + 1] * dpois((i -
              j), (i - j) * al)
     }
     cq[i + 1] <-  - si
     }
     fsu[1] <- ppois(kg1, (1 + kg1 - g1) * al)
     for(l in 1:Ns) {
          sl <- 0
          sg <- 0
          for(m in 1:l) {
              sl <- sl + cq[m] * dpois(l - m, (
                  l - m + g2) * al)
              sg <- sg + cq[m] * dpois(l - m, (
                  l - m + dlt) * al)
          }
     fsl[l] <- sl
     G0[l] <- sg
     }
     for(n in 2:Ns) {
          sl <- 0
          for(i in (kg1 + 1):(kg1 + n - 1)) {
              si <- 0
              for(l in 0:(kg1 + n - 1 - i))
                  {
                  sj <- 0
                  for(j in 0:(kg1 + n - i -
                          1 - l)) {
                      sj <- sj + dpois(j, (
                          j + n + kg1 - i) *
```

```
                                  al)
                         }
                     si <- cq[l + 1] * sj
                 }
                 sl <- sl + dpois(i, (i - kg1) *
                     al) * si
            }
            fsu[n] <- ppois(n - 1 + kg1, n * al) -
                 sl
            }
            fnu[1] <- 1 - fsu[1]
            for(n in 2:Ns) {
            fnu[n] <- fsu[n - 1] - fsu[n]
            }
            fn[1:kg1] <- fsl[1:kg1]
            for(i in (kg1 + 1):Ns) {
            fn[i] <- fsl[i] + fnu[i - kg1]
            sij <- 0
            for(j in (kg1 + 1):i) {
                 sij <- sij + fnu[j - kg1] * G0[
                     i - j + 1]
            }
            fn[i] <- fn[i] - sij
            }
            av <- sum(fn * c(1:Ns))
            out <- list(a = psum(fn), b = av, c = sum(fsl),
            d = psum(fsl))
            out
            }
```

Function to compute the distribution of the stopping variable N in Table 10.2. Input variables: g1, g2 = the parameters γ_1 and γ_2 defined after (10.1.38); al = $\lambda = 1/\mu$; Ns = number of probabilities to compute.

Author Index

Topic Index

WILEY SERIES IN PROBABILITY AND STATISTICS

ESTABLISHED BY WALTER A. SHEWHART AND SAMUEL S. WILKS

The ***Wiley Series in Probability and Statistics*** is well established and authoritative. It covers many topics of current research interest in both pure and applied statistics and probability theory. Written by leading statisticians and institutions, the titles span both state-of-the-art developments in the field and classical methods.

Reflecting the wide range of current research in statistics, the series encompasses applied, methodological and theoretical statistics, ranging from applications and new techniques made possible by advances in computerized practice to rigorous treatment of theoretical approaches.

This series provides essential and invaluable reading for all statisticians, whether in academia, industry, government, or research.

† ABRAHAM and LEDOLTER · Statistical Methods for Forecasting
AGRESTI · Analysis of Ordinal Categorical Data
AGRESTI · An Introduction to Categorical Data Analysis, *Second Edition*
AGRESTI · Categorical Data Analysis, *Second Edition*
ALTMAN, GILL, and McDONALD · Numerical Issues in Statistical Computing for the Social Scientist
AMARATUNGA and CABRERA · Exploration and Analysis of DNA Microarray and Protein Array Data
ANDĚL · Mathematics of Chance
ANDERSON · An Introduction to Multivariate Statistical Analysis, *Third Edition*
* ANDERSON · The Statistical Analysis of Time Series
ANDERSON, AUQUIER, HAUCK, OAKES, VANDAELE, and WEISBERG · Statistical Methods for Comparative Studies
ANDERSON and LOYNES · The Teaching of Practical Statistics
ARMITAGE and DAVID (editors) · Advances in Biometry
ARNOLD, BALAKRISHNAN, and NAGARAJA · Records
* ARTHANARI and DODGE · Mathematical Programming in Statistics
* BAILEY · The Elements of Stochastic Processes with Applications to the Natural Sciences
BALAKRISHNAN and KOUTRAS · Runs and Scans with Applications
BALAKRISHNAN and NG · Precedence-Type Tests and Applications
BARNETT · Comparative Statistical Inference, *Third Edition*
BARNETT · Environmental Statistics
BARNETT and LEWIS · Outliers in Statistical Data, *Third Edition*
BARTOSZYNSKI and NIEWIADOMSKA-BUGAJ · Probability and Statistical Inference
BASILEVSKY · Statistical Factor Analysis and Related Methods: Theory and Applications
BASU and RIGDON · Statistical Methods for the Reliability of Repairable Systems
BATES and WATTS · Nonlinear Regression Analysis and Its Applications
BECHHOFER, SANTNER, and GOLDSMAN · Design and Analysis of Experiments for Statistical Selection, Screening, and Multiple Comparisons

*Now available in a lower priced paperback edition in the Wiley Classics Library.
†Now available in a lower priced paperback edition in the Wiley–Interscience Paperback Series.

BELSLEY · Conditioning Diagnostics: Collinearity and Weak Data in Regression

† BELSLEY, KUH, and WELSCH · Regression Diagnostics: Identifying Influential Data and Sources of Collinearity

BENDAT and PIERSOL · Random Data: Analysis and Measurement Procedures, *Third Edition*

BERRY, CHALONER, and GEWEKE · Bayesian Analysis in Statistics and Econometrics: Essays in Honor of Arnold Zellner

BERNARDO and SMITH · Bayesian Theory

BHAT and MILLER · Elements of Applied Stochastic Processes, *Third Edition*

BHATTACHARYA and WAYMIRE · Stochastic Processes with Applications

BILLINGSLEY · Convergence of Probability Measures, *Second Edition*

BILLINGSLEY · Probability and Measure, *Third Edition*

BIRKES and DODGE · Alternative Methods of Regression

BISWAS, DATTA, FINE, and SEGAL · Statistical Advances in the Biomedical Sciences: Clinical Trials, Epidemiology, Survival Analysis, and Bioinformatics

BLISCHKE AND MURTHY (editors) · Case Studies in Reliability and Maintenance

BLISCHKE AND MURTHY · Reliability: Modeling, Prediction, and Optimization

BLOOMFIELD · Fourier Analysis of Time Series: An Introduction, *Second Edition*

BOLLEN · Structural Equations with Latent Variables

BOLLEN and CURRAN · Latent Curve Models: A Structural Equation Perspective

BOROVKOV · Ergodicity and Stability of Stochastic Processes

BOULEAU · Numerical Methods for Stochastic Processes

BOX · Bayesian Inference in Statistical Analysis

BOX · R. A. Fisher, the Life of a Scientist

BOX and DRAPER · Response Surfaces, Mixtures, and Ridge Analyses, *Second Edition*

* BOX and DRAPER · Evolutionary Operation: A Statistical Method for Process Improvement

BOX and FRIENDS · Improving Almost Anything, *Revised Edition*

BOX, HUNTER, and HUNTER · Statistics for Experimenters: Design, Innovation, and Discovery, *Second Editon*

BOX, JENKINS, and REINSEL · Time Series Analysis: Forcasting and Control, *Fourth Edition*

BOX and LUCEÑO · Statistical Control by Monitoring and Feedback Adjustment

BRANDIMARTE · Numerical Methods in Finance: A MATLAB-Based Introduction

† BROWN and HOLLANDER · Statistics: A Biomedical Introduction

BRUNNER, DOMHOF, and LANGER · Nonparametric Analysis of Longitudinal Data in Factorial Experiments

BUCKLEW · Large Deviation Techniques in Decision, Simulation, and Estimation

CAIROLI and DALANG · Sequential Stochastic Optimization

CASTILLO, HADI, BALAKRISHNAN, and SARABIA · Extreme Value and Related Models with Applications in Engineering and Science

CHAN · Time Series: Applications to Finance

CHARALAMBIDES · Combinatorial Methods in Discrete Distributions

CHATTERJEE and HADI · Regression Analysis by Example, *Fourth Edition*

CHATTERJEE and HADI · Sensitivity Analysis in Linear Regression

CHERNICK · Bootstrap Methods: A Guide for Practitioners and Researchers, *Second Edition*

CHERNICK and FRIIS · Introductory Biostatistics for the Health Sciences

CHILÈS and DELFINER · Geostatistics: Modeling Spatial Uncertainty

CHOW and LIU · Design and Analysis of Clinical Trials: Concepts and Methodologies, *Second Edition*

CLARKE · Linear Models: The Theory and Application of Analysis of Variance

CLARKE and DISNEY · Probability and Random Processes: A First Course with Applications, *Second Edition*

*Now available in a lower priced paperback edition in the Wiley Classics Library.

†Now available in a lower priced paperback edition in the Wiley–Interscience Paperback Series.

* COCHRAN and COX · Experimental Designs, *Second Edition*
CONGDON · Applied Bayesian Modelling
CONGDON · Bayesian Models for Categorical Data
CONGDON · Bayesian Statistical Modelling
CONOVER · Practical Nonparametric Statistics, *Third Edition*
COOK · Regression Graphics
COOK and WEISBERG · Applied Regression Including Computing and Graphics
COOK and WEISBERG · An Introduction to Regression Graphics
CORNELL · Experiments with Mixtures, Designs, Models, and the Analysis of Mixture Data, *Third Edition*
COVER and THOMAS · Elements of Information Theory
COX · A Handbook of Introductory Statistical Methods
* COX · Planning of Experiments
CRESSIE · Statistics for Spatial Data, *Revised Edition*
CSÖRGŐ and HORVÁTH · Limit Theorems in Change Point Analysis
DANIEL · Applications of Statistics to Industrial Experimentation
DANIEL · Biostatistics: A Foundation for Analysis in the Health Sciences, *Eighth Edition*
* DANIEL · Fitting Equations to Data: Computer Analysis of Multifactor Data, *Second Edition*
DASU and JOHNSON · Exploratory Data Mining and Data Cleaning
DAVID and NAGARAJA · Order Statistics, *Third Edition*
* DEGROOT, FIENBERG, and KADANE · Statistics and the Law
DEL CASTILLO · Statistical Process Adjustment for Quality Control
DEMARIS · Regression with Social Data: Modeling Continuous and Limited Response Variables
DEMIDENKO · Mixed Models: Theory and Applications
DENISON, HOLMES, MALLICK and SMITH · Bayesian Methods for Nonlinear Classification and Regression
DETTE and STUDDEN · The Theory of Canonical Moments with Applications in Statistics, Probability, and Analysis
DEY and MUKERJEE · Fractional Factorial Plans
DILLON and GOLDSTEIN · Multivariate Analysis: Methods and Applications
DODGE · Alternative Methods of Regression
* DODGE and ROMIG · Sampling Inspection Tables, *Second Edition*
* DOOB · Stochastic Processes
DOWDY, WEARDEN, and CHILKO · Statistics for Research, *Third Edition*
DRAPER and SMITH · Applied Regression Analysis, *Third Edition*
DRYDEN and MARDIA · Statistical Shape Analysis
DUDEWICZ and MISHRA · Modern Mathematical Statistics
DUNN and CLARK · Basic Statistics: A Primer for the Biomedical Sciences, *Third Edition*
DUPUIS and ELLIS · A Weak Convergence Approach to the Theory of Large Deviations
EDLER and KITSOS · Recent Advances in Quantitative Methods in Cancer and Human Health Risk Assessment
* ELANDT-JOHNSON and JOHNSON · Survival Models and Data Analysis
ENDERS · Applied Econometric Time Series
† ETHIER and KURTZ · Markov Processes: Characterization and Convergence
EVANS, HASTINGS, and PEACOCK · Statistical Distributions, *Third Edition*
FELLER · An Introduction to Probability Theory and Its Applications, Volume I, *Third Edition,* Revised; Volume II, *Second Edition*
FISHER and VAN BELLE · Biostatistics: A Methodology for the Health Sciences
FITZMAURICE, LAIRD, and WARE · Applied Longitudinal Analysis
* FLEISS · The Design and Analysis of Clinical Experiments

*Now available in a lower priced paperback edition in the Wiley Classics Library.
†Now available in a lower priced paperback edition in the Wiley–Interscience Paperback Series.

FLEISS · Statistical Methods for Rates and Proportions, *Third Edition*
† FLEMING and HARRINGTON · Counting Processes and Survival Analysis
FULLER · Introduction to Statistical Time Series, *Second Edition*
† FULLER · Measurement Error Models
GALLANT · Nonlinear Statistical Models
GEISSER · Modes of Parametric Statistical Inference
GELMAN and MENG · Applied Bayesian Modeling and Causal Inference from Incomplete-Data Perspectives
GEWEKE · Contemporary Bayesian Econometrics and Statistics
GHOSH, MUKHOPADHYAY, and SEN · Sequential Estimation
GIESBRECHT and GUMPERTZ · Planning, Construction, and Statistical Analysis of Comparative Experiments
GIFI · Nonlinear Multivariate Analysis
GIVENS and HOETING · Computational Statistics
GLASSERMAN and YAO · Monotone Structure in Discrete-Event Systems
GNANADESIKAN · Methods for Statistical Data Analysis of Multivariate Observations, *Second Edition*
GOLDSTEIN and LEWIS · Assessment: Problems, Development, and Statistical Issues
GREENWOOD and NIKULIN · A Guide to Chi-Squared Testing
GROSS, SHORTLE, THOMPSON, and HARRIS · Fundamentals of Queueing Theory, *Fourth Edition*
GROSS, SHORTLE, THOMPSON, and HARRIS · Solutions Manual to Accompany Fundamentals of Queueing Theory, *Fourth Edition*
* HAHN and SHAPIRO · Statistical Models in Engineering
HAHN and MEEKER · Statistical Intervals: A Guide for Practitioners
HALD · A History of Probability and Statistics and their Applications Before 1750
HALD · A History of Mathematical Statistics from 1750 to 1930
† HAMPEL · Robust Statistics: The Approach Based on Influence Functions
HANNAN and DEISTLER · The Statistical Theory of Linear Systems
HARTUNG, KNAPP, and SINHA · Statistical Meta-Analysis with Applications
HEIBERGER · Computation for the Analysis of Designed Experiments
HEDAYAT and SINHA · Design and Inference in Finite Population Sampling
HEDEKER and GIBBONS · Longitudinal Data Analysis
HELLER · MACSYMA for Statisticians
HINKELMANN and KEMPTHORNE · Design and Analysis of Experiments, Volume 1: Introduction to Experimental Design, *Second Edition*
HINKELMANN and KEMPTHORNE · Design and Analysis of Experiments, Volume 2: Advanced Experimental Design
HOAGLIN, MOSTELLER, and TUKEY · Fundamentals of Exploratory Analysis of Variance
* HOAGLIN, MOSTELLER, and TUKEY · Exploring Data Tables, Trends and Shapes
* HOAGLIN, MOSTELLER, and TUKEY · Understanding Robust and Exploratory Data Analysis
HOCHBERG and TAMHANE · Multiple Comparison Procedures
HOCKING · Methods and Applications of Linear Models: Regression and the Analysis of Variance, *Second Edition*
HOEL · Introduction to Mathematical Statistics, *Fifth Edition*
HOGG and KLUGMAN · Loss Distributions
HOLLANDER and WOLFE · Nonparametric Statistical Methods, *Second Edition*
HOSMER and LEMESHOW · Applied Logistic Regression, *Second Edition*
HOSMER, LEMESHOW, and MAY · Applied Survival Analysis: Regression Modeling of Time-to-Event Data, *Second Edition*
† HUBER and RONCHETTI · Robust Statistics, *Second Edition*

*Now available in a lower priced paperback edition in the Wiley Classics Library.
†Now available in a lower priced paperback edition in the Wiley–Interscience Paperback Series.

HUBERTY · Applied Discriminant Analysis
HUBERTY and OLEJNIK · Applied MANOVA and Discriminant Analysis, *Second Edition*
HUNT and KENNEDY · Financial Derivatives in Theory and Practice, *Revised Edition*
HURD and MIAMEE · Periodically Correlated Random Sequences: Spectral Theory and Practice
HUSKOVA, BERAN, and DUPAC · Collected Works of Jaroslav Hajek—with Commentary
HUZURBAZAR · Flowgraph Models for Multistate Time-to-Event Data
IMAN and CONOVER · A Modern Approach to Statistics
† JACKSON · A User's Guide to Principle Components
JOHN · Statistical Methods in Engineering and Quality Assurance
JOHNSON · Multivariate Statistical Simulation
JOHNSON and BALAKRISHNAN · Advances in the Theory and Practice of Statistics: A Volume in Honor of Samuel Kotz
JOHNSON and BHATTACHARYYA · Statistics: Principles and Methods, *Fifth Edition*
JOHNSON and KOTZ · Distributions in Statistics
JOHNSON and KOTZ (editors) · Leading Personalities in Statistical Sciences: From the Seventeenth Century to the Present
JOHNSON, KOTZ, and BALAKRISHNAN · Continuous Univariate Distributions, Volume 1, *Second Edition*
JOHNSON, KOTZ, and BALAKRISHNAN · Continuous Univariate Distributions, Volume 2, *Second Edition*
JOHNSON, KOTZ, and BALAKRISHNAN · Discrete Multivariate Distributions
JOHNSON, KEMP, and KOTZ · Univariate Discrete Distributions, *Third Edition*
JUDGE, GRIFFITHS, HILL, LÜTKEPOHL, and LEE · The Theory and Practice of Econometrics, *Second Edition*
JUREČKOVÁ and SEN · Robust Statistical Procedures: Aymptotics and Interrelations
JUREK and MASON · Operator-Limit Distributions in Probability Theory
KADANE · Bayesian Methods and Ethics in a Clinical Trial Design
KADANE AND SCHUM · A Probabilistic Analysis of the Sacco and Vanzetti Evidence
KALBFLEISCH and PRENTICE · The Statistical Analysis of Failure Time Data, *Second Edition*
KARIYA and KURATA · Generalized Least Squares
KASS and VOS · Geometrical Foundations of Asymptotic Inference
† KAUFMAN and ROUSSEEUW · Finding Groups in Data: An Introduction to Cluster Analysis
KEDEM and FOKIANOS · Regression Models for Time Series Analysis
KENDALL, BARDEN, CARNE, and LE · Shape and Shape Theory
KHURI · Advanced Calculus with Applications in Statistics, *Second Edition*
KHURI, MATHEW, and SINHA · Statistical Tests for Mixed Linear Models
KLEIBER and KOTZ · Statistical Size Distributions in Economics and Actuarial Sciences
KLUGMAN, PANJER, and WILLMOT · Loss Models: From Data to Decisions, *Third Edition*
KLUGMAN, PANJER, and WILLMOT · Solutions Manual to Accompany Loss Models: From Data to Decisions, *Third Edition*
KOTZ, BALAKRISHNAN, and JOHNSON · Continuous Multivariate Distributions, Volume 1, *Second Edition*
KOVALENKO, KUZNETZOV, and PEGG · Mathematical Theory of Reliability of Time-Dependent Systems with Practical Applications
KOWALSKI and TU · Modern Applied U-Statistics
KROONENBERG · Applied Multiway Data Analysis
KVAM and VIDAKOVIC · Nonparametric Statistics with Applications to Science and Engineering

*Now available in a lower priced paperback edition in the Wiley Classics Library.
†Now available in a lower priced paperback edition in the Wiley–Interscience Paperback Series.

LACHIN · Biostatistical Methods: The Assessment of Relative Risks
LAD · Operational Subjective Statistical Methods: A Mathematical, Philosophical, and Historical Introduction
LAMPERTI · Probability: A Survey of the Mathematical Theory, *Second Edition*
LANGE, RYAN, BILLARD, BRILLINGER, CONQUEST, and GREENHOUSE · Case Studies in Biometry
LARSON · Introduction to Probability Theory and Statistical Inference, *Third Edition*
LAWLESS · Statistical Models and Methods for Lifetime Data, *Second Edition*
LAWSON · Statistical Methods in Spatial Epidemiology
LE · Applied Categorical Data Analysis
LE · Applied Survival Analysis
LEE and WANG · Statistical Methods for Survival Data Analysis, *Third Edition*
LEPAGE and BILLARD · Exploring the Limits of Bootstrap
LEYLAND and GOLDSTEIN (editors) · Multilevel Modelling of Health Statistics
LIAO · Statistical Group Comparison
LINDVALL · Lectures on the Coupling Method
LIN · Introductory Stochastic Analysis for Finance and Insurance
LINHART and ZUCCHINI · Model Selection
LITTLE and RUBIN · Statistical Analysis with Missing Data, *Second Edition*
LLOYD · The Statistical Analysis of Categorical Data
LOWEN and TEICH · Fractal-Based Point Processes
MAGNUS and NEUDECKER · Matrix Differential Calculus with Applications in Statistics and Econometrics, *Revised Edition*
MALLER and ZHOU · Survival Analysis with Long Term Survivors
MALLOWS · Design, Data, and Analysis by Some Friends of Cuthbert Daniel
MANN, SCHAFER, and SINGPURWALLA · Methods for Statistical Analysis of Reliability and Life Data
MANTON, WOODBURY, and TOLLEY · Statistical Applications Using Fuzzy Sets
MARCHETTE · Random Graphs for Statistical Pattern Recognition
MARDIA and JUPP · Directional Statistics
MASON, GUNST, and HESS · Statistical Design and Analysis of Experiments with Applications to Engineering and Science, *Second Edition*
McCULLOCH, SEARLE, and NEUHAUS · Generalized, Linear, and Mixed Models, *Second Edition*
McFADDEN · Management of Data in Clinical Trials, *Second Edition*
* McLACHLAN · Discriminant Analysis and Statistical Pattern Recognition
McLACHLAN, DO, and AMBROISE · Analyzing Microarray Gene Expression Data
McLACHLAN and KRISHNAN · The EM Algorithm and Extensions, *Second Edition*
McLACHLAN and PEEL · Finite Mixture Models
McNEIL · Epidemiological Research Methods
MEEKER and ESCOBAR · Statistical Methods for Reliability Data
MEERSCHAERT and SCHEFFLER · Limit Distributions for Sums of Independent Random Vectors: Heavy Tails in Theory and Practice
MICKEY, DUNN, and CLARK · Applied Statistics: Analysis of Variance and Regression, *Third Edition*
* MILLER · Survival Analysis, *Second Edition*
MONTGOMERY, JENNINGS, and KULAHCI · Introduction to Time Series Analysis and Forecasting
MONTGOMERY, PECK, and VINING · Introduction to Linear Regression Analysis, *Fourth Edition*
MORGENTHALER and TUKEY · Configural Polysampling: A Route to Practical Robustness
MUIRHEAD · Aspects of Multivariate Statistical Theory

*Now available in a lower priced paperback edition in the Wiley Classics Library.
†Now available in a lower priced paperback edition in the Wiley–Interscience Paperback Series.

MULLER and STOYAN · Comparison Methods for Stochastic Models and Risks
MURRAY · X-STAT 2.0 Statistical Experimentation, Design Data Analysis, and Nonlinear Optimization
MURTHY, XIE, and JIANG · Weibull Models
MYERS, MONTGOMERY, and ANDERSON-COOK · Response Surface Methodology: Process and Product Optimization Using Designed Experiments, *Third Edition*
MYERS, MONTGOMERY, and VINING · Generalized Linear Models. With Applications in Engineering and the Sciences
† NELSON · Accelerated Testing, Statistical Models, Test Plans, and Data Analyses
† NELSON · Applied Life Data Analysis
NEWMAN · Biostatistical Methods in Epidemiology
OCHI · Applied Probability and Stochastic Processes in Engineering and Physical Sciences
OKABE, BOOTS, SUGIHARA, and CHIU · Spatial Tesselations: Concepts and Applications of Voronoi Diagrams, *Second Edition*
OLIVER and SMITH · Influence Diagrams, Belief Nets and Decision Analysis
PALTA · Quantitative Methods in Population Health: Extensions of Ordinary Regressions
PANJER · Operational Risk: Modeling and Analytics
PANKRATZ · Forecasting with Dynamic Regression Models
PANKRATZ · Forecasting with Univariate Box-Jenkins Models: Concepts and Cases
* PARZEN · Modern Probability Theory and Its Applications
PEÑA, TIAO, and TSAY · A Course in Time Series Analysis
PIANTADOSI · Clinical Trials: A Methodologic Perspective
PORT · Theoretical Probability for Applications
POURAHMADI · Foundations of Time Series Analysis and Prediction Theory
POWELL · Approximate Dynamic Programming: Solving the Curses of Dimensionality
PRESS · Bayesian Statistics: Principles, Models, and Applications
PRESS · Subjective and Objective Bayesian Statistics, *Second Edition*
PRESS and TANUR · The Subjectivity of Scientists and the Bayesian Approach
PUKELSHEIM · Optimal Experimental Design
PURI, VILAPLANA, and WERTZ · New Perspectives in Theoretical and Applied Statistics
† PUTERMAN · Markov Decision Processes: Discrete Stochastic Dynamic Programming
QIU · Image Processing and Jump Regression Analysis
* RAO · Linear Statistical Inference and Its Applications, *Second Edition*
RAUSAND and HØYLAND · System Reliability Theory: Models, Statistical Methods, and Applications, *Second Edition*
RENCHER · Linear Models in Statistics
RENCHER · Methods of Multivariate Analysis, *Second Edition*
RENCHER · Multivariate Statistical Inference with Applications
* RIPLEY · Spatial Statistics
* RIPLEY · Stochastic Simulation
ROBINSON · Practical Strategies for Experimenting
ROHATGI and SALEH · An Introduction to Probability and Statistics, *Second Edition*
ROLSKI, SCHMIDLI, SCHMIDT, and TEUGELS · Stochastic Processes for Insurance and Finance
ROSENBERGER and LACHIN · Randomization in Clinical Trials: Theory and Practice
ROSS · Introduction to Probability and Statistics for Engineers and Scientists
ROSSI, ALLENBY, and McCULLOCH · Bayesian Statistics and Marketing
† ROUSSEEUW and LEROY · Robust Regression and Outlier Detection
* RUBIN · Multiple Imputation for Nonresponse in Surveys
RUBINSTEIN and KROESE · Simulation and the Monte Carlo Method, *Second Edition*
RUBINSTEIN and MELAMED · Modern Simulation and Modeling
RYAN · Modern Engineering Statistics

*Now available in a lower priced paperback edition in the Wiley Classics Library.
†Now available in a lower priced paperback edition in the Wiley–Interscience Paperback Series.

RYAN · Modern Experimental Design
RYAN · Modern Regression Methods, *Second Edition*
RYAN · Statistical Methods for Quality Improvement, *Second Edition*
SALEH · Theory of Preliminary Test and Stein-Type Estimation with Applications
* SCHEFFE · The Analysis of Variance
SCHIMEK · Smoothing and Regression: Approaches, Computation, and Application
SCHOTT · Matrix Analysis for Statistics, *Second Edition*
SCHOUTENS · Levy Processes in Finance: Pricing Financial Derivatives
SCHUSS · Theory and Applications of Stochastic Differential Equations
SCOTT · Multivariate Density Estimation: Theory, Practice, and Visualization
† SEARLE · Linear Models for Unbalanced Data
† SEARLE · Matrix Algebra Useful for Statistics
† SEARLE, CASELLA, and McCULLOCH · Variance Components
SEARLE and WILLETT · Matrix Algebra for Applied Economics
SEBER · A Matrix Handbook For Statisticians
† SEBER · Multivariate Observations
SEBER and LEE · Linear Regression Analysis, *Second Edition*
† SEBER and WILD · Nonlinear Regression
SENNOTT · Stochastic Dynamic Programming and the Control of Queueing Systems
* SERFLING · Approximation Theorems of Mathematical Statistics
SHAFER and VOVK · Probability and Finance: It's Only a Game!
SILVAPULLE and SEN · Constrained Statistical Inference: Inequality, Order, and Shape Restrictions
SMALL and McLEISH · Hilbert Space Methods in Probability and Statistical Inference
SRIVASTAVA · Methods of Multivariate Statistics
STAPLETON · Linear Statistical Models
STAPLETON · Models for Probability and Statistical Inference: Theory and Applications
STAUDTE and SHEATHER · Robust Estimation and Testing
STOYAN, KENDALL, and MECKE · Stochastic Geometry and Its Applications, *Second Edition*
STOYAN and STOYAN · Fractals, Random Shapes and Point Fields: Methods of Geometrical Statistics
STREET and BURGESS · The Construction of Optimal Stated Choice Experiments: Theory and Methods
STYAN · The Collected Papers of T. W. Anderson: 1943–1985
SUTTON, ABRAMS, JONES, SHELDON, and SONG · Methods for Meta-Analysis in Medical Research
TAKEZAWA · Introduction to Nonparametric Regression
TAMHANE · Statistical Analysis of Designed Experiments: Theory and Applications
TANAKA · Time Series Analysis: Nonstationary and Noninvertible Distribution Theory
THOMPSON · Empirical Model Building
THOMPSON · Sampling, *Second Edition*
THOMPSON · Simulation: A Modeler's Approach
THOMPSON and SEBER · Adaptive Sampling
THOMPSON, WILLIAMS, and FINDLAY · Models for Investors in Real World Markets
TIAO, BISGAARD, HILL, PEÑA, and STIGLER (editors) · Box on Quality and Discovery: with Design, Control, and Robustness
TIERNEY · LISP-STAT: An Object-Oriented Environment for Statistical Computing and Dynamic Graphics
TSAY · Analysis of Financial Time Series, *Second Edition*
UPTON and FINGLETON · Spatial Data Analysis by Example, Volume II: Categorical and Directional Data
† VAN BELLE · Statistical Rules of Thumb, *Second Edition*

*Now available in a lower priced paperback edition in the Wiley Classics Library.
†Now available in a lower priced paperback edition in the Wiley–Interscience Paperback Series.

VAN BELLE, FISHER, HEAGERTY, and LUMLEY · Biostatistics: A Methodology for the Health Sciences, *Second Edition*
VESTRUP · The Theory of Measures and Integration
VIDAKOVIC · Statistical Modeling by Wavelets
VINOD and REAGLE · Preparing for the Worst: Incorporating Downside Risk in Stock Market Investments
WALLER and GOTWAY · Applied Spatial Statistics for Public Health Data
WEERAHANDI · Generalized Inference in Repeated Measures: Exact Methods in MANOVA and Mixed Models
WEISBERG · Applied Linear Regression, *Third Edition*
WELSH · Aspects of Statistical Inference
WESTFALL and YOUNG · Resampling-Based Multiple Testing: Examples and Methods for *p*-Value Adjustment
WHITTAKER · Graphical Models in Applied Multivariate Statistics
WINKER · Optimization Heuristics in Economics: Applications of Threshold Accepting
WONNACOTT and WONNACOTT · Econometrics, *Second Edition*
WOODING · Planning Pharmaceutical Clinical Trials: Basic Statistical Principles
WOODWORTH · Biostatistics: A Bayesian Introduction
WOOLSON and CLARKE · Statistical Methods for the Analysis of Biomedical Data, *Second Edition*
WU and HAMADA · Experiments: Planning, Analysis, and Parameter Design Optimization
WU and ZHANG · Nonparametric Regression Methods for Longitudinal Data Analysis
YANG · The Construction Theory of Denumerable Markov Processes
YOUNG, VALERO-MORA, and FRIENDLY · Visual Statistics: Seeing Data with Dynamic Interactive Graphics
ZACKS · Stage-Wise Adaptive Designs
ZELTERMAN · Discrete Distributions—Applications in the Health Sciences
* ZELLNER · An Introduction to Bayesian Inference in Econometrics
ZHOU, OBUCHOWSKI, and McCLISH · Statistical Methods in Diagnostic Medicine

*Now available in a lower priced paperback edition in the Wiley Classics Library.
†Now available in a lower priced paperback edition in the Wiley–Interscience Paperback Series.

Printed and bound by CPI Group (UK) Ltd, Croydon, CR0 4YY
16/09/2026
14963457-0004